T0203156

Participation: Optimising Outcomes in Childhood-Onset Neurodisability

Clinics in Developmental Medicine

Participation: Optimising Outcomes in Childhood-Onset Neurodisability

Edited by

Christine Imms

Professor, Centre for Disability and Development Research,
the Australian Catholic University,
Melbourne, Australia

Dido Green

Professor, Occupational Therapy, Department of Rehabilitation,
Jönköping University, Jönköping, Sweden;
Professor, Occupational Therapy, Brunel University, London; and
Research Therapist, Royal Free London Hospital
NHS Foundation Trust,
London UK

2020
Mac Keith Press

© 2020 Mac Keith Press

Managing Director: Ann-Marie Halligan
Senior Publishing Manager: Sally Wilkinson
Publishing Co-ordinator: Lucy White
Project Management: Riverside Publishing Solutions Ltd

First published in this edition in 2020 by Mac Keith Press
2nd Floor, Rankin Building, 139–143 Bermondsey Street, London, SE1 3UW

British Library Cataloguing-in-Publication data
A catalogue record for this book is available from the British Library

Cover illustration by Adam Green from the photograph 'From Overcoming to Enjoying'.
Cover designer: Marten Sealby

ISBN: 978-1-911612-16-2

Typeset by Riverside Publishing Solutions Ltd
Printed by Jellyfish Solutions Ltd

Contents

Author Appointments

Brooke Adair
Senior Field Coordinator, Generation Victoria, Murdoch Children's Research Institute, Melbourne, Australia.

Mattijs Alsem
Rehabilitation Physician, Department of Rehabilitation, Amsterdam UMC, Academisch Medisch Centrum, Amsterdam, The Netherlands.

Dana Anaby
Associate Professor, School of Physical and Occupational Therapy, McGill University, Montreal, Canada.

Orit Bart
Senior Lecturer, Occupational Therapy Department, Stanley Steyer School of Health Professions, Sackler Faculty of Medicine, Tel Aviv University, Israel.

Beata Batorowicz
Assistant Professor, School of Rehabilitation Therapy, Health Sciences, Queen's University, Kingston, Ontario, Canada.

Stefania Bibolar
Children's Occupational Therapist, Maria Beatrice Centre, Romania.

Juan Bornman
Professor, Centre for Augmentative and Alternative Communication, University of Pretoria, Pretoria, South Africa.

Chris Bradbeer
Principal, Stonefields Primary School Auckland, and Doctoral Candidate, Melbourne Graduate School of Education, University of Melbourne, Australia.

Karen Bunning
Reader, Developmental Disabilities, School of Health Sciences, University of East Anglia, Norwich Research Park, UK.

Nicole Cassar
Aboriginal Consultant, Australia.

Benjamin Cleveland
Senior Lecturer, Faculty of Architecture, Building and Planning, University of Melbourne, Australia.

Bernard Dan
Professor, Université Libre de Bruxelles and Inkendaal Rehabilitation Hospital, Brussels, Belgium.

Carolyn Dunford
Senior Lecturer, Brunel University, London, UK.

Naru Fukuchi
Vice President, Miyagi Disaster Mental Health Care Centre, Miyagi, Japan.

Joseph K. Gona
Kuhenza for the Children's Foundation, Gede, Kenya.

Mats Granlund
Professor, CHILD Research Group and Swedish Institute for Disability Research, School of Health Sciences, Jonkoping University, Jonkoping, Sweden.

Dido Green
Professor, Occupational Therapy, Department of Rehabilitation, Jönköping University, Jönköping, Sweden; Professor, Occupational Therapy, Brunel University, London; and Research Therapist, Royal Free London Hospital NHS Foundation Trust, London UK.

Ai-Wen Hwang
Associate Professor, Graduate Institute of Early Intervention, College of Medicine, Chang Gung University, Taoyuan, Taiwan; and Department of Physical Medicine and Rehabilitation, Chang Gung Memorial Hospital, Linkou, Taiwan.

Christine Imms
Professor, Centre for Disability and Development Research, the Australian Catholic University, Melbourne, Australia.

Wesley Imms   Associate Professor, Melbourne Graduate School of Education, University of Melbourne, Australia.

Reidun Jahnsen   Professor, Research Centre for Habilitation and Rehabilitation Models and Services (CHARM) University of Oslo; Head of the Research Department, Beitostoelen Healthsports Center, and Director of the Norwegian CP surveillance program (CPOP), Department of Clinical Neurosciences for Children, Oslo University Hospital, Oslo, Norway.

Jessica M Jarvis   Postdoctoral Research Associate, Department of Occupational Therapy, College of Applied Health Sciences, University of Illinois at Chicago, Chicago, Illinois, USA.

Pranay Jindal   Physiotherapy Specialist, Neonatal Intensive Care Unit, Women's Wellness and Research Center, Hamad Medical Corporation, Doha, Qatar.

Marjolijn Ketelaar   Associate Professor, Center of Excellence for Rehabilitation Medicine, UMC Utrecht Brain Center, University Medical Centre Utrecht, and De Hoogstraat Rehabilitation, Utrecht, The Netherlands.

Mary A Khetani   Associate Professor, Department of Occupational Therapy, College of Applied Health Sciences, University of Illinois at Chicago, Chicago, Illinois, USA.

Gillian King   Distinguished Senior Scientist, Bloorview Research Institute; Professor, Occupational Science and Occupational Therapy, University of Toronto; Canada Research Chair in Optimal Care for Children with Disabilities, Canada.

Martijn Klem   Parent, BOSK, Association of People with Congenital Disabilities, Utrecht, The Netherlands.

Jessica Kramer   Associate Professor, Department of Occupational Therapy, College of Public Health and Health Professions, University of Florida, Gainesville, Florida, USA.

Citlali López-Ortiz Assistant Professor, Neuroscience of Dance in Health and Disability Laboratory, Department of Kinesiology and Community Health, Department of Dance, Center for Health, Aging, and Disability, Neuroscience Program, Illinois Informatics Institute, Beckman Institute for Advanced Science and Technology, University of Illinois, Urbana-Champaign; Joffrey Ballet Academy, The Official School of the Joffrey Ballet; New York, USA.

Yen-Thanh Mac   Medical Advisor, No Ordinary Journey Foundation, Calgary, Canada.

Annette Majnemer   Professor, School of Physical & Occupational Therapy; Vice Dean – Education, Faculty of Medicine, McGill University; Senior Scientist, Research Institute of the McGill University Health Centre, Montreal, Canada.

Motohide Miyahara   Associate Professor, School of Physical Education, Sport and Exercise Sciences, University of Otago, New Zealand and Visiting Research Fellow, Department of Neuropsychiatry, School of Medicine, Hirosaki University, Aomori, Japan.

Liana Nagy   Lecturer in Occupational Therapy, Oxford Brookes University, UK.

Charles R Newton   Professor, Centre for Geographic Medicine Research (Coast), Kenya Medical Research Institute, Kilifi Kenya. Department of Psychiatry, Oxford University, Oxford, UK.

Bridget O'Connor PhD Candidate, Centre for Disability and Development Research, the Australian Catholic University, Melbourne, Australia.

Karine Pelc Paediatric Neurologist, Université libre de Bruxelles and Inkendaal Rehabilitation Hospital, Brussels, Belgium.

Peter Rosenbaum Professor of Paediatrics, McMaster University; CanChild Centre for Childhood Disability Research; Hamilton, Ontario, Canada.

Limor Rosenberg Senior Teacher, Occupational Therapy Department, Stanley Steyer School of Health Professions, Sackler Faculty of Medicine, Tel Aviv University, Israel.

Manabu Saito Associate Professor, Department of Neuropsychiatry, Graduate School of Medicine, Hirosaki University, Aomori, Japan.

Loretta Sheppard Associate Professor, Occupational Therapy, National School of Allied Health, Australian Catholic University, Melbourne, Australia.

Nora Shields Professor of Physiotherapy, La Trobe University, Melbourne, Australia.

Michele Shusterman Parent and Founder, President of CP NOW non-profit & CP Daily Living blog, South Carolina, USA.

Martine Smith Associate Professor Speech Language Pathology, Department of Clinical Speech and Language Studies, University of Dublin, Trinity College, Ireland.

Dirk-Wouter Smits Postdoctoral Research Fellow, Center of Excellence for Rehabilitation Medicine; UMC Utrecht Brain Center, University Medical Centre Utrecht, and De Hoogstraat Rehabilitation, Utrecht, The Netherlands.

Michel Sylin Professor, Université libre de Bruxelles, Centre de recherche en psychologie des organisations et des institutions, Brussels, Belgium.

Karen van Meeteren Parent, Center of Excellence for Rehabilitation Medicine, UMC Utrecht Brain Center, University Medical Centre Utrecht, and De Hoogstraat Rehabilitation, Utrecht, The Netherlands; and Co-founder, 'OuderInzicht', Parent Organization for Improvement of Parent Involvement in Research, Amsterdam, The Netherlands.

Bengt Westerberg Hon Dr, Minister of Social Affairs and Deputy Prime Minister of the Swedish National Government 1991–94. MP 1984–94, Chair of the Board of the Swedish Institute of Disability Research, Sweden.

Claire Willis Research Fellow, School of Allied Health, La Trobe University, Melbourne, Australia.

Farzaneh Yazdani Senior Lecturer in Occupational Therapy, Oxford Brookes University, Oxford UK.

Jenny Ziviani Professor, School of Health and Rehabilitation Sciences, The University of Queensland, Brisbane, Australia.

Preface

WHAT THIS BOOK IS ABOUT

Why this Book?

Participation: Optimising Outcomes in Childhood-Onset Neurodisability comes nearly 20 years after the publication of the International Classification of Functioning, Disability and Health (ICF; World Health Organization 2001) which proved a catalyst for an altered focus in health and education, for those with lifelong impairments. We have seen a major shift in thinking from the focus of disability on the child and associated impairments to a broader understanding of the roles and opportunities that are available for meaningful participation in life irrespective of measurable impairments. This is the right time to reflect on and explore the crucial notion of participation. Participation is what people do every day – but how we support, promote, maximise or otherwise enable participation will depend entirely on how we understand what it is, and how we value who is able to take part in the multitude of life situations. Society's attitudes towards impairment, disability and participation have evolved over time, and will – and should – continue to change. However, while we aim to consign exclusion and segregation of those with impairments to the pages of history, we are not there yet.

A central goal of this book is: to gather the experiences and knowledge of participation of those with childhood onset neurodisabilty from around the world; to identify and highlight the salient features of participation from multiple perspectives and across varying cultures and contexts; and to endeavour to identify key methods for enabling positive health-promoting participation.

What is it About?

The focus of this book is *participation*. Participation is conceptualised as both attendance and involvement in life situations; by attendance, we mean having a physical or virtual presence, by involvement we mean the experience of participation while attending (Imms et al. 2017). Participation is considered distinct from the ability of an individual to be independent, to have the skills and attributes to perform activities as expected, and is distinct from the ability to make choices or be self-determined. Although competence and autonomy are key issues, and strongly related to participation outcomes, they are not the same as participation. Autonomy does contribute importantly to ensuring an individual is involved, not just present in a situation. In this book the reader is encouraged to consider how to enable individuals to attend the varied life situations that are part of their personal, familial and cultural world, and once there, to be involved – to be 'part of it'. This might include connecting emotionally, or cognitively, or in the doing, in ways that are meaningful and satisfying to those in the situation.

Who is Our Intended Audience?

We wrote this book for practitioners and researchers who work in the field of childhood-onset neurodisability; in health, community and educational settings. This is a complex field that involves engagement with individuals, and their families, whose conditions arise early in life and impact the central nervous system; including those with diagnoses such as cerebral palsy, autism, intellectual impairment and a myriad of other conditions that present in childhood. Practitioners will be working with individuals and their families, as well as those in their communities, to enable increased opportunities and better outcomes. The book takes a non-categorical approach – we are not focused on the 'diagnosis': participation is for all, across contexts irrespective of diagnostic labels. There are scenarios and vignettes that provide stories and exemplars to engage and challenge the reader. These vignettes aim to bring life to underlying concepts and contexts and provide applications for assessment and intervention.

This book may also help those with childhood onset impairments, their parents and other interested community members to develop their own ideas and methods for goal-setting and collaboration with professionals, as well as with day-to-day participation. There are a variety of 'voices' in the book – we have sought contributions from around the world – and each continent is represented to some degree. We have sought stories from children and about children, and from families and from professionals. Some of the stories are so challenging they are heartbreaking. We hope that the reader will use these to drive an agenda for fundamental change in our communities towards attendance and involvement for all. A paradigm shift is required in our thinking; participation must be placed at the forefront of our ambitions as both means and outcomes in the way we work and live.

How is the Book Structured?

The five parts of the book are sequenced to deliver and illustrate:

  i) Information that aids understanding of the concept of participation;
 ii) Where participation occurs and how contexts and settings influence participation;
iii) How to measure the changing levels of participation;
 iv) What we know about interventions that promote participation; and
  v) Considerations for future directions.

Each part of the book contains several chapters by authors known for their expertise in the field and who bring research and practice knowledge to the topic.

In addition, each part contains several vignettes. This compilation of 'stories' are contributions from authors from across the world. They were asked to give vivid expression to the participatory experiences of those with childhood-onset disability from within their own country or cultural setting. The vignettes are linked to the chapters by connecting statements within the text and by a brief introduction at the beginning of the vignette to draw your attention to key ideas in the chapter that are exemplified in the vignette. The intent of the vignettes is to provide food for thought and to support the reader's future actions. Some stories may describe experiences novel to the reader and thus bring alternative perspectives to prompt one's creativity in developing solutions to any barriers to participation. Some stories may strike a chord and make for uncomfortable reading, and these too can be used to prompt a reconsideration of *how* and *what* we do in practice.

The book can be read either sequentially – as we have considered carefully how the information builds across the parts and chapters – or each part and each chapter can be read in isolation if a particular element is of interest or concern. The aim of this book is to both challenge and motivate the reader and thereby encourage a change in our approach and attitude to childhood onset neurodisability. There is much work to be done together to realise everyone's rights, hopes and dreams.

At the end of the book we will look again at where we are, where we hope the field is going and how we may progress understanding and developments to optimise opportunities for participation.

REFERENCES

Imms C, Granlund M, Wilson PH, Steenbergen B, Rosenbaum PL, Gordon AM (2017) Participation, both a means and an end: a conceptual analysis of processes and outcomes in childhood disability. *Dev Med Child Neurol* **59**: 16–25.

World Health Organization (2001) *International Classification of Functioning, Disability and Health (ICF)* [Online]. World Health Organization. Available: www.who.int/icf [Accessed January 2002].

Christine Imms and Dido Green
August 2019

Acknowledgements

All books are a journey from first thoughts to realisation. This book was inspired and motivated by our appreciation of the many children, young people and their families whose lives we have briefly shared, and whose paths through life we value. We thank them all, including those who have provided considered feedback on many of the drafts of chapters.

We express our gratitude to our colleagues at Jönköping University, Sweden, Royal Free London NHS Foundation Trust UK, and the Australian Catholic University, who supported the editors during the preparation of this book, and to the staff of Mac Keith Press for their encouragement, guidance and patience throughout. We are also sincerely appreciative of the authorship groups who contributed to the book – the work here represents a serious and ongoing commitment to changing the landscape of the journeys of those with childhood-onset disability and the important people in their lives.

Heartfelt thanks are also extended to our families for their tolerance of the many late night and early morning meetings across continents which allowed this work to develop. Special appreciation goes to our husbands: Wes Imms for unstinting support and long nights of discussion that provoked thoughtful changes in direction and fruitful connections across fields of endeavour and Adam Green for his diligence in proofreading many chapters. The cover illustration is a graphic design by Adam Green of the photograph 'From Overcoming to Enjoying'. We are grateful to the photographer, Mai Anh Le, for permission to adapt the photo and Adam for his artistry.

Christine Imms and Dido Green

PART I

Conceptual Issues
in Participation

Samuel's Magic Talking Machine!

Juan Bornman

Hi! My name is Samuel. I live in a house with my mom, dad and younger sister, Rebecca. We call her Becky. I have cerebral palsy. This means that the parts of my brain that help me to do things like walk, run and talk were hurt before I was born. When I try to use my legs, my brain doesn't send the message to the muscles to move, so I get around in a wheelchair. Some of my friends at school use crutches that help them to walk. I am very lucky. The part of my brain that helps me to think and learn new things is fine! So, I can think just like you, and I know what I like or don't like.

Some days I get really angry and sad when people don't understand what I am trying to tell them. I try my best to say the words, but my lips and tongue can't make the movements that I want them to make. Somewhere between my brain and my mouth the words come out all wrong. So, although my speech sounds funny and you might not understand me, I can understand everything that you say to me!

People sometimes stare at me when my mom pushes me in my wheelchair at the shops. I see in their eyes that they feel sorry for me and that they think I don't have a brain because I can't speak. They talk to mom as if I don't exist and as if I can't hear them. Most people think that because I can't speak clearly, they can't speak to me. This makes me feel very lonely!

I like it when my sister's friends come to play. They are very nice to me, but I wish that I could also have new friends to come and play. I could show them my computer! But it is hard to make friends when people don't understand you when you speak.

Every morning my mom picks me up from my bed and helps me into my wheelchair. She helps me to get dressed and to have breakfast. My arms have jerky movements that I can't control and this makes it hard to hold a spoon or pen or to be neat when I am playing. Sometimes I can hold the spoon or cup by myself, but not when we're in a hurry to get ready for school! Mom drives me to school.

Last year, my parents took me to meet some people at the university who would show me some other ways to 'talk'! I did not believe that there were other ways to talk other than by saying things with your mouth! I was very excited but also really nervous. They asked my parents some questions about me and played with lots of different toys and paged through books with me. Then they showed me the most wonderful things I have ever seen! A talking machine!

On the top part of the machine there is a lot of pictures of different things. Look here – if I press this button with the 'ball' picture on, the voice says: 'Please play ball with me'. If I press this button of a boy shaking his head, my machine says 'No, I don't want that one'. Don't you agree that it is super cool? I still learn new pictures and new words every day, so my machine can grow with me.

So next time when you see me at the shops, come over and chat with me! I might even be able to go to your school one day! It hurts more to be ignored or stared at than to be asked questions about myself. If you talk to me, it shows me that you care!

The Nature of Participation

Christine Imms

In his descriptions of the joy and wonder experienced on discovering talking machines, Samuel gives us a window into the loneliness of being misunderstood, ignored and excluded from social connection. In Samuel's story, participation is being 'visible' so that you really are present in the situation and being spoken to, so you can be involved in a communicative exchange. In his story, enabling participation is about caring and making a human connection. Samuel lives in South Africa, but his 'story' is experienced across the world: it exemplifies the imperative for us to be focused on participation for all children and especially those with neurodisability.

> LINK TO VIGNETTE 1.1
> *'Samuel's Magic Talking Machine!', p. 3.*

In this chapter, I explore the nature of participation from a theoretical perspective and from the perspective of those who have given voice to knowledge about participation through their involvement in research. People give voice to their perspective when: (1) they contribute data to research studies – this typically includes those who have impairments or their caregivers; (2) when they design, conduct and interpret research findings – this is typically researchers and/or practitioners, and (3) when policy is formed and used to determine services provided – this typically occurs at the level of government or organisational management. More recently we have been working to include the voice of consumers (parents and/or those with impairments) in all aspects of research, practice and policy decision making. Given the diversity of interests in participation, there is a wide variety of perspectives to be considered and this increases the complexity of our knowledge base and of how we might respond. This chapter therefore aims to provide a common language for the book to inform our future practice, research and policy making.

THEORETICAL FRAMEWORKS

Over the past 30+ years, rehabilitation models have moved towards an ecological rather than strictly medical-model approach to thinking about how performance and change in performance, occurs in people. Consistent with this, the World Health Organization's (WHO) International Classification of Functioning, Disability and Health (ICF, see Fig. 1.1) (WHO 2001) provides a universal framework for describing health outcomes with consideration of the multidimensional influences on an individual's functioning and disability. This bio-psycho-social framework considers the transactional influences among body functions (physiology) and structures (anatomy), activity (ability to execute tasks and actions), participation (involvement in life situations), as well as contextual factors related to the environment (e.g. family, school, home, community settings) and personal factors (e.g. age, sex, preferences). The ICF, therefore, provides a detailed framework for all people to consider the influence of a variety of potential factors, as well as the dynamic interplay among factors, on a person's health and development across the lifespan.

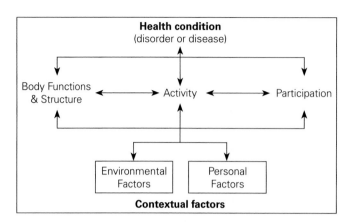

Figure 1.1 Interactions between the components of International Classification of Functioning, Disability and Health. Reprinted from WHO (2001) with permission from the World Health Organization.

The publication of the ICF led to an international shift in the healthcare focus for those with a disability. This shift moved us from emphasising assessment of, and interventions to 'fix' body functions and structures, to a position today where successful participation in everyday life is seen as the ultimate outcome of health services for those in need of special support, such as children with neurodisability. This shift takes a welcome broader view about how to influence long term wellbeing. For children with neurological impairments, who experience a range of life-long impairments and activity limitations associated with their condition, this perspective means that healthcare interventions must consider how to achieve three key outcomes: minimise the children's impairments; maximise their activity performance; and optimise participation outcomes. The order in which we should approach these goals may be contested or depends on the personal goals of the individuals with whom we work. In this book, we place the need to optimise participation in prime focus. We argue that detailed, nuanced knowledge about how to support and effectively influence the participation outcomes of people living with childhood-onset disability is required. We need this knowledge to achieve universal equity and human rights outcomes, as well as the best possible outcomes for individuals.

While the ICF shifted some people's focus to participation outcomes in practice and research, the framework did not provide a well-defined conceptualisation of participation, and for 15 years, researchers have approached the task of establishing knowledge about participation outcomes from disparate perspectives. These disparities mean that building a shared understanding from which to guide practice is very difficult. Between 2015 and 2017, our team undertook a series of systematic reviews (Adair et al. 2015, 2018; Imms et al. 2016) and conceptual work (Imms et al. 2017) derived from 15+ years of childhood-onset disability research and theory, to establish a common language and propose a conceptual framework. The family of participation related constructs (fPRC; see Fig. 1.2) uses the ICF as a foundation and proposes that a more detailed understanding of the participation construct and its relationship with the intrinsic elements of the person (activity competence, sense of self and preferences), the activity setting or context, and the broader environment, are required to enable clarity in future participation focused work.

THE PARTICIPATION CONSTRUCT

Within the fPRC, participation is described as having two conceptual elements: (1) attendance, defined as 'being there' and measured as frequency of attending and/or the range or diversity of activities; and (2) involvement, defined as the experience of participation while attending. Involvement might include elements of engagement, persistence, social connection, and level of affect. This separation of the participation construct into two essential components is crucial to support the clarity of our understanding of people's

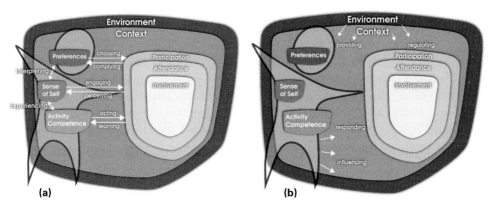

Figure 1.2   The family of participation related constructs: **(a)** person-focused processes, **(b)** environment-focused processes (Imms et al. 2017). A colour version of this figure can be seen in the plate section.

experiences and the effect of interventions. When defined as 'involvement in a life situation' (WHO 2001) the word 'involvement' can be interpreted to mean being able to attend or being able to engage, or both. In addition, the idea of participation was equated with performance. Consequently, the approach to participation research and practice has lacked clarity. Distinctions between attendance and involvement will provide important avenues for further knowledge generation and support how we approach practice.

Participation in life situations has two essential elements; attendance and involvement.

There is already a body of evidence about the attendance element of the participation construct in childhood disability. The attendance dimension is an objective phenomenon: it can therefore be measured through time-use devices, diaries and surveys, and by observation, self or proxy report (see Chapter 12). Using these processes, and new tools as they are developed, will allow us to continue to build our knowledge about patterns of attendance, or changes in attendance over the life course and to build knowledge about the effects on attendance of new legislation, changed practice policies, community expectations as well as health and educational interventions.

The involvement dimension of the participation construct is more complex than the attendance dimension. The definition of involvement in the fPRC is 'the experience of participation while attending that may include elements of engagement, motivation, persistence, social connection, and affect' (Imms et al. 2017, p. 18). This definition was derived from a thematic analysis of research literature and requires further refinement. In some research, the terms involvement and engagement are used interchangeably, in some they are used in ways that imply different meanings. In some languages, there is only one word for involvement/engagement. In English the words may be used to define each other. The important point here is that when we wish to undertake research, or focus on supporting change in a specific area, we need to clearly define and communicate our constructs.

The involvement dimension is also complicated because, at least in part, it is a personally experienced phenomenon that may not be observable; or may be misinterpreted when apparently observed. In addition, complexity is driven by the potential for involvement to be considered at multiple ecological levels. For example, we might consider involvement at a neural level – what is occurring in the brain at the time of participation. At this level we may be able to measure effects of attention, focus or curiosity (each of which may or may not be good proxies for involvement) using contemporary neuroimaging techniques. Involvement can also be considered at the level of the individual in the moment – conceptualised as how the individual interacts within a specific context, defined as the activity, objects, place, people (if present) over time (Batorowicz et al. 2016). This idea of involvement is likely of particular interest to therapists and educators who aim to extend the learning and experiences of young people with impairments. At a broader societal level, participation can be seen as 'a process where young people, as active citizens, take part in, express views on, and have decision-making power about issues that affect them' (Farthing 2012, p. 73). Farthing's definition can be applied at the personal healthcare perspective (e.g. involvement in healthcare decisions) as well as at a socio-political level where youth participate through exercising their democratic right to vote, for example. Involvement at this systems level appears much closer to aspects of self-determination, autonomy and preference – which in the fPRC, are participation related constructs, not participation. However, dividing where one construct finishes and another starts, may be somewhat artificial.

THE INTRINSIC ELEMENTS OF THE fPRC

Three intrinsic elements of the fPRC, activity competence, sense-of-self and preferences, have often been used in research as proxies for participation (Adair et al. 2018). However, the fPRC clarifies their distinctness; the intrinsic elements are crucially related to participation, but not synonymous with participation. These elements are both antecedents of future participation and consequences of current or past participation.

Activity competence is defined as the extent to which an individual can perform an activity to an expected level or in an expected manner (Imms et al. 2017). This element is typically the focus of developmental, functional and other performance-based assessments. These skills and abilities may be considered from the perspective of the best possible competence, typically assessed under ideal or test conditions and sometimes referred to as capacity. Activity competence may also be assessed as usual performance, as the skills demonstrated in natural environments, or as capability – the amount of ability that the individual can use in natural environments (Morris 2009). Regardless of these distinctions, the key element under consideration in the construct of activity competence is the individual's skill when doing the activity. For this reason, it is very important that activity competence not be used as a proxy for participation. If competence is deemed synonymous or strongly related to participation, then individuals with less communicative, cognitive or physical ability are by definition excluded from many aspects of participation. While this may in fact be true, it should not in principle be true. Consistent with the declarations of human rights, rights of children and disabled persons (UN General Assembly 1948, 1989, 2007), all people have the right to attend and be involved in the daily activities of their communities and societies.

Activity competence should not be used as a proxy for participation.

The sense-of-self construct within the fPRC, considers aspects of self-determination, self-esteem, self-confidence and experiences of satisfaction with participation. These notions relate to the development of perceptions of self: Who am I? Am I capable? Can I exercise choice and control? These elements of self are critical to identity formation and wellbeing, and are both influenced by, and influence future participation experiences (Imms et al. 2017). Self-determination theory describes internal and external mechanism for self-regulation, with self-determined behaviour based on internal motivations, as opposed to externally controlled regulation (Ryan and Deci 2000). Self-determined experiences are strongly associated with 'greater persistence, more positive feelings, higher quality performance and better mental health' (Ryan and Deci 2000, p. 1). Self-determination then, is an important attribute to promote. Self-determination theory describes three psychological needs – relatedness, competence and autonomy – as important conditions to be met for the development of self-determination (Ryan and Deci 2000).

Participation may be enhanced when individuals' needs for autonomy, relatedness and competence are met (see Chapter 2).

Preferences are those activities that hold meaning, are important or are given precedence over other activities in a person's life. Preferences can explain participation choices of individuals, families and societies, and are therefore important to understand (Skille and Osteras 2011). Development of personal preferences is influenced by past participation experiences, and the individual's interpretation of those experiences. Positive experiences are more likely to drive motivation for future repeated participation, than negative. In practice, preferences can be elicited as a component of intervention or educational goal setting (What do you want, or need, to do?), or through exploring the activity setting in which individuals prefer to situate their participation. Not all activity participation is preference based; we all take part in some non-discretionary activities, and this can be more so for children. Complying or coping with participation choices made by others, such as going to school, taking part in family social events whether we enjoy them or not, is part of the participation experience.

The final intrinsic element of the framework are the self-regulatory processes that guide the individuals thinking, emotions and actions. These executive processes are understood to bring together, or create some level of cohesion between, the intrinsic elements of sense-of-self, activity competence and preference.

THE EXTRINSIC ELEMENTS OF THE fPRC

The elements of the fPRC that are extrinsic to the person are the context or close setting in which participation occurs, and the broader social and physical environment. Context is conceptualised using Batorowicz et al.'s (2016) definition as involving the people, place, objects, activity and time in which participation is situated. Of note though, in the fPRC an individual can participate by themselves – not only in the presence of other people. This close activity setting is critical to the experience of attendance and involvement. Exploration of the extent to which individuals have access to (i.e. can attend) and are accommodated and accepted within (i.e. can be involved) activity settings can occur through the study of the person in context.

The broader environment is considered from the perspective of the physical (e.g. climate, terrain, built environment) and social (e.g. community, cultural, institutional processes and practices) elements in which people live. These environmental factors can be considered from an objective, observable perspective – they are the elements that are consistent across people in the same environment. How an individual perceives these elements though, is subjective. For example, an organisation such as a community gymnasium may provide physical access for those who use wheeled mobility and have policies to support inclusion; however, unless the individual perceives the facility to be accessible, at least to some extent, then attendance is compromised.

THE HYPOTHESISED PROCESSES WITHIN THE fPRC

The bidirectional arrows in the fPRC framework highlight the transactional nature of participatory change over the life course. Thus, any of the intrinsic or extrinsic elements may be targeted as agents of change to participation, and correspondingly, participation may be an agent of change to the intrinsic or extrinsic elements. The framework proposes that it is in the exchange among the variables that occurs iteratively over time that builds the participatory experiences and capacities of individuals.

Participation is transactional: we need to attend to the arrows in the fPRC to understand and promote healthy transactions.

A transactional perspective means that we attend to the influences of the individual on the nature of the context and environment, as well as attending to how the environment and context afford and/or regulate participation opportunity and experience. A transactional perspective means that we consider the complex exchanges that occur within an individual during the participatory experience in context, and on how those experiences are interpreted and processed after the event (King et al. 2018). It is the experience and interpretation of the experience that has the potential to drive future participation preferences and choices, as well as later involvement when complying with the choices of others. Across the vignettes presented in this book, perspectives on participation of people with neurodisability are presented from varying cultural settings. Multiple experiences, and interpretations of experience, are provided through these vignettes; they provide powerful information about where and how to focus our efforts to enable participation.

> LINK TO VIGNETTE 1.2
> *'You Have to Walk and Talk to Go to School', p. 12.*

CONCLUSION

The fPRC has been described in this chapter and offered as a framework and common language from which to explore participation in childhood-onset neurodisability. Authors of subsequent chapters explore this further or situate their work in related theoretical perspectives. In addition, we seek to bring varied cultural perspectives to the understanding of participation in this book, and the range of vignettes provided serve to spotlight differences and challenge our future thinking.

SUMMARY OF KEY IDEAS

- Participation is a complex idea involving transactional exchanges among multiple intrinsic and extrinsic elements over time.
- Participation in life situations has two essential elements: (1) attendance, defined as 'being there' and measured as frequency of attending and/or the range or diversity of activities; and (2) involvement, defined as the experience of participation while attending.

REFERENCES

Adair B, Ullenhag A, Keen D, Granlund M, Imms C (2015) The effect of interventions aimed at improving participation outcomes for children with disabilities: a systematic review. *Dev Med Child Neurol* **57**: 1093–1104.

Adair B, Ullenhag A, Rosenbaum P, Granlund M, Keen D, Imms C (2018) Measures used to quantify participation in childhood disability and their alignment with the family of participation-related constructs: a systematic review. *Dev Med Child Neurol* **60**: 1101–1116.

Batorowicz B, King G, Mishra L, Missiuna C (2016) An integrated model of social environment and social context for pediatric rehabilitation. *Disabil Rehabil* **38**: 1204–1215.

Farthing R (2012) Why youth participation? Some justifications and critiques of youth participation using New Labour's youth policies as a case study. *Youth Policy* **109**: 71–97.

Imms C, Adair B, Keen D, Ullenhag A, Rosenbaum P, Granlund M (2016) "Participation": a systematic review of language, definitions, and constructs used in intervention research with children with disabilities. *Dev Med Child Neurol* **58**: 29–38.

Imms C, Granlund M, Wilson PH, Steenbergen B, Rosenbaum PL, Gordon AM (2017) Participation, both a means and an end: a conceptual analysis of processes and outcomes in childhood disability. *Dev Med Child Neurol* **59**: 16–25.

King G, Imms C, Stewart D, Freeman M, Nguyen T (2018) A transactional framework for pediatric rehabilitation: shifting the focus to situated contexts, transactional processes, and adaptive developmental outcomes. *Disabil Rehabil* **40**: 1829–1841.

Morris C (2009) Measuring participation in childhood disability: how does the capability approach improve our understanding? *Dev Med Child Neurol* **51**: 92–94.

Ryan RM, Deci EL (2000) Self-determination theory and the facilitation of intrinsic motivation, social development, and well-being. *Am Psychol* **55**: 68–78.

Skille E, Osteras J (2011) What does sport mean to you? Fun and other preferences for adolescents' sport participation. *Crit Public Health* **21**: 359–372.

UN General Assembly (1948) Universal Declaration of Human Rights (217 [III] A). Paris: UN General Assembly.

UN General Assembly (1989) Convention on the Rights of the Child. *United Nations, Treaty Ser* **1577**: 3.

UN General Assembly (2007) Convention on the Rights of Persons with Disability: Resolution (A/RES/61/106). Paris: UN General Assembly.

WHO (2001) *International Classification of Functioning, Disability and Health: Short Version.* https://apps.who.int/iris/bitstream/handle/10665/42407/9241545429.pdf?sequence=1&isAllowed=yISBN 9241545429 Fig. 1. Interactions between the components of ICF, p 18.

In the following scenario participation is conceptualised as independence. Requirements of the context mean children need to be able to walk and talk to go to school, and concepts of disability and cultural preferences for privacy and 'hiding' away of disability influence expectations and goal setting. As you read, consider the challenges of bringing multiple aspects of the context or setting together with family and child preferences and how these impact participation outcomes.

You Have to Walk and Talk to Go to School (India)

Pranay Jindal

In India, parents want their children with cerebral palsy to actively participate in various areas of life, but face many sociocultural and infrastructural barriers in doing so (Jindal et al. 2018). Most children stay at home with family members playing with toys, watching TV and listening to music (Jindal et al. 2018). For mobility, most children crawled at home or were carried by parents. Personal beliefs of parents hindered their child's independence in walking. One mother said:

> I don't want a wheelchair. I just can't imagine my son in a wheelchair. At least, I want them to walk. If they are given wheelchair, whole life, they will be in wheelchair only (6 years, GMFCS V) (Jindal et al. 2018).

To promote activity and independence in daily activities, parents were reluctant to use motorised wheelchairs, walkers and adaptive devices. In a society where the infrastructure is less accessible, parents placed a strong emphasis on walking; using ankle foot orthosis (AFOs) to enhance children's capacity to walk. Social stigma about using a wheelchair and other assistive technology hinders home and community participation of children in India. One father said (child, 6 years, GMFCS IV) (Jindal et al. 2018):

> Wheelchair is the last option. In US and Canada, they don't have that stigma in the society. Here it is different. There are relatives and all these people in the society, at least, you will want him to walk to some extent.

Social stigma, lack of financial help to buy powered wheelchairs and inaccessible infrastructure may have forced parents to use AFOs, as they were less costly and, hidden underneath clothes, were associated with less stigma.

Most Indian parents had the expectation that their child would recover one day and would be able to live a near normal life. Many Indian children did not attend school as they had hospital appointments for various therapy sessions, or the child was not able to sit and/or walk (Jindal et al. 2018). Since ambulatory level and ability to speak (Anish et al. 2013) are generally used as admission criteria by Indian schools, many parents were waiting for the child to walk or sit independently for school admittance. One father reported (child, 3.5 years, GMFCS IV) (Jindal et al. 2018):

> He is not able to walk, so I thought we will wait up to 5 or 6 months. He is sitting properly now, but sometimes he slides. So, someone has to be there in school to watch him.

Another father explained the reason for not sending his child to school as (child, 6 years, GMFCS IV) (Jindal et al. 2018):

> If he gets to a sitting position, then we can put him in a school. Unfortunately, here we don't have that kind of special schools [sic] which you might have in other places like Canada. Normal schools cannot make such changes.

Indian children had fewer supports to facilitate engagement and were not physically active at school; however, they were socially included in sedentary activities. A father said (child, 7 years, GMFCS IV) (Jindal et al. 2018):

> In the physical training period, the teacher will take him to ground, but he cannot involve in all activities because he cannot stand. But they will take him to the ground, and he will also enjoy. They are not leaving him alone.

Presently in India, multiple interconnected factors hinder children's participation in various areas of life (Jindal et al. 2019). Changes at attitudinal, policy and infrastructural levels are needed to optimise the participation of children with cerebral palsy.

REFERENCES

Anish TS, Ramachandran R, Sivaram P, Mohandas S, Sasidharan A, Sreelakshmi PR (2013) Elementary school enrolment and its determinants among children with cerebral palsy in Thiruvananthapuram district, Kerala, India. *J Neurosci Rural Pract* **4**(Suppl 1): S40–S44.

Jindal P, MacDermid JC, Rosenbaum P, DiRezze B, Narayan A (2018) Perspectives on rehabilitation of children with cerebral palsy: exploring a cross-cultural view of parents from India and Canada using the international classification of functioning, disability and health. *Disabil Rehabil* **40**: 2745–2755.

Participation: Theoretical Underpinnings to Inform and Guide Interventions

Gillian King, Jenny Ziviani and Christine Imms

There is nothing as practical as a good theory
— Unknown, but ascribed to Lewin (1943)

OVERVIEW AND AIM OF THE CHAPTER

In Chapter 1, the International Classification of Functioning, Disability and Health (ICF; WHO 2001), and the family of Participation Related Constructs (fPRC; Imms et al. 2017) were introduced. In this chapter, we delve deeper into theories that underpin and inform our notions of participation. Theories are powerful when they assist practitioners to understand what 'sits behind' practice and research, and enable the identification of mechanisms that most effectively elicit change.

In participation-based practice, attention to theory will help us to uncover what might otherwise be overlooked. For example, we might miss important aspects of the person, such as their history, life and goals that are beyond, or outside, the current purview of our practice. Consistent with person-centred practice principles, these aspects of the person need to be acknowledged, understood and respected because they are inextricably linked with personally meaningful participation.

Participation is a fundamental right for all (UN General Assembly 1948), yet people with disability still experience participation restrictions and exclusion. The ICF and the fPRC have assisted and guided our thinking – but we also need to understand the theoretical premises that support these frameworks, to understand the active ingredients that promote change.

As practitioners, we are most concerned with the idea of change – how it happens, its pace and shape (linear or non-linear) – because understanding how change occurs will help us decide what to do and how to act. In the field of childhood disability, our focus is on theories of behaviour, learning and development. These theories specify constructs, principles and assumptions about how change occurs that guide our thinking and can inform our actions to drive change in practice. Change is complex, but theories help us to understand these complexities – they give us the scope and fluidity in thinking about what is needed in clinical practice, allowing us to provide flexible, needs-based, transparent services (Hodgetts et al. 2013). These are services that will assist people to live the lives they desire.

The word 'participation' became part of our paediatric rehabilitation language following publication of the ICF in 2001, but the idea of participation was 'alive and well' before that. This is evident through many well-studied aspects of human behaviour from varied disciplines and traditions; including motivation, cognition, social cognition, ecological/context-based learning and lifespan development. These varied bodies of work provide some universal constructs and theories related to human needs, cognition and self-identity. Theories also tell us about the importance of environments and settings, which are associated with expectations and norms for behaviour. As well, theories tell us that development and learning occur as functions of time.

In this chapter we focus on theories that deal with behaviour, learning or development of the individual (rather than the group). We aim to identify theoretical orientations that will add insight into how we study and promote participation in the presence of childhood onset disability.

SCENARIO AND INTRODUCTION TO THE THEORETICAL ORIENTATIONS

SAMI'S STORY

Sami is 7 years old. He, his mother Maya, and younger brother Zain (aged 6), have just arrived in Melbourne, Australia from Syria after 12 months of travel and hardship. Maya speaks some English, Sami has only a few words in English and he has dysarthria so it is often difficult for people who do not know him to understand what he is saying. He is enrolled to start school – but the term has already started without him. He will go to a local school that is wheelchair accessible, which is important because he has cerebral palsy and his gross motor function is classified at Gross Motor Function Classification System (GMFCS) level IV: Sami can take a few steps if fully supported, but otherwise he uses his new electric wheelchair. The family have no close relatives in Melbourne but are linked to their religious community. Sami and Zain are very close friends as well as being brothers. Maya tells us that Zain has always looked out for Sami, speaking for him if needed when visiting with the large extended family in Syria, and playing with him at home. The boys' favourite activity is soccer and now Sami can chase the ball with his electric wheelchair, instead of being pushed in a manual chair as he was in Syria. Sami has not had regular healthcare for some years, and he has missed a lot of school. His mother Maya wants to know how best to help him assimilate at school and in the community.

This story outlines various aspects of Sami's life, including his disability, family, current life situation, activities, past experiences, and his mother's hopes for him. The five theoretical orientations in Table 2.1 focus on different aspects that can be considered in relation to Sami's life, and bring to the fore different ideas about how change comes about. Each orientation deals with the person-in-environment, but with different key constructs, explanatory assumptions (causal propositions), and relative emphases and scope. Practitioners can use one, or several, of these theoretical orientations to guide their thinking and reasoning about 'what to do'. If you think about operating a zoom camera, the theories guide the practitioner to focus on one aspect of the whole picture at any one time. The practitioner can also zoom out to get the bigger picture of Sami's life, then focus in again on another aspect, considering what that might mean for how, when, and where to intervene. The different orientations can therefore be used to consider intervention in the complex system of factors that comprise participation – the constructs and processes in the fPRC. Thus, the fPRC constructs can be 'seen' from various theoretical vantage points. The theoretical lenses guide the practitioner's thinking and action so that practice is theory-informed as well as evidence-based.

Different theoretical orientations provide varying perspectives on how change occurs.

Table 2.1 Theoretical orientations, key constructs and principles, and examples of theories

Theoretical orientation and lens	Link to fPRC	Key constructs and principles	Theory example
1. Needs-based motivational theories Motivational lens	Links to activity competence and sense-of-self	**Level of analysis:** personal **Key constructs:** motivation, needs **Driving principles:** Innate psychological needs underpin motivation to initiate and sustain goal pursuits	**Self-determination theory** (Ryan and Deci 2000) • Concerned with the extent to which three basic psychological *needs* are nurtured in the social context. These needs are: autonomy – feeling agency and choice; competence – belief that one has the ability to pursue one's goals; and relatedness – the need to want to interact with and be connected to others • The extent to which needs are fulfilled influences self-determined motivation (Standage et al. 2003)
2. Expectancy-value theories Cognitive lens	Links to preferences	**Level of analysis:** personal **Key constructs:** beliefs, values, norms, expectancies, behavioural intentions **Driving principles:** An individual's expectations, as well as values or beliefs, affect behaviour and the choices s/he makes	**Theory of planned behaviour** (Ajzen 1985) • Human behaviour is guided by *beliefs* about (1) the likely outcomes of the behaviour and evaluations of these outcomes (behavioural beliefs); (2) the normative expectations of others and motivation to comply with these expectations (normative beliefs); and (3) the presence of factors that may facilitate or impede performance of the behaviour and the perceived power of these factors (control beliefs) • Attitude toward the behaviour, subjective norms and perception of behavioural control lead to the formation of a *behavioural intention*
3. Social cognitive learning theories Psychosocial lens	Links to sense of self and self-regulation	**Level of analysis:** personal (in relation to others and the environment) **Key constructs:** cognition, learning, outcome expectancies, self-efficacy, identification (re self), self-regulation **Driving principles:** Cognition (beliefs) underlies behaviour People learn by observing others in the context of social interactions, experiences and outside media influences Human behaviour is caused by three influences: personal self-efficacy, the response received after the behaviour is performed and aspects of the setting that influence ability to successfully complete a behaviour	**Social cognitive theory** (Bandura 2001) • Individuals are self-developing, self-regulating, self-reflecting and proactive, rather than being just shaped by environments or inner forces (an *agentic perspective*) • Human agency is characterised by intentionality and forethought, self-regulation and self-reflection about one's capabilities, functioning and the meaning and purpose of one's life pursuits (Bandura 2001) • People make judgments about their capabilities, anticipate the probable effects of different events and courses of action, size up socio-structural opportunities and constraints, and regulate their behaviour accordingly • Self-efficacy, belief systems and self-regulation are linked to self-development, adaptation and self-renewal

(Continued)

Table 2.1   (Continued...)

Theoretical orientation and lens	Link to fPRC	Key constructs and principles	Theory example
4. Ecological/ context-based learning theories Ecological lens	Links to the role of context/ environment	**Level of analysis:** ecological **Key constructs:** learning, context, engagement, identity **Driving principles:** People learn and develop self-identity through actual, practical experience with a subject through participation in the social world; this points to the importance of the active engagement of the learner with the material and in context. Learning is not purely a cognitive process; learning is an integral and inseparable aspect of social practice. Learning is situated in a specific context and particular social and physical environment	**Situated learning theory** (Aadal and Kirkevold 2011; Lave and Wenger 1991) • Focuses on the relationship between learning and the social situation in which it occurs; focus is on the types of social engagements that provide the proper context for learning to take place • Legitimate peripheral participation leads to membership in a community of practice • Participation always entails situated negotiation and renegotiation of meaning in the world • People understand and experience the world through the constant interactions by which they reconstruct their *identity* (i.e. changing one's identity)
5. Lifespan developmental systems theories Systems-based, developmental and socio-ecological lens	Links to the fPRC as a dynamic system	**Level of analysis:** socio-ecological **Key constructs:** person-environment transactions, relational change, homeostasis, human plasticity, interdependence **Driving principles:** An individual requires access to an environment, is interdependent with other humans, has an innate tendency to preserve and expand life and has capacity for behavioural variability. 'Systems thinking' refers to a framework or set of theoretical principles for understanding the dynamic interrelations among various personal and environmental factors; emphasises reciprocal and dynamic person-environment transactions; pays explicit attention to the social, institutional and cultural contexts of people-environment relations There are changing relationships between the individual and his/her life context over time (Lerner 1998)	**Positive youth development perspective** (Lerner et al. 2006) • Systemic (bidirectional, fused) relations between individuals and contexts provide the basis of human behaviour and developmental change • Changes across the lifespan are propelled by dynamic relations between individuals and the multiple levels of the ecology of human development • Human development is relatively plastic and is based on individual-context relations, legitimising an optimistic view of the potential for positive change (bringing in a strengths-based model)

Table 2.1 displays an overview of five theoretical orientations pertinent to participation. This table links the orientations to the fPRC framework and provides one example of a theory reflecting each orientation.

NEEDS-BASED MOTIVATIONAL THEORIES: SELF-DETERMINATION THEORY

Literature

Self-determination theory (Ryan and Deci 2000), a meta-theory of motivation, provides a basis for considering key motivational processes that influence the desire to participate and sustain involvement in life situations. Autonomy, the psychological need for agency and choice, provides a way of understanding the extent to which goals are internally or externally regulated. Collaborative goal setting in therapy contexts is a practical example of harnessing this mechanism (Poulsen et al. 2015). Competence, the psychological need to feel one has the ability to strive towards one's goals, is nurtured through experiences that scaffold a sense of accomplishment. Competence support is well acknowledged in many interventions for children with disabilities and can be enhanced through both skill development and environmental accommodations (Miller et al. 2016). Finally, Relatedness, the psychological need to feel connected to and cared for by others, can be seen to manifest in the therapist–client relationship (King 2017) and in the sense of belonging that children can experience in community leisure, home and academic environments.

Application to Sami's Story

Developing an appreciation of Sami's personal interests and strengths provides a basis from which to start exploring the way he may optimally engage with both school and religious organisations. He may have had limited opportunities to develop his interests and self-awareness in the past, so exposure to novel and stimulating activities may provide the basis for exploration. Being able to share an interest with peers, teachers and religious leaders can provide the means whereby he starts to feel better connected and cared for in his new environment. He may also lack confidence in his abilities to act upon his environment because of his disabilities and limited opportunities. Scaffolding of the social and physical environment may help him start to grow in confidence.

How might the broader Syrian and school community be enlisted to provide Sami with a sense of social connectedness?

EXPECTANCY-VALUE THEORIES: THEORY OF PLANNED BEHAVIOUR

Literature

Expectancy-value theories such as the theory of Planned Behaviour (Ajzen 1985) focus on various cognitive variables, including beliefs and expectancies. Expectancy-value theories have been used to understand how expectancies and values underlie the activity choices of children with and without disabilities. This includes the trade-offs they make in choosing whether or not to participate in social activities (Stewart et al. 2012) and how interests and perceived costs determine children's engagement in activities at recess (Watkinson et al. 2005). These theories suggest the importance of creating value and meaning for therapy activities through authentic connections to activities, as seen in the literature on youth development (Dawes and Larson 2011) and therapy engagement (King et al. 2019). This theoretical orientation illuminates the importance of cognitions in addition to preferences in the fPRC, including, for example, behavioural intentions. Implementation intentions ('I intend to perform goal-directed behaviour y when I encounter situation z') serve to connect intentions to action and are a powerful self-regulatory tool for overcoming the typical obstacles encountered in the initiation of goal-directed actions. Extensive research shows the importance of implementation intentions on goal attainment (Gollwitzer and Sheeran 2006).

Application to Sami's Story

Sami's mother Maya wants to know how to best help Sami assimilate at school and in the community. Expectancy-value theories draw our attention to her expectations, beliefs and values. What are Maya's expectations regarding school and community involvement for her son? What are her beliefs, what does she value, and what does she hope for? When she mentions 'assimilation', does this mean Sami doing well in school and being involved in a religious community? Does it involve Sami making friends or feeling less anxious when speaking to others? The trauma experienced by the family in their 12-month journey may play a role here, as well as Syrian culture, which emphasises interdependence and the collective rather than the individual. The service provider might focus on understanding what Maya and Sami both want and expect, which may enhance their engagement in the therapy process and contribute to positive outcomes.

What would you do if Maya and Sami express different goals regarding 'assimilation'; if it means something different to each of them?

SOCIAL COGNITIVE LEARNING THEORY

Literature

Social cognitive learning theories such as Bandura's Social Cognitive Theory (2001) focus on cognitive variables operating in a social context, providing a **psychosocial lens** to therapy. People learn about their capacities and self-identity from observing and interacting with others in a social context. There is relatively little literature focusing on self-constructs in paediatric rehabilitation, although self-efficacy has been examined in interventions ranging from virtual play (Reid 2002) to family-centred care (King and Chiarello 2014). The role of self-regulation of cognitive and social behaviour has been examined in the literature on acquired brain injury (Ylvisaker and Feeney 2002). This theoretical orientation illuminates the importance of a range of self-constructs, linking to 'sense of self' and self-regulation in the fPRC, including self-understanding and reflective self-processes. This orientation expands our understanding of the importance of the self in participation.

Application to Sami's Story

From this lens, the social environment of Maya and Sami becomes the emphasis. Maya is particularly interested in Sami's participation at school and in the community. Social cognitive learning theories draw our attention to how these environments and activity settings can provide learning opportunities for Sami. What activity settings might accommodate Sami's interests and abilities, and offer opportunity for involvement? How might Sami's limited English vocabulary and dysarthria affect his participation and enjoyment of participation opportunities? Does Sami feel anxious or frustrated when speaking to others he doesn't know well, given that they often have difficulty in understanding what he is saying? The value of the community to Syrians indicates that group experiences may be particularly beneficial. The service provider might focus on helping Maya to find a support group of Syrian parents, or to find community recreational groups for the children, particularly ones where parents can be involved.

How would you work to provide Sami with experiences where he can develop his sense of self as an agentic and proactive human being; driving what he does but also in making sense of his world?

ECOLOGICAL/CONTEXT-BASED LEARNING THEORIES: SITUATED LEARNING THEORY

Literature

Ecological approaches view learning as inextricably linked to the context in which it occurs. Situated Learning Theory posits that people acquire knowledge and skills in settings that 'make sense' – that is, the everyday settings in which the skills and behaviours are used to engage with objects and people (Dunst et al. 2010). This theoretical orientation links with the notion of participation in context in the fPRC.

Dunst and colleagues' research and development of Contextually Mediated Practices™ in early intervention is grounded in situated learning theory (Dunst et al. 2010). This practice model proposes that everyday family and community life provide the opportunity for learning that children need for development (Dunst et al. 2000). Contextually Mediated Practices™ is based on four principles: (1) culturally meaningful everyday experiences are sources of child learning and mastery of competencies; (2) experiences and opportunities should strengthen children's self-initiated and self-directed learning to promote both development of competence and recognition of their own abilities; (3) parent- or caregiver-mediated child learning is effective when it strengthens parent confidence and competence in supporting everyday child learning; and (4) the role of practitioners is to support parent capacity and confidence (Morgan et al. 2016). This approach prioritises the identification of interest-based everyday activity settings. It also alerts the parent or caregiver to the rich learning opportunities within those settings. Capitalising on available existing opportunities is an effective method of increasing both child and parent confidence and competence.

Application to Sami's Story

Maya's interest in Sami's assimilation at school can be supported through assisting her to identify activities in which to situate Sami's learning of knowledge, skills and practices relevant to the school setting. For example, assisting Maya and Zain to seek out naturally occurring opportunities for Sami to experience repeated social interactions with others in the community (e.g. in the shops and at the mosque) may increase his communication success with peers at school. Sami's strong interest in soccer is another avenue for supporting a wide range of learning in 'soccer-rich' environments, such as seeking to join an all-ability local soccer club, being an active spectator at games or collecting soccer paraphernalia. This preference-based learning can act as positive behavioural support in the development of a range of skills (Dunst et al. 2010). Situated learning theory can also be used to support in-school learning opportunities by identifying multiple opportunities for exploration and mastery in social and non-social activities, as learning is dependent on having a sufficient number of opportunities to participate.

How can the school-based team (teachers, aides, therapists) be supported to identify and enable repeated positive opportunities for learning for Sami? What goals could be prioritised for this?

LIFESPAN DEVELOPMENTAL SYSTEMS THEORIES: POSITIVE YOUTH DEVELOPMENT PERSPECTIVE

Literature

Lifespan development theories conceptualise development as occurring within a dynamic transactional system characterised by individual-on-context and context-on-individual influences (Halfon et al. 2014; Lerner 2005). Developmental systems theories encompass the notion of plasticity, or capacity for change over time, and diversity of development within and between individuals (Lerner 2005).

The positive youth development perspective has two core premises (Lerner 2005). The first is that youth-context alignment promotes positive youth development. Achieving contextual alignment requires marshalling personal and contextual developmental assets, such as human (skills and abilities of people in their roles), physical/institutional, collective activity (engagement between people) and accessibility (ability of the individual to use the assets). Community-based programmes are a vital source of developmental assets and optimal youth development programmes are characterised by three key features: (1) they are positive and sustained; (2) provide for adult–youth relationships; and (3) provide skill building activities and opportunity to use the skills in community activities (Lerner 2005).

The second premise is that positive youth development is characterised by five Cs, competence, confidence, connection, character and caring/compassion, representing functionally valued behaviours that promote well-being in time. These five Cs lead to thriving over time, as characterised by the sixth C, contribution: contribution to self (maintaining one's health and ability to be an active agent in one's own development), contribution to family, contribution to community and contribution to civic society. Contribution has a strong connection to the notion of participation.

Application to Sami's Story

Sami's story highlights strengths in some developmental assets, such as collective activity within the immediate family and access to safe learning environments, but a loss of other contextual assets through the move from Syria to Australia. Using a developmental systems theory lens suggests that focusing on strengths within the individual and seeking and supporting contextual assets will lead to greater youth-context alignment, and that this will in turn support the development of the five Cs. Importantly in youth development theory is the perspective that promoting wellbeing in the here-and-now, by attending to health needs, access to quality education and community connectedness can lead to thriving over time.

Which assets might you identify as being most critical to enable or support Sami?

BRINGING THE IDEAS TOGETHER

The theoretical orientations we have discussed provide a range of perspectives by which to explain participation and how changes in participation may occur. The orientations point to key operative factors, suggesting where and how to intervene to promote participation. In the case of Sami, the orientations variously focused on his motivation, family beliefs and valued activities, learning opportunities, natural opportunities for everyday learning– and the importance of context–person alignment. The theories foreground different explanatory concepts, highlighting various yet overlapping causal or pivotal aspects involved in understanding behaviour, learning and development.

Considering these theoretical perspectives in relation to the fPRC can facilitate the operationalisation of participation interventions. Therapists informally hypothesise, test and evaluate their interventions through clinical reasoning. Therapists can choose from the orientations to see what each brings to their intervention with a given client and family. Each lens directs attention to different entry points for intervention and considers different mechanisms of change. In addition, however, the theories have common implications for practice. They all point to:

- the importance of understanding and being responsive to the client's situation and circumstances;
- the value of listening with intent to clients;
- treating people with respect and dignity; and
- acknowledging clients' perspectives, strengths and priorities.

LINK TO VIGNETTE 2.1
'Annie's in Charge of the Baking', p. 25.

Thus, the theoretical orientations endorse the value and use of family-centred/person-centred care principles. From a humanistic perspective, the client and family are considered to have motivations (desire to have relationships, and be autonomous and competent), beliefs and expectations that affect their actions, and a sense of self (worth, concept, identity) whose coherence is important to maintain. Our examination of the relevance of various theoretical orientations in explaining participation and the operation of the fPRC framework indicates the importance of the practitioner's sensitivity, experience and expertise, and relational skills in bringing about client change (King 2017). The implications for practice include the importance of client/family-centred and culturally sensitive care, respect for diversity, the importance of being transparent about expectations and openly negotiating roles, and fostering experience-based learning in natural environments and over time.

There is undoubted value in adopting clear theoretical perspectives that illuminate the underlying assumptions of how we understand and apply the concept of participation in practice. In this chapter, we did not consider the application of other theories to the field of participation, including theories of group dynamics/behaviour, such as Zimmerman's empowerment theory (Zimmerman and Warschausky 1998), and sociological/sociocultural theories, such as role theory. These theories help us to understand acculturation and transition to new groups (King et al. 2018). Essentially, the field could do more with the 'group' aspect of participation – the 'social inclusion' perspective that has long been contrasted with 'participation'.

SUMMARY OF KEY IDEAS

The reflective practitioner draws on theory-informed evidence. Intentional practice aimed at enabling positive participation outcomes can be informed by a range of theoretical lens:

- **Needs-based motivational theories** focus on how to motivate children through their personal interests, choices, experience of competence and connectedness.
- **Expectancy-value theories** focus on cognitive variables such as beliefs, behaviour, and intentions.
- **Social cognitive learning theories** consider the sense of self and view the person as agentic.
- **Ecological/context-based learning theories** stress the importance of context and natural learning opportunities in everyday life.
- **Lifespan developmental systems theories** stress the alignment of person-context for wellbeing and participation.

REFERENCES

Aadal L, Kirkevold M (2011) Integrating situated learning theory and neuropsychological research to facilitate patient participation and learning in traumatic brain injury rehabilitation patients. *Brain Inj* 25: 717–728.

Ajzen I (1985) From intentions to actions: A theory of planned behavior. In: Kuhl J (Ed), *Action Control*. Heidelberg, Berlin: Springer-Verlage.

Bandura A (2001) Social cognitive theory: an agentic perspective. *Annu Rev Psychol* **52**: 1–26.

Dawes NP, Larson R (2011) How youth get engaged: grounded-theory research on motivational development in organized youth programs. *Dev Psychol* **47**: 259–269.

Dunst CJ, Hamby D, Trivette CM, Raab M, Bruder MB (2000) Everyday family and community life and children's naturally occurring learning opportunities. *J Early Interv* 23: 151–164.

Dunst CJ, Raab M, Trivette CM, Swanson J (2010) Community based everyday child learning opportunities. In: Mcwilliam RA (Ed) *Working with Families of Young Children with Special Needs*. New York: The Guilford Press.

Gollwitzer PM, Sheeran P (2006) Implementation intentions and goal achievement: A meta-analysis of effects and processes. *Adv Exp Soc Psychol* **38**: 69–119.

Halfon N, Larson K, Lu M, Tullis E, Russ S (2014) Lifecourse health development: past, present and future. *Matern Child Health J* **18**: 344–365.

Hodgetts S, Nicholas D, Zwaigenbaum L, McConnell D (2013) Parents' and professionals' perceptions of family-centered care for children with autism spectrum disorder across service sectors. *Soc Sci Med* **96**: 138–146.

Imms C, Granlund M, Wilson PH, Steenbergen B, Rosenbaum PL, Gordon AM (2017) Participation, both a means and an end: a conceptual analysis of processes and outcomes in childhood disability. *Dev Med Child Neurol* **59**: 16–25.

King G (2017) The role of the therapist in therapeutic change: how knowledge from mental health can inform pediatric rehabilitation. *Phys Occup Ther Pediatr* **37**: 121–138.

King G, Chiarello L (2014) Family-centered care for children with cerebral palsy: conceptual and practical considerations to advance care and practice. *J Child Neurol* **29**: 1046–1054.

King G, Imms C, Stewart D, Freeman M, Nguyen T (2018) A transactional framework for pediatric rehabilitation: shifting the focus to situated contexts, transactional processes, and adaptive developmental outcomes. *Disabil Rehabil* **40**: 1829–1841.

King G, Chiarello L, Ideishi R et al. (2019) The nature, value, and experience of engagement in pediatric rehabilitation: Perspectives of youth, caregivers, and service providers. *Developmental Neurorehabilitation.* **23**: 18–30.

Lave J, Wenger E (1991) *Situated Learning: Legitimate Peripheral Participation.* Cambridge University Press, Cambridge.

Lerner RM (1998) Theories of human development: Contemporary perspectives. In: Lerner RM (Ed) *Handbook of Child Psychology*, 5th ed. New York: John Wiley & Sons.

Lerner RM (2005) Promoting positive youth development: Theoretical and empirical bases. *Workshop on the Science of Adolescent Health and Development.* Washington DC: National Research Council/Institute of Medicine: National Academy of Sciences.

Lerner RM, Lerner JV, Almerigi J et al. (2006) Towards a new vision and vocabulary about adolescence: Theoretical, empirical, and applied bases of a 'Positive Youth Development' perspective. In: Balter L, Tamis-Lemonda CS (Eds) *Child Psychology: A Handbook of Contemporary Issues.* New York: Psychology Press/Taylor & Francis.

Lewin K (1943) Psychology and the process of group living. *J Soc Psychol* **17**: 113–131.

Miller L, Ziviani J, Ware RS, Boyd RN (2016) Does context matter? Mastery motivation and therapy engagement of children with cerebral palsy. *Phys Occup Ther Pediatr* **36**: 155–170.

Morgan C, Novak I, Dale RC, Guzzetta A, Badawi N (2016) Single blind randomised controlled trial of GAME (Goals – Activity – Motor Enrichment) in infants at high risk of cerebral palsy. *Res Dev Disabil* **55**: 256–267.

Poulsen A, Ziviani J, Cuskelly M (2015) The science of goal setting. In: Poulsen A, Ziviani J, Cuskelly M (Eds) *Motivation and Goal Setting: Engaging Children and Parents in Therapy.* London: Jessica Kingsley.

Reid DT (2002) Benefits of a virtual play rehabilitation environment for children with cerebral palsy on perceptions of self-efficacy: a pilot study. *Pediatr Rehabil* **5**: 141–148.

Ryan RM, Deci EL (2000) Self-determination theory and the facilitation of intrinsic motivation, social development, and well-being. *Am Psychol* **55**: 68–78.

Standage M, Duda JL, Ntoumanis N (2003) A model of contextual motivation in physical education: using constructs from self-determination and achievement goal theories to predict physical activity intentions. *J Educ Psychol* **95**: 97–110.

Stewart DA, Lawless JJ, Shimmell LJ et al. (2012) Social participation of adolescents with cerebral palsy: trade-offs and choices. *Phys Occup Ther Pediatr* **32**: 167–179.

UN General Assembly (1948) Universal Declaration of Human Rights (217 [III] A). Paris: UN General Assembly.

Watkinson EJ, Dwyer SA, Nielsen AB (2005) Children theorize about reasons for recess engagement: does expectancy-value theory apply? *Adapt Phys Activ Q* **22**: 179–197.

WHO (2001) *International Classification of Functioning, Disability and Health: Short Version.* Geneva: World Health Organization.

Ylvisaker M, Feeney T (2002) Executive functions, self-regulation, and learned optimism in paediatric rehabilitation: a review and implications for intervention. *Pediatr Rehabil* **5**: 51–70.

Zimmerman MA, Warschausky S (1998) Empowerment theory for rehabilitation research: conceptual and methodological issues. *Rehabil Psychol* **43**: 3–16.

Annie's journey from acute to postacute rehabilitation in preparation for transition from hospital to home highlights some of the challenges in providing opportunities for participation. From the lens of self-determination theory, accessing and enabling key motivational processes for autonomy and agency, competence and skill development and relatedness and connection with family – while they too are in transition – can be challenging in these situations. As you read, consider how the nature of participation changed – for both the therapist and Annie. In this vignette, participation is enacted as agency or influence and self-determination theory may help explain the shifts that are made to reconstruct roles and responsibilities through providing opportunities for choice and decision making.

Annie's in Charge of the Baking (UK)

Carolyn Dunford

Annie is a 16-year-old girl with an acquired brain injury due to an arterial venous malformation. She has retained the majority of her cognitive skills but is dependent on a ventilator to breathe, a wheelchair for mobility and the assistance of two people for personal care. Annie is receiving 6 months of intensive residential rehabilitation in a specialist centre for children and young people with severe acquired brain injuries. Annie is keen to participate in a wide range of activities during her rehabilitation but is particularly keen to start baking again.

Enabling meaningful participation in postacute residential rehabilitation settings can be challenging as visits to home and school are limited. Therapists find out as much as possible about the child and family's unique profile to ensure rehabilitation is as relevant as possible. In addition to the complexity of the setting, the nature of participation can change following severe injury, due to limitations caused by the newly acquired disability.

The family dynamics are also in a state of transition; family members may have been told that the child was unlikely to survive and are adjusting to the reality of them being alive with a severe disability. The parent–child relationship needs renegotiation with the young person finding themselves suddenly dependent again, often for basic personal care. Furthermore, there will have been a big impact on any siblings as the child with the brain injury requires much of the parents' care and emotional energy and siblings often feel neglected and are adjusting to a different relationship with their disabled sibling.

The occupational therapist, Lucy, considered how Annie could participate in baking given her physical disabilities including very limited hand movements. Lucy brought all the ingredients to the kitchen in the house where Annie had her room. It was holiday time and Annie stated she wanted her brother and grandparents who were visiting to be included. Annie had selected a biscuit recipe she was familiar with.

Lucy had thought the way for Annie to participate was for her to feel the texture of the baking mixture and to operate the food processor which had been adapted for switch use.

Annie had other ideas. She did not want to put her hands in the mixture or use the adapted equipment rather she wanted to instruct her brother and grandparents in what they needed to do to make the biscuits. Annie was using her strengths, her cognitive and verbal skills, to make the biscuit making happen in the way she wanted it to. Her brother Tom was used to being bossed about by his older sister but had not been involved with her in baking before. Tom really wanted to help his sister and was pleased to have found a way to be involved. Her grandparents watched on and soon realised they could help by following Annie's instructions and letting her be in charge.

Lucy reflected on how she had made assumptions about participating with the baking activity requiring Annie's physical involvement. She had not considered how you can participate, and in fact control an activity without having the motor skills to perform the task, by directing others. Annie's rehabilitation goals included many non-discretionary activities that she needed to do such as learning to drive her electric wheelchair and using eye-gaze technology for word processing at school and to access social media. Annie felt she had lost control in so many areas of her life so selecting a discretionary activity such as baking and deciding her method of participating gave her a sense of agency over one meaningful life situation.

Impact of Childhood Neurodisability on Participation

Claire Willis and Mats Granlund

INTRODUCTION

Participation, defined as 'involvement in a life situation' (WHO 2001), is a complex multidimensional concept that has both an attendance and involvement component (Imms et al. 2017, Chapter 1). Life situations have been described as frequently occurring routines or activities that are complex and directed towards meaningful goals (Adolfsson et al. 2011). Participation in activities within life situations for individuals with disabilities varies; in environmental setting, such as home, school/work, community and leisure; in activity type, range and frequency; and in levels of engagement and enjoyment. In addition to these individual variations, the content and structure of life situations shift with changes in age, activity preference, life roles, context and culture. It is this constellation of elements that we call patterns of participation.

Patterns of participation can be considered from the perspective of the two dimensions of participation: being there, and being involved (or engaged) while being there. To date, most measures of participation focus on attendance, with less focus on involvement or engagement (Adair et al. 2018). These objective indicators of attendance are important in identifying areas of need and difference within populations, to assist in guiding targets for service provision and policy development. However, involvement in any life situation is (on an individual level) associated with engagement and meaning. We know that the two dimensions are related, as people attend activities more frequently if they are more engaged in the activity (Lygnegård et al. 2019). However, attendance and involvement patterns can also vary independently of each other. Understanding the association between these dimensions is imperative for accurately identifying patterns and challenges, and addressing participation goals.

Patterns of participation (and restrictions) vary with chronological age and environmental setting (King et al. 2009). The activity preferences (and subsequently, participation patterns) of very young children with disabilities are vastly different than those of school-aged children, adolescents and adults. Home, school, work, leisure and community settings present diverse tasks and experiences that will similarly vary according to age and activity type. Participation patterns within each age group and environmental setting can be further dependent on sex, perceived and actual functional ability of an individual, and environmental factors such as family support. These significant influences and individual differences indicate the importance of opportunity, support and preference; particularly

Age influences the life roles and activity preferences of individuals, both of which will shift throughout the life course.

as children may acquire particular activity preferences and participation patterns very early in life (Imms et al. 2016).

We must also acknowledge that participation patterns across age groups and environmental settings are influenced by variations in socio-economics, culture, and services, systems and policies between regions and countries. For example, in a low-income environment, children are expected to take on household tasks at an earlier age than those living in a high-income environment, and often fulfil the role as the primary income earner in the family. While needs such as food and clothing are frequently investigated and emphasised, we have limited knowledge of higher order needs (e.g.

LINK TO VIGNETTE 1.2
'You Have to Walk and Talk to Go to School', p. 12.

belonging, self-actualisation) of individuals with disabilities in low and middle-income settings (Lygnegård et al. 2013). Similarities and differences in participation patterns within and between countries can provide insights into the extent to which nations uphold disability rights constitutions, value the participation of people with disabilities, and highlight how children and families perceive and choose their opportunities.

There are several elements that together describe patterns of participation for individuals with a disability. This information enables us to identify participation opportunities and challenges, tailor programmes to meet the needs of diverse ages and environmental settings, and develop effective approaches for use across differing systems and cultural settings. In this chapter we will discuss patterns of participation based on age groups, that is, very young children, school-aged children, adolescents, young adults and adults. Observed across a life time perspective, individuals with a disability are first active participants in the home setting, gradually transferring to activity settings at school, in the community, and leisure pursuits. We then perhaps come full circle, with older adults participating less in community settings, and more in the home. Within each age cluster, we will describe patterns of participation from the perspective of both attendance and involvement across relevant environmental settings. Finally, we will deliver conclusions regarding the bidirectional interactions between participation patterns and influencing factors across the lifespan, highlighting knowledge gaps and future directions.

PARTICIPATION PATTERNS ACROSS THE LIFESPAN
Very Young Children

The first years of a child's life are characterised by rapid changes in common activity types. This is due to children obtaining new skills as a result of developmental changes associated with learning and growth, and to the expectations of parents and society regarding life roles and school entry. In a child's first 12–24 months of life, the home environment (including the family) is the most prominent environmental setting. Childcare settings, kindergartens and preschools are often introduced as second pertinent environmental settings before children attend formal school. Both home and preschool settings are characterised by recurring routines and activities that make up the fabric of everyday life. Participation in activities within these settings has a significant impact on a child's functioning and development, if children attend the activities frequently and with a high degree of involvement (Aydogan 2012). A relatively small number of studies have investigated the participation patterns of very young children with disabilities in the home and preschool settings (see Chapter 5).

Our most comprehensive knowledge of participation patterns of young children comes from the recent development of the Young Children's Participation and Environment Measure (YC-PEM, Chapter 12).

Di Marino et al. (2018) used the YC-PEM to capture attendance and involvement in home activities, day-care setting, and in the community for young children with disabilities (n = 90). While the average level of involvement was the same across environmental settings, there was significant variation in attendance. The highest frequency of attendance was reported for activities in the home, followed by day-care settings. Although the greatest restrictions were observed in activities in the community, parents also desired the least amount of change in this setting. While the community environment may present with greater challenges, health professionals should be aware that parents may also have different expectations about community engagement for their children at this age.

Studies investigating the participation patterns of children with disabilities in preschool settings typically define and measure 'inclusion' and comprise all children in need of special supports. Inclusion has been operationalised in terms of a child's attendance and level of engagement in activities (Lillvist 2010), or as social interaction between children (Guralnick et al. 2008). While there are inconsistent results describing attendance in preschool activities and the frequency of social interactions for children with and without a need for special support, there is agreement that the characteristics of the activities that the two groups of children attend, differ. Children in need of special support (primarily children with disabilities) spend more time with adults and less time with peers and are less engaged in complex activities such as role play. These differences are especially pronounced in free-play and child-initiated activities, activities known for supporting the development of self-regulation and initiation skills in young children (Reszka et al. 2012). Consideration of the activity context (i.e. place, activity, people and objects) in the preschool environment, may be necessary to optimise patterns of attendance and involvement for young children with disabilities.

Recent emphasis has been placed on the environment in supporting participation of young children in relevant life situations. Although there is evidence to suggest that child-related factors (e.g. medical fragility, complex behaviours) can make it difficult for families to build sustainable daily routines (Axelsson et al. 2013), environmental factors demonstrate a more pronounced and consistent contribution in explaining participation patterns (Di Marino et al. 2018). Specifically, environmental helpfulness (resources, support) and family functioning influence participation patterns across home, preschool and community settings – a finding also demonstrated in studies of school-age children and adolescents (Lygnegård et al. 2019; King et al. 2009). Redirecting focus to modifying the environment (family functioning, support and access to resources), should support intervention planning for very young children, in collaboration with their families.

School-Age Children

In addition to the transition from preschool to school, school-age children begin to engage in leisure activities in community settings. Increasing importance is placed on participating in activities with peers, rather than solely with family members (Ullenhag et al. 2014). Research by King et al. (2009) has reported that children with disabilities transition at a slower rate from participation in activities in the home to the community, and from activities with family members to activities with peers. A successful transition seems to be dependent on family factors, such as family coherence and family social networks. However, the fit between the child's capability, that is, the ability to perform activities with different levels of support, and environmental facilitators, are also important to consider. Hwang et al. (2015) described that children with more profound impairments attend fewer activities outside the home than children with more mild impairments. Interestingly, the gap between what activities the children could perform with support (capability) and the activities actually attended, was larger for children with mild

It is the cumulative effect of several factors, rather than a single factor, that influence participation. What are the interacting factors influencing participation for a child you know?

impairments, compared to those with more profound impairments. Children with mild impairments may perceive more participation restrictions outside of the home (relative to their capability) as a result of the more frequent exposure to activities in this setting. Professionals may therefore need to obtain information about attendance and involvement across a wide spectrum of activities and settings (especially outside home), together with understanding preferences of the child and family, before developing interventions to optimise participation. This is particularly relevant when considering factors that impact participation in these settings, as it is the cumulative effect of several factors, rather than emphasis of a single factor, that influence outcomes (Imms et al. 2017). Professionals should be aware of the shifting influential factors dependent on activity type, in addition to child preferences and family resources.

Adolescents and Young Adults (Youth)

Adolescence is a life stage characterised by explorations of independence and identity, relationships and sexuality, and social life. It is also a phase of multiple transitions across health, education and employment, as young people move into adulthood.

School continues to be a major life setting, supporting multiple aspects of adolescent development in addition to educational growth. Within the classroom, students with more profound impairments are often not present in classes for a substantial proportion of instructional time, with these absences observed to be highest at the end of a class period (Feldman et al. 2016). As conversations and interactions with peers typically occur shortly after class begins and just before it concludes, restrictions in classroom participation may also influence involvement in social interactions and peer relationships. Outside of the classroom, students with disabilities display lower rates of participation in break activities and in school-based teams and clubs than their typically developing peers. Efforts to facilitate participation opportunities in these contexts may be particularly valuable during high school, for their role in supporting positive adolescent development.

While youth with disabilities have similar leisure time activity preferences as their age-matched peers, they experience significantly lower levels of participation in these contexts. Youth with disabilities attend more unstructured, informal activities alone at home, and less structured, community-based activities with friends (Tonkin et al. 2014). Across all leisure time activities, the greatest participation restrictions are observed in active leisure and physical activities. Children and youth with disabilities participate in significantly less moderate-to-vigorous intensity physical activity and are less likely to meet recommended physical activity guidelines, than their typically developing peers (Carlon et al. 2013). Research exploring the subjective experience of leisure participation has uncovered that meaningful interactions with others contributes substantially to creating positive and engaging experiences for youth with disabilities in these settings (Powrie et al. 2015; Willis et al. 2017). Relationships with family, peers and the wider community may need to be considered as key ingredients to attaining leisure participation goals and influencing healthy, sustained participation patterns.

Within the context of peer relationships, romantic relationships develop. Compared to typically developing youth, those with physical disabilities have less experience of romantic relationships, intimate relationships evolve at later ages, and they are less likely to reach sexual milestones as adolescents (Wiegerink et al. 2010). While these patterns have shown to be strongly associated with participation in peer group activities and dating, they were only weakly associated with physical impairment or sex. Similar patterns have been reported in young people with intellectual disability, describing limited social networks but also detailing greater misunderstandings about sexuality (Jahoda and Pownall 2014). Creating opportunities to participate in peer-based activities and ensuring families and health professionals are proactive in providing suitable information may support young adults with disabilities to engage in safe and age-appropriate romantic relationships.

For young adults, work participation is important for providing financial independence, but also for social interaction and a sense of self-esteem. Studies among young adults with cerebral palsy have described paid work to be among their most frequently identified problems, and that they consider problems related to work very important (Livingston et al. 2011). Compared with the general population of the same age, low proportions of young adults with disabilities are employed or studying, and a relatively high proportion are unemployed. While lower gross motor function capacity and younger age have been associated with unemployment, those who do achieve employment have shown to be able to maintain employment over several years (Verhoef et al. 2014).

> *Peer relationships, meaningful leisure pursuits and employment are important to youth with disabilities.*

Adults and Older Adults

Data from the United Kingdom has shown that among people with cerebral palsy who survived to age 20, 85% lived to age 50 (Hemming et al. 2006). It has been reported that up to 80% of adults with cerebral palsy completed high school, 25% completed university, between 25–55% were employed, over 60% were living independently in the community, and about a third were involved in long-term relationships (Frisch and Msall 2003). Compared with adults without disability, adults with cerebral palsy have significantly greater rates of lifestyle diseases, smaller social networks and greater experiences of loneliness (Peterson et al. 2013; Verdonschot et al. 2009). Although adults with cerebral palsy are living longer, we have limited evidence describing approaches facilitating meaningful participation and supporting positive ageing.

Although restrictions in participation have been described across employment, independent living, and social and leisure activities for adults with disabilities, there appears to be some variation in outcomes. Ambulant individuals with hemiplegic cerebral palsy demonstrate leisure participation patterns and daily physical activity levels comparable to healthy adults (van der Slot et al. 2007). In contrast, adults with bilateral spastic cerebral palsy, especially those with low-level gross motor functioning, display significantly lower durations and intensities of physical activity than healthy adults of the same age (Nieuwenhuijsen et al. 2009). Similarly, adults with cerebral palsy with intellectual disability reported lower frequencies of living independently and having children (van der Dussen et al. 2001). There is also some evidence to suggest that the activity participation of adults with intellectual disabilities may not necessarily reflect their personal interests. Adults with lower levels of functioning and/or multiple impairments may represent a cohort with a greater need for participation support, within which person-centred goal setting should form the foundation.

CONCLUSION

Considered from a life course perspective, this chapter describes the participation patterns of individuals with neurodisability. There are significant challenges experienced by people with neurodisabilities in both attendance and involvement dimensions across all environmental settings throughout the lifespan. However, participating in activities preferred by the individual, and experiencing positive participatory contexts and environments, are highly valued and prioritised by children, youth and adults, and their families. Knowledge of attendance and involvement patterns, *and* the interactions between attributes of the individual, activity context and the environment, are essential for the comprehensive understanding of an individual's participation.

Perhaps our most pertinent conclusion is not a statement, but a question: How can we support children and adults with neurodisability to define optimal participation, on an individual basis, in the here and now? Without this knowledge, how do individuals, families, clinicians and the community accurately interpret and effectively utilise evidence describing participation patterns? For body structure and function and activity outcomes, there are discrete values (e.g. cardiovascular fitness) or developmental curves (e.g. gross motor function, body mass index) that define age-expected and/or individual outcomes. But are such quantifications appropriate for interpreting participation patterns, or deciding whether they are optimal for an individual? Palisano et al. (2012, p. 1 042) have previously defined optimal participation as 'a subjective, personally determined construct, related to the meaning that is associated with and derived from an individual's physical, social, and self-engagement in activity and life situations'. The family of Participation-Related Constructs builds on this, proposing the attendance and involvement components, and transactional processes between these elements and a person's preferences, sense of self, activity competence, context and the environment (Imms et al. 2017, Chapter 1). What constitutes optimal participation needs to be individually and contextually defined (and measured), not only at one point in time, but continually over the life course.

With this is mind, we must recognise the gaps in our knowledge of participation patterns, influencing processes, and subsequent outcomes. We have limited knowledge of how involvement changes over time, due largely to the challenges associated with conceptualising and measuring this dimension longitudinally. Our understandings of the transaction(s) between individuals, their participation, context and the environment are only beginning to evolve (see Part II). This knowledge will help us identify not only *what* changes over time, but *how*, to better inform targeted interventions. With the intimate link between participation and context, it is essential to highlight that our understandings of participation patterns are derived largely from children with disabilities in high-income Western countries. It is imperative we determine patterns across varying socio-economic and cultural environments and identify the needs and preferences of individuals and communities if we are to facilitate meaningful participation outcomes in these settings. Finally, medical advances and concurrent policy initiatives enabling greater access to rehabilitation services have resulted in children with disabilities surviving (and thriving) into adolescence and adulthood. Observing long-term participation outcomes over the life course is essential if we are to support healthy and fulfilling lives for an ageing disability population.

LINK TO VIGNETTE 3.1
'The Battle Hymn of the Tiger Mom', p. 35.

SUMMARY OF KEY IDEAS

- Participation patterns of individuals with neurodisability are best appraised by the individual.
- Identifying patterns of both attendance and involvement is vital for accurately identifying and addressing participation goals.
- Both participation dimensions are influenced by age, intrinsic person-factors and the environment; as such, participation patterns will shift over time both in content and form.
- While participation is a lifespan issue, much less is known about the experiences of adults with childhood-onset neurodisability.
- Children, youth and adults with disabilities have similar participation preferences to their age-matched peers.
- Supportive relationships, family functioning and access to resources are key aspects of the environment that influence participation patterns across home, school and community settings for children, youth and adults.
- Children, youth and adults with higher support needs may represent a cohort with a greater need for intervention: Person/family-centred goal setting should form its foundation.

REFERENCES

Adair B, Ullenhag A, Rosenbaum P, Granlund M, Keen D, Imms C (2018) Measures used to quantify participation in childhood disability and their alignment with the family of participation-related constructs: a systematic review. *Dev Med Child Neurol* **60**: 1101–1116.

Adolfsson M, Malmqvist J, Pless M, Granuld M (2011) Identifying child functioning from an ICF-CY perspective: everyday life situations explored in measures of participation. *Disabil Rehabil* **33**: 1230–1244.

Axelsson AK., Granlund M, Wilder J (2013) Engagement in family activities: A comparative study of children with profound intellectual and multiple disabilities and children with typical development. *Child Care Health Dev* **39**(4): 523–534.

Aydogan C (2012) *Influences of Instructional and Emotional Classroom Environments and Learning Engagement on Low-Income Children's Achievement in the Pre-Kindergarten Year*. Doctoral Dissertation. Nashville, Tenesse: Vanderbilt University.

Carlon SL, Taylor NF, Dodd KJ, Shields N (2013) Differences in habitual physical activity levels of young people with cerebral palsy and their typically developing peers: a systematic review. *Disabil Rehabil* **35**: 647–655.

Di Marino E, Tremblay S, Khetani M, Anaby D (2018) The effect of child, family and environmental factors on the participation of young children with disabilities. *Disabil Health J* **11**: 36–42.

Feldman R, Carter EW, Asmus J, Brock ME (2016) Presence, proximity, and peer interactions of adolescents with severe disabilities in general education classrooms. *Except Child* **82**: 192–208.

Frisch D, Msall ME (2013) Health, functioning, and participation of adolescents and adults with cerebral palsy: a review of outcomes research. *Dev Disabil Res Rev* **18**: 84–94.

Guralnick MJ, Neville B, Hammond MA, Connor RT (2008) Continuity and change from full-inclusion early childhood programs through the early elementary period. *J Early Interv* **30**: 237–250.

Hemming K, Hutton JL, Pharoah PO (2006) Long-term survival for a cohort of adults with cerebral palsy. *Dev Med Child Neurol* **48**: 90–95.

Hwang A-W, Yen C-F, Liou T-H et al. (2015) Participation of children with disabilities in Taiwan: the gap between independence and frequency. *PLoS One* **10**: e0126693.

Imms C, Froude E, Adair B, Shields N (2016) A descriptive study of the participation of children and adolescents in activities outside school. *BMC Pediatr* **16**: 84.

Imms C, Granlund M, Wilson PH, Steenbergen B, Rosenbaum PL, Gordon AM (2017) Participation, both a means and an end: a conceptual analysis of processes and outcomes in childhood disability. *Dev Med Child Neurol* **59**: 16–25.

Jahoda A, Pownall J (2014) Sexual understanding, sources of information and social networks; the reports of young people with intellectual disabilities and their non-disabled peers. *J Intellect Disabil Res* **58**: 430–441.

King G, McDougall J, Dewit D, Petrenchik T, Hurley P, Law M (2009) Predictors of change over time in the activity participation of children and youth with physical disabilities. *Child Health Care* **38**: 321–351.

Lillvist A (2010) Observations of social competence of children in need of special support based on traditional disability categories versus a functional approach. *Early Child Dev Care* **180**: 1129–1142.

Livingston MH, Stewart D, Rosenbaum PL, Russell DJ (2011) Exploring issues of participation among adolescents with cerebral palsy: what's important to them? *Phys Occup Ther Pediatr* **31**: 275–287.

Lygnegård F, Donohue D, Bornman J, Granlund M, Huus K (2013) A systematic review of generic and special needs of children with disabilities living in poverty settings in low-and middle-income countries. *J Policy Pract* **12**: 296–315.

Lygnegård F, Almqvist L, Granlund M, Huus K (2019) Participation profiles in domestic life and peer relations as experienced by adolescents with and without impairments and long-term health conditions. *Dev Neurorehabil* **22**: 27–38.

Nieuwenhuijsen C, van der Slot WM, Beelen A et al. (2009) Inactive lifestyle in adults with bilateral spastic cerebral palsy. *J Rehabil Med* **41**: 375–381.

Palisano RJ, Chiarello LA, King GA, Novak I, Stoner T, Fiss A (2012) Participation-based therapy for children with physical disabilities. *Disabil Rehabil* **34**: 1041–1052.

Peterson MD, Gordon PM, Hurvitz EA (2013) Chronic disease risk among adults with cerebral palsy: the role of premature sarcopoenia, obesity and sedentary behaviour. *Obes Rev* **14**: 171–182.

Powrie B, Kolehmainen N, Turpin M, Ziviani J, Copley J (2015) The meaning of leisure for children and young people with physical disabilities: a systematic evidence synthesis. *Dev Med Child Neurol* **57**: 993–1010.

Reszka SS, Odom SL, Hume KA (2012) Ecological features of preschools and the social engagement of children with autism. *J Early Interv* **34**: 40–56.

Tonkin BL, Ogilvie BD, Greenwood SA, Law MC, Anaby DR (2014) The participation of children and youth with disabilities in activities outside of school: A scoping review. *Can J Occup Ther* **81**: 226–236.

Ullenhag A, Krumlinde-Sundholm L, Granlund M, Almqvist L (2014) Differences in patterns of participation in leisure activities in Swedish children with and without disabilities. *Disabil Rehabil* **36**: 464–471.

van der Dussen L, Nieuwstraten W, Roebroeck M, Stam HJ (2001) Functional level of young adults with cerebral palsy. *Clin Rehabil* **15**: 84–91.

van der Slot WM, Roebroeck ME, Landkroon AP, Terburg M, Berg-Emons RJ, Stam HJ (2007) Everyday physical activity and community participation of adults with hemiplegic cerebral palsy. *Disabil Rehabil* **29**: 179–189.

Verdonschot MM, de Witte LP, Reichrath E, Buntinx WH, Curfs LM (2009) Community participation of people with an intellectual disability: a review of empirical findings. *J Intellect Disabil Res* **53**: 303–318.

Verhoef JA, Bramsen I, Miedema HS, Stam HJ, Roebroeck ME, Transition and Lifespan Research Group South West Netherlands (2014) Development of work participation in young adults with cerebral palsy: a longitudinal study. *J Rehabil Med* **46**: 648–655.

Wiegerink DJ, Roebroeck ME, van der Slot WM et al. (2010) Importance of peers and dating in the development of romantic relationships and sexual activity of young adults with cerebral palsy. *Dev Med Child Neurol* **52**: 576–582.

Willis C, Girdler S, Thompson M, Rosenberg M, Reid S, Elliott C (2017) Elements contributing to meaningful participation for children and youth with disabilities: a scoping review. *Disabil Rehabil* **39**: 1771–1784.

WHO (2001) *International Classification of Functioning Disability and Health (ICF)*. Geneva: World Health Organization.

Concepts of participation and their translation to different cultures will influence how both attendance and involvement are perceived. This vignette illustrates the dilemmas and intergenerational shifts that occur when translating Western concepts to different cultures. When reading this vignette, consider how cultural expectations may shape concepts of participation and how these may influence expectations and patterns of participation across the lifespan.

The Battle Hymn of the Tiger Mom (Taiwan)

Ai-Wen Hwang

There is an old saying in Taiwan 'To hope one's boy will become a dragon, to hope one's girl will become a phoenix' (望子成龍，望女成鳳). It means every parent hopes their children will have a bright future that reflects Taiwanese culture; involving high expectations for children, especially excellence in academic competition, ranking and performance. Socially, most parents consider children good if they are tolerant, obedient (服從), persevere and are easy to get along with in a group (Hwang 2016). Parenting behaviour tends to be one of over protection but also strict and demanding, exemplified in the *The Battle Hymn of the Tiger Mom* (Chua 2011) – written by a mother who is an American citizen of Chinese origin. Likewise, traditional Taiwanese teaching style is always judgmental, and this attitude is passed on in children's relationships with others, including peer interactions, marriage relationships or other relationships across life. Most parents and teachers in Taiwan consider children have the right to be protected in ways that parents or teachers consider good for the children. From a positive point of view, these are strong Taiwanese characteristics, in that we believe 'no pain, no gain'. In other words, the best outcomes should be achieved through painful processes such as training and therapies that parents sometimes insist on to ensure children's success and excellence.

The term 'participation', though is very new in Taiwan; it was introduced following the launch of the Implementation Act of the Convention on the Rights of the Child in Taiwan in 2014. This provides a Western style of child rights advocacy in Taiwan. Researchers have been struggling to find specific wording in traditional Chinese for 'participation' and to identify measures of children's participation. In an effort to understand what the word 'participation' (參與 in Chinese) means to children – with or without neuro-disability – and parents in Taiwan, we asked them directly. What follows is what we learned.

This is part of the conversation between a **3.5-year-old girl with typical development**, and the interviewer.

[Interviewer]:   Do you know what is participation?
[YiXuan Wang]:   I don't know!
[I]:   Do you know what it is take part in some activities?

[Y W]:	Yes!
[I]:	Have you been taking part in what activities?
[Y W]:	Yes, such as sports with peers…
[I]:	How do you feel when you take part in the activities?
[Y W]:	Very happy!
[I]:	Why did you feel very happy?
[Y W]:	Because I am with my friends, we do it together!
[I]:	What if you should do it alone?
[Y W]:	I will not be happy at all!
[I]:	Could you say more about how you do the sports? You do it with friends by yourself and do what you want to do?
[Y W]:	No, I do it carefully and I should avoid some mistakes and dangerous around, and there are teachers watching us…. We use muscles, power, strength….
[I]:	Is there other activity that you do and feel you are more taking part in?
[Y W]:	Yes, such as blowing bubbles with family! (Response by YiXuan Wang)

For school age children, the term 'participation' is not familiar until they are 10 years old. The following is a quote from **a 10-year-old girl with typical development**:

> Participation means take part in, get involved, and do things with others. It must be more than two people for participation. Sometimes listening to others or watching others doing things is one kind of participation. (Said by Kuan-Fang Chen)

> 要兩個人以上的才叫參與；有時候聽別人講話或看人做事情也是參與；我不想理別人的時候，就不叫參與。(陳冠方 口述)

This 10-year-old typical child can express multiple contexts when defining 'participation', and the concept of 'self' emerges such as 'I want…, I don't…'. Furthermore, participation is not limited to physically participating; paying attention (engaging) to what others do also counts.

This quote is from **a 10-year-old boy with autism spectrum disorder (ASD)**, who was able to express this with a lot of assistance from his mother:

> Participation is involved happily and comfortably in diverse life situations, such as in classroom or doing recreation. I love to participate very much – that will promote my relationship with others. To tell the truth, I used to do things alone. To participate needs opportunities. The hard work is to find a feasible way to participate. The true opportunities need to be explored. I feel I am not participating when others accept me deliberately. I value the time that I am accepted by others, freely and happily. (Said by Derek Wang)

> 參與就是加入，快樂自在的加入生活各種情況。可能是加入上課 (或是休閒。超級喜歡參與，可增加我的人際關係。講實在，習慣自己做。自己喜歡參與可是需要機會。辛苦是想可行的方式。真正的機會是需要被看到。因為解釋或是刻意接納，只是混進去，不是真正的參與。就像我在學校一樣，珍惜交匯的時間，正向珍惜就是快樂的參與。 (王亮凱 口述)

This 10-year-old boy with ASD was also eager to be with others. The idea of preference emerges. Furthermore, the boy has the concept about using participation as a strategy to promote activity competence, such as more participation to enhance the relationship with others.

Based on personal communications with Taiwanese parents, parents of children at this age view their children's participation as gaining good scores academically, paying attention to teachers, and not being discriminated against or excluded by peers.

A 14-year-old girl with typical development said:

Participation means that I join an activity that I feel I am getting involved in, not being neglected, and is meaningful for me. For example, in some classes, teachers are not good at teaching and don't care about students, and it would make me bored. It's no sense of participation for me.

對我來說，如果那個活動是讓我感覺到有融入，不會被忽略，而且活動的結果是有意義的就是一種參與。像有些學校的課程，老師講的沒有特別好也沒辦法關心到每個學生，就會讓我想發呆，沒什麼參與感。

For a 14-year-old girl with cerebral palsy:

Participation is to be the same with my classmates. For example, I don't want to wear the orthosis that my therapist required me to wear because it make me look strange. I believe that I can walk well without orthosis.

參與"的感覺就是要和同學們一樣啦!治療師要我穿著支架走路，我不穿也可以走，這樣別人才不會覺得奇怪!我想跟家一樣就好。

For this age, the peer identity and self-confidence are obvious. The teenagers can also judge the quality of environment that will benefit or bore them and try to resolve or manage the conflicts between their wants and adults' expectation.

For a 20-year-old young adult with typical development:

Participation is being respected. If my expression is not heard, such as some questions for government and no response, I feel I am not participating in any political issues.

我覺得參與就是在一件事或活動裡，自己的想法有被尊重還有參考，這樣對我來說就是參與。參與的話喔，我覺得像座談會或者研討會特別讓人有參與感吧，畢竟每個人的發言都會被拿出來討論。

Taiwanese parents consider that young adults who have good jobs, especially if they are making more money, as having greater participation in society. They are also interested in comparing their children's work performance with those of the children of other parents.

We can see that the contexts in the quotes extend from family, schools, to larger society across ages regardless of whether children have a disability or not. Parents' concept of their children's participation extends from children's well-being and safety, to school and work performance. In contrast, the children's opinions appear to reflect terms in the fPRC and seem to express their fulfilment in life. But parents retain traditional cultural characteristics such as focusing on academic or work performance. Parents in Taiwan are also concerned about their 'good parenting'. When they are taught the importance of children's participation for later adulthood outcomes, they will begin to look for ways to 'train' their children using 'structured courses, such as training on play, self-care, and making friends' to increase children's participation. We can expect a positive transformation and transaction between parents and children in Taiwan for children's development in participation based on our cultural strengths.

REFERENCES

Chua A (2011) *Battle Hymn of the Tiger Mother*. New York: Penguin Press.

Hwang A-W (2013–2016) "Participation" in children with physical disabilities and in typically developed children: a longitudinal study. [Project No: NSC 102-2628-B-182-001-MY3]. Taiwan: Ministry of Science and Technology.

Note: All identified quotes are provided with full permission. Some individuals who have been quoted in this vignette asked to be identified by name.

PART II
Contexts for Participation

Defining Contexts of Participation: A Conceptual Overview

Dido Green

Behaviour is meaningless without a social context
– Frith (1986)

The changing nature of participation across the lifespan will be explored within this section; covering roles and contexts of participation within the family and community and in relation to developmental, social and cultural outcomes. This section will explore the transactional and dynamic relationships of the person in differing contexts.

Taking a closer look at disability in childhood – its nature and experience for children and their families – we see a number of areas where families and professional groups may provide differing perspectives to empower and facilitate active engagement in meaningful activities. This section includes chapters reflecting intrinsic (person in place) and extrinsic (social, physical, attitudinal) influences on specific contexts for activity performance and also broader social environmental impacts on participation. We also consider the institutional and socio-political effects, including political advocacy and societal 'nudges' that influence participatory objectives and rights and responsibilities of individuals and society.

Societal notions of disability contribute strongly to attitudinal influences on specific contexts for participation; not least by setting the scene for cultural expectations that impact directly and indirectly on the aspirations of many children and young people with disabilities. Societal models of disability have been shifting in the 'Western World' towards a construct in which it is the physical, political and societal experiences of people who have the impairment that give rise to disability and discrimination rather than any specific combination of impairments (Reeve 2004).

The 'affirmation model of disability' acknowledges that the experience of living with impairment(s) is part of a disabled person's life and identity (Swain and French 2000). Swain and French (p. 569) define this as:

> A non tragic view of disability and impairment which encompasses positive social identities, both individual and collective, for disabled people grounded in the benefits of lifestyle and life experience of being impaired and disabled.

Separating the person from their environment is an artificial divide for all people, but the conceptual separation is particularly problematic for children and young people who have grown up living and experiencing the constraints and enablers of their physical and social environments.

The boundaries between the capacities of an individual, specific contexts of participation and the affordances of an environment are not always easy to distinguish.

The International Classification of Functioning, Disability and Health (ICF; WHO 2001) and other social models of disability provide frameworks in which disability is no longer situated within the individual but is defined by the contexts of participation. The ICF provides a common language for health professionals to communicate but, importantly, it has broadened its focus beyond that of a person's impairments to incorporate the numerous biopsychosocial factors impacting on participation across multiple contexts. In this respect experiences will influence expectations and provide the drivers for future actions. It follows, then, that to understand the impact of disability on participation in diverse settings, the interactions that exist between the person, activity and environmental factors need to be considered. There is, therefore, a challenge in defining contexts of participation in which the person and environment cannot be seen as separate entities but in fluctuating and dynamic iterations that reflect the qualities of the context and also the perceptions, capacities and expectations of the individual. A framework for considering participatory contexts thus needs to shift from a focus on individual impairments and capacities distinct from environmental barriers and enablers, to a more fluid construct that reflects the transactional nature of the person–activity–environment interfaces (King et al. 2018).

Contexts are defined as a dynamic construct accounting for the variability of individuals in on-going transactional relationships with changing landscapes.

Context in its broadest sense is an amorphous construct that defines multiple interacting variables in the setting for activity participation which includes: the individual; the place as a physical, social or virtual space; activity and objects; and, time including the immediate and lifespan temporal elements of the person and activity (Batorowicz et al. 2016; Imms et al. 2016).

EXTRINSIC AND INTRINSIC CONTEXTS

The family of participation related constructs (fPRC; see Chapter 1) will be used as a basis for understanding the contexts of participation. Batorowicz et al. (2016), distinguishes between the environment and context to consider how the setting affects a person's participation and vice versa, with a particular focus on the social environment. Within the fPRC, the environment is considered as external, referring to more objective social and physical structures in which we live; while context is defined from the perspective of the person participating, incorporating the lived subjective experience of the individual (Imms et al. 2017). The ICF (WHO 2001) outlines attitudinal influences of the social environment; the 'attitudinal world' which influences the subjective experience of participation as well as societal structures that enable opportunities for participation.

While the ICF defines personal factors as attributes of the person distinct from the health condition, such as sex, race or background of an individual's life and living, these factors may influence health and behaviour (WHO 2001). A more expanded perspective shows personal factors including individuals' capacities, experiences and aspirations interacting with, and influenced by, contexts of participation and the activities (and objects); both in relation to meaningfulness and preferences as well as self perception of ability. The reciprocal interaction among children or young people, the contexts in which the activities are being undertaken and their broader environmental influences shape participation preferences. For example, medications that reduce pain may increase tolerance to physical activity, in turn improving skill and potentially enhancing enjoyment and contributing to a future desire to seek out and engage in a particular sport or leisure activity.

The environment therefore, is a platform for participation, shaped by personal factors and influencing motivational components underpinning the drivers for participation. Both the extrinsic factors of the environment and intrinsic factors within the person provide and mould the contexts for participation; thus contexts of participation are inherently individual in nature. Environmental dimensions may be considered in regard to their *availability, accessibility, affordability, accommodability* and *acceptability* (Maxwell et al. 2012) from both objective and subjective perspectives by all in the situation. Perceptions of environmental affordances that may act as prompts and set a context for participation are coloured by experiences and memories. This has been illustrated in research exploring the relationship between the expressed desire of children with cerebral palsy to participate in physical activity versus the actual uptake of physical activity programmes (Jaber et al. 2017) and also in the experiences of children using communication devices (Batorowicz et al. 2014).

The interrelatedness between supportive (social) relationships, availability of opportunities and services and perspectives of the individual have been seen as critical determinants of preferences and thus the goals relating to leisure participation in the community (Willis et al. 2017). This dynamic interaction between the person and environment is also evident in the home environment in which capacities of the child are interrelated with caregiver perceptions of environmental supports (Albrecht and Khetani 2017). Across cultures there are dilemmas and challenges in supporting attitudinal change to enable participation. This may be at a fundamental level as exposed by Mama Shuku's story in Vignette 4.1, or be more subtle societal influences on expectations for behaviour. Understanding the transactional, as well as individual nature, of these interactions is an important first step to providing interventions and services (Terwiel et al. 2017) and particularly, to supporting participation across contexts.

> LINK TO VIGNETTE 4.1
> *'I Will Not Kill My Child', p. 46.*

Figure 4.1 illustrates the transactional influences of intrinsic and extrinsic factors; representing the dynamic nature of the process in relation to perceived relativity of time. Much as gravitational forces change across time and differ in place, personal factors are influenced by experiences and our memories of these, motivating us towards or away from engaging in different activities and contexts.

TEMPORAL DIMENSIONS OF PARTICIPATION

The nature and complexity of children's environments change considerably across developmental stages of infancy, early childhood, middle childhood and adolescence through to early and later adulthood (see Chapter 3). For children, including those with disabilities, some of these changes are universal, transcending cultures, and some more influenced by the cultural and spiritual dimensions of the environment and expectations for competence and independence. Perceptions of time will also differ between and across individuals, dependent on experience, to influence expectations and motivations and goal setting behaviour (Green 2017).

Children with disabilities, experience additional contexts in which they participate, relating to the multiple 'health' environments that they encounter. These may include extensive in-patient, and often intensive care, hospital settings to community based clinical or therapy services. In these settings, the engagement over and above attendance in therapy and rehabilitation may have a substantial influence on outcomes (Miller et al. 2015). Taking this concept forward, we raise the issue of 'research participation' as we endeavour to include children and young people not just as research participants but as individuals who can help define the direction of research and participate as researchers to shape the evidence base underpinning the interventions they may receive (Morris et al. 2011).

The chapters in this section delve into the impact of disability on participation and influences which vary according to context from perspectives of the individual and their family, taking into consideration

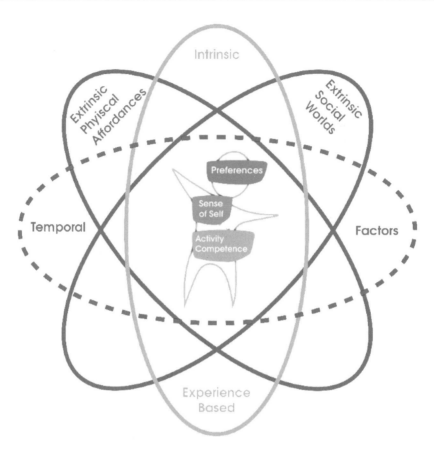

Figure 4.1 Transactional influences of the family of participation related constructs over time. Figure adapted from the fPRC, Imms et al. (2017), with permission. A colour version of this figure can be seen in the plate section.

cultural influences. Personal contexts will be considered from the viewpoint of the person participating and relate to the people, place, activity, objects and time (lifespan) in which participation is set. Contexts of family, school and leisure, and broader environmental influences on participation will be explored, presenting some dilemmas and challenges to supporting attitudinal change and translating that to practice. The impact of these varying contexts will also be considered in relation to the expectations and opportunities that influence the aspirations of young people with disabilities. The challenges in understanding and defining contexts will be addressed from the perspective of the individual as well as communities, in efforts to move away from understanding participation from the limitations of what can currently be measured.

SUMMARY OF KEY IDEAS

- Contexts represent a dynamic construct defining multiple interacting variables for the setting of activity participation that includes the individual, the place, activity, objects and time.
- Contexts for participation are set within broader physical, social, societal and political environments with differing temporal influences.
- Separating person from context is artificial in reality; disability is an outcome of inadequate context–person fit.

REFERENCES

Albrecht EC, Khetani MA (2017) Environmental impact on young children's participation in home-based activities. *Dev Med Child Neurol* **59**: 388–394.

Batorowicz B, Campbell F, von Tetzchner S, King G, Missiuna C (2014) Social participation of school-aged children who use communication aids: the views of children and parents. *Augment Altern Commun* **30**: 237–251.

Batorowicz B, King G, Mishra L, Missiuna C (2016) An integrated model of social environment and social context for pediatric rehabilitation. *Disabil Rehabil* **38**: 1204–1215.

Frith U (1986) A developmental framework for developmental dyslexia. *Ann Dyslexia* **36**: 67–81.

Green D (2017) Time and relativity in therapeutic rehabilitation. *Dev Med Child Neurol* **59**: 112–112.

Imms C, Adair B, Keen D, Ullenhag A, Rosenbaum P, Granlund M (2016) "Participation": a systematic review of language, definitions, and constructs used in intervention research with children with disabilities. *Dev Med Child Neurol* **58**: 29–38.

Imms C, Granlund M, Wilson PH, Steenbergen B, Rosenbaum PL, Gordon AM (2017) Participation, both a means and an end: a conceptual analysis of processes and outcomes in childhood disability. *Dev Med Child Neurol* **59**: 16–25.

Jaber M, Farr W, Morris C, Bremner S, Male I, Green D (2017) Barriers and facilitators to physical activity participation and engagement in Wii Fit home-therapy programmes for children with cerebral palsy. *Dev Med Child Neurol* **59**(S2): 22.

King G, Imms C, Stewart D, Freeman M, Nguyen T (2018) A transactional framework for pediatric rehabilitation: shifting the focus to situated contexts, transactional processes, and adaptive developmental outcomes. *Disabil Rehabil* **40**: 1829–1841.

Maxwell G, Alves I, Granlund M (2012) Participation and environmental aspects in education and the ICF and the ICF-CY: findings from a systematic literature review. *Dev Neurorehabil* **15**: 63–78.

Miller L, Ziviani J, Ware RS, Boyd RN (2015) Mastery motivation: a way of understanding therapy outcomes for children with unilateral cerebral palsy. *Disabil Rehabil* **37**: 1439–1445.

Morris C, Shilling V, McHugh C, Wyatt K (2011) Why it is crucial to involve families in all stages of childhood disability research. *Dev Med Child Neurol* **53**(8): 769–771.

Reeve D (2004) Chapter 6: Psycho-emotional dimensions of disability and the social model In: Barnes C, Mercer G *Implementing the Social Model of Disability: Theory and Research* (Eds). Leeds: The Disability Press, pp. 83–100.

Swain J, French S (2000) Towards an affirmation model of disability. *Disabil Soc* **15**: 569–582.

Terwiel M, Alsem MW, Siebes RC, Bieleman K, Verhoef M, Ketelaar M (2017) Family-centred service: differences in what parents of children with cerebral palsy rate important. *Child Care Health Dev* **43**: 663–669.

Willis C, Girdler S, Thompson M, Rosenberg M, Reid S, Elliott C (2017) Elements contributing to meaningful participation for children and youth with disabilities: a scoping review. *Disabil Rehabil* **39**: 1771–1784.

WHO (2001) *International Classification of Functioning Disability and Health (ICF)*. Geneva: World Health Organization.

Mama Shuku's story is a search for inclusion. This vignette highlights the tensions between a fundamental right to 'be', in conflict with cultural beliefs and social expectations, providing an example of how the broader social environment regulates the behaviour in her close context. The story also represents the desperation born of exclusion and the impact on the health and wellbeing of all involved.

I Will Not Kill My Child (Kenya)

Joseph K Gona and Charles R Newton

Mama Shuku (not her real name), from rural Kilifi County in Kenya, has a child with severe cerebral palsy. In this culture, a child with such a neurodevelopmental disability is considered 'a curse' within the community. Such a child is believed to cause calamities in the community.

Mama Shuku had initially lived in Bamba, a place where she was born and married. But when she had this child with cerebral palsy, she was divorced by her husband. After the divorce, she was chased from that village as her child was thought to be the cause of long droughts in the area.

I gave birth to this child after struggling with labour pains for two days. I was taken to Bamba health centre and when I gave birth, my child was like this. I was asked to take the child for exercises, but the hospital was very far away. I could not afford the daily travel expenses. My husband divorced me as he thought I was the cause of the child being born like that. I went back to my parents. After staying there for some time, allegations came up saying that my child was a 'kijego' (curse) and that my child was a possible cause of long droughts in the area. Other children were warned not to come close to my child. Eventually I was chased from my own village. I went to Kibarani, another village, very far from my own village.

However, in Kibarani village things were no different from her own village. The sight of her child by community members raised speculations and rumours leading Mama Shuku to relocate to another village.

When I arrived at Kibarani village, I expected a friendly atmosphere and that my heart could have some peace. But I was totally wrong. Same issues that my child could bring evil happenings followed me to this village. I was shocked when one morning the area sub chief came to the place I had rented and asked me to leave as the villagers were plotting to come and drive me out of the village. I did not know where to go but I had to leave for the safety of my child.

I met Mama Shuku outside her thatched hut. She was deep in thought. As I sat down to interview her, tears started flowing down her cheeks.

This is the third time I'm being asked to leave a village. I arrived at Kithengwani village after being chased from Kibarani village. Where do I go now? Will my child ever have a friend to play with? When will this child be accepted as any child in this community? What sin did I commit? I will not kill my child. I will carry this burden to the end.

I watched as Mama Shuku sobbed. She seemed to have lost hope of a better life both for herself and her child.

Unpacking Contexts for Participation in Activities that Comprise Family Life: Self and Family

Jessica M Jarvis and Mary A Khetani

Participating in activities provides children and youth with opportunities to acquire knowledge, skills and relationships that are meaningful and culturally valued (Fiese et al. 2002). Prior studies have identified discretionary (e.g. listening to music) and non-discretionary (e.g. household chores) activities that are essential to sustaining daily life (Coster and Khetani 2008). These activities are represented in current assessments of participation, and range from cleaning up to celebrations at home.

Families orchestrate many of the opportunities for their children's participation in organised sets and sequences of activities. Families have a fundamental role in creating opportunities for children and youth to participate in valued activities for the purpose(s) of: (1) sustenance and physical health; (2) developing skills and capacities; and (3) enjoyment and well-being (Larson and Miller-Bishoff 2014). Participation, especially for children and youth, is embedded within the family context. Therefore, it is important to consider the family unit when evaluating and optimising a child's participation (Fiese et al. 2002).

Families of children with disabilities may experience greater difficulty in establishing family routines that provide meaningful opportunities for their child to participate in activities at home (Axelsson et al. 2013). These challenges can negatively impact the child's development of motor, cognitive, emotional and social capacities. Trevlas and colleagues (2003) found a positive association between young children's participation in play routines and their movement. Similarly, Phillips and Hogan (2015) reported that young children who participated in recreation with low frequency and diversity (i.e. number of activities a child participates in) were 1.5–2 times more likely to have poor social competence.

There are a range of intrinsic and extrinsic factors that may contribute to a family's ability to establish and maintain meaningful routines that include their children (Pfeiffer et al. 2017). Figure 5.1 provides an example of these factors in relation to a child's participation in play. Understanding these factors and their influence is crucial for clinicians to effectively partner with families to promote participation for children and youth within the context of the family and home (Khetani et al. 2013).

This chapter provides a contemporary overview of intrinsic and extrinsic factors that form the context for children and youth to participate in activities that comprise family life. While family life typically includes activities that take place in the home and community during early childhood, family life tends to

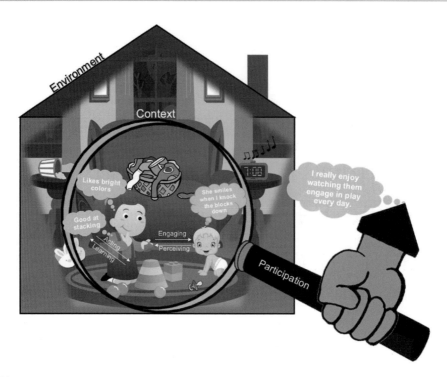

Figure 5.1   Participation-related constructs specific to indoor play and games. A colour version of this figure can be seen in the plate section.

refer to life in the home context as children age and participate in school and community activities without family members present (Bagatell 2016). As this chapter focuses on the family context for children across a broad age range, we maintain a focus on activities that take place at home. This decision does not imply that family life is constrained to the home context, but rather highlights the continued importance of the child's home in shaping opportunities for their participation with family members.

INTRINSIC FACTORS SHAPING PARTICIPATION IN ACTIVITIES THAT COMPRISE FAMILY LIFE

Caregivers and their children have expectations, preferences, attitudes and self-efficacy that influence participation in activities of family life (Soref et al. 2012). These intrinsic factors are often dynamic in nature and influence each other (Imms et al. 2017) as they shape children's participation in the activities that comprise family life.

Intrinsic Factors Specific to Caregivers

Caregivers' ideologies may significantly shape their preferences and self-efficacy for orchestrating family life. Caregiver belief systems shape their decisions about the family routines that are valued, as well as expectations of their child when participating in these valued routines (Kellegrew 2000; see Chapter 8 for details of societal attitudes to and acceptance of disability). These expectations, in turn, influence how caregivers interact with their child during family routines and rituals, and their preferences for directing services and supports to help their child participate in activities of family life (Harkness et al. 2011). Prior studies suggest that children's engagement in non-discretionary household chores is often prioritised by caregivers of young children with developmental delays because it is expected to help their children develop vocational skills (Law et al. 2013).

LINK TO VIGNETTE 5.1
'The Mothers' Wishes and Dreams', p. 55.

Since cultural belief systems can shape caregiver expectations for children's participation in family life, studies have focused on culturally adapting participation assessments to examine cross-cultural differences in how children and youth participate in activities (Åström et al. 2018). This knowledge can support culturally responsive rehabilitative care directed towards improving participation outcomes. However, most studies to date are not specific to family life, and few studies have accounted for acculturation status to overcome the challenge of ascribing normative standards to participation for a cultural group (Bult et al. 2010).

Caregiver self-efficacy to support their child's participation can also impact the opportunities that children and youth have to participate in family life (Soref et al. 2012). Availability of educational materials for caregivers, a common element of caregiver education within a rehabilitation service model, has been associated with increased participation for their child within the home (Sood et al. 2014).

Intrinsic Factors Specific to Children

Family routines are often established in light of child preferences, such as their preference for predictability in activities that comprise home life (Bagatell 2016). For example, families may expand the length of a bedtime routine because their toddler prefers the predictability of story or relaxation routines with multiple caregivers individually. Alternatively, families may shorten a breakfast routine at home because of their youth's preference to participate in a morning snack with peers as part of the school day.

Children's preferences may be influenced by a variety of factors, such as the child's prior success in performing relevant activity tasks, their prior exposure to activities at home, and societal norms/attitudes and policies about participation (Skille and Øterås 2011; Imms et al. 2017). For example, a preschooler may want to help his father with preparing snacks because of his prior success in choosing his snack from the family's pantry. In contrast to his twin sister, he might avoid helping his mother with preparing dinner. He used to believe he could perform cooking tasks at a higher skill level, but recently injured his finger when participating in this activity in the family kitchen (Soref et al. 2012). In contrast, his adolescent brother might avoid meal preparation with his mother altogether, not because of his age but rather his perception that he is only expected to help prepare meals that involve the family's barbecue or outdoor grill.

Children's preferences can influence how often they participate in the activity and how engaged they are during that activity (Imms et al. 2017).

A child's preferences and perceptions of activity competency for performing activities shape their sense of self (Imms et al. 2017). Sense of self shapes and motivates the child's participation which, in turn, then shapes their sense of self over time (Ray and Henry 2011). In the family of participation-related constructs (fPRC) framework, self-regulation is described as the 'glue' that binds a child's preferences, sense of self, and activity competence to enable participation. Self-regulation refers to how a child thinks about and directs their actions when participating in family routines (Howard et al. 2018).

It is important to recognise that children's preferences may change over time, such as during transitions when youth with disabilities demonstrate an increasing desire to shift their participation in employment, educational and leisure activities from within the home to school and community contexts. Youth with disabilities may work to develop self-determination skills to seek and obtain needed resources to participate in these activities (Wehmeyer et al. 2013). Most studies have examined the impact of self-determination interventions within a community context. However, since many youth with disabilities continue to live at home into adulthood (Johnson and Kastner 2005), the impact of shifting preferences for participation on family life merits study.

EXTRINSIC FACTORS SHAPING PARTICIPATION IN ACTIVITIES THAT COMPRISE FAMILY LIFE

Extrinsic factors refer to external factors within the child's home environment that can shape their participation in activities. Common contemporary developmental and rehabilitation frameworks describe multiple dimensions of a child's home environment, ranging from the physical and sensory features of the environment (Sood et al. 2014), to the demands of the activities, and the social relationships and attitudes of individuals who are present at home (Hansen et al. 2016).

There is a growing body of evidence on how environmental factors influence a child's participation in family life. Anaby and colleagues (2014) used a multidimensional environmental assessment (i.e. physical, sensory, social, attitudinal and institutional features) in a model that explained 50–51% of the variance in home participation. Albrecht and Khetani (2017) extended the use of this multidimensional environmental assessment, with findings that suggest caregiver perceptions of home environmental support mediate the association between child and family factors and the child's home participation. The significant role of environmental support on participation has been replicated in subsequent studies involving other cultural contexts and target populations (Di Marino et al. 2018), including children recovering from critical illness (Khetani et al. 2018a) though there is need for more research and education on environmental interventions (Jarvis et al. 2019). In the remainder of this section, we highlight current knowledge about various dimensions of the home environment that may be modifiable targets for home-based and participation-focused intervention.

Physical Features of the Home Environment

Physical features of the child's home environment can help or hinder the child's participation. These factors 'include the housing structure and home density, physical items in the home, quality and characteristics of the home, predictability of daily routines, and availability of resources' (Sood et al. 2014). Freitas and colleagues (2013) found the physical environment of the home (i.e. space to move freely, availability of toys and materials, and caregiver time spent with the child) was associated with increased child participation.

Sensory Features of the Home Environment

The sensory features of the child's environment also impact a child's participation in activities of family life, regardless of diagnosis or disability (Schaaf et al. 2011; Roberts et al. 2018). Children at risk for sensory processing difficulty may need modifications to the sensory environment in the home, include limiting stimuli (e.g. turning the sound off on a toy, removing clothing tags) or increasing stimuli (e.g. providing a fidget toy, giving firm hugs) (Pfeiffer et al. 2017).

Social Relationships Within the Home Environment

Families with established support systems fare better in adapting to the challenges of managing home life, reporting lower stress and caregiving burden and better adjustment to parenthood (Raina et al. 2004). Caregivers with informal support from friends and family were more likely to report confidence in caring for their child's needs, and in partnering with professionals to advocate for their child's needs and service quality (Davey et al. 2015).

Attitudes and Actions of Individuals at Home

Positive attitudes have been associated with children's home participation, though most studies to date relate to participation outside of the home (e.g. peer attitudes impacting children's participation in the community) (Anaby et al. 2013). Qualitative studies with families of children with disabilities have examined relevant correlates of participation in family life. Lawlor and colleagues, for example, found that families who exhibit positive attitudes towards their child (e.g. advocating for the child) facilitate increased participation for their child (Lawlor et al. 2006).

Services Within the Home Environment

Rehabilitation services, particularly during early childhood, are commonly implemented at home. These services are family-centred when they attend to diverse family circumstances, beliefs and preferences, and provide choices and information to support shared decision-making (Bamm and Rosenbaum 2008). Formal services using a family-centred care approach (i.e. linking families to resources, social supports, information and services) have been associated with improved family functioning and positive social outcomes for young children with disabilities (Di Marino et al. 2018).

Despite its importance, to our knowledge, there is less evidence linking family-centred care to participation outcomes. Khetani and colleagues (2018b) used electronic data capture to establish an association between intensity of early intervention service use and home participation outcomes. Estimates of service use via record extraction does not afford for estimating caregiver and provider perceptions about care qualities (e.g. family-centredness) that are hypothesised to impact participation. Future studies should include items on caregiver perceptions of service use as it impacts home participation or adopt established caregiver and provider assessments of service quality (e.g. measure of processes of care) (Cunningham and Rosenbaum 2014).

Most of the evidence on service use and participation outcomes is specific to habilitation focused service contexts (e.g. early intervention). However, hospitalisation is a service use that may indirectly impact both family life, via its impact on intrinsic factors (e.g. shaping caregiver expectations) and extrinsic factors (e.g. time and finances to support family life). Children with chronic illnesses or special healthcare needs may experience repeated or lengthy hospitalisations throughout their life (Boyd and Hunsberger 1998). Hospitalisations can disrupt the family routine, interfere with caregivers' work, and be emotionally distressing for children and their families (Nakamura et al. 2014). A recent study found that when children are discharged following an admission due to critical illness, the slowest area of recovery is caregiver ability to shift the responsibility for performing complex activities of daily living to their child (Choong et al. 2018). This responsibility in caring for their child may help to explain caregiver perceptions of difficulty resuming family life following discharge.

Helping caregivers develop participation-focused strategies to facilitate family routines is an important aspect of rehabilitation services, particularly when transitioning home from hospital.

Consistent family routines allow for a strong sense of family identity, cohesion and enhanced family well-being (Bagatell 2016), and the disruption of these routines can impact the intrinsic factors that shape the child's participation.

Family Resources

Families typically rely on resources to gain access to activities that comprise family life, though most of the supporting evidence comes from studies on community participation (Law et al. 2013; Soref et al. 2012). For example, caregivers' education level and socio-economic status have been associated with patterns in service use and community participation outcomes among families of young children with developmental disabilities and delays (Freitas et al. 2013; Khetani et al. 2013). Similarly, family income may influence children's participation (e.g. hindering access to programmes) (Carlson et al. 2010). Some studies have shown that caregivers earning less annual income report their child participates less frequently and is less involved in community activities (Khetani et al. 2013; Anaby et al. 2014). However, Rosenberg and colleagues found that income significantly affected diversity and intensity (i.e. the range and frequency of activity participation) only (Soref et al. 2012).

CONCLUSION

Contextual factors that influence a child's participation in family life are complex and dynamic. Researchers have established the range of relevant intrinsic and extrinsic factors that enable children's participation, to improve the lived experiences of children with and without neurodisability. Greater understanding of these factors will enhance the way we assess and intervene on children's participation in activities that comprise family life.

SUMMARY OF KEY IDEAS

- The activities children participate in are often nested within family life; considering the context of family life is crucial to evaluating and optimising children's participation.
- Understanding intrinsic and extrinsic family factors is crucial for clinicians to effectively partner with families in minimising participation disparities.
- There is strong evidence for home environments impacting children's home participation and great need for research and education on environmental interventions.

ACKNOWLEDGEMENTS

We thank Dianna Bosak and Weronika Zuczek, research assistants in the Children's Participation in Environment Research Lab, for assisting with assembling the figure and references and providing critical feedback to illustrate key points.

REFERENCES

Albrecht EC, Khetani MA (2017) Environmental impact on young children's participation in home-based activities. *Dev Med Child Neurol* **59**: 388–394.

Anaby D, Hand C, Bradley L et al. (2013) The effect of the environment on participation of children and youth with disabilities: a scoping review. *Disabil Rehabil* **35**: 1589–1598.

Anaby D, Law M, Coster W et al. (2014) The mediating role of the environment in explaining participation of children and youth with and without disabilities across home, school, and community. *Arch Phys Med Rehabil* **95**: 908–917.

Åström FM, Khetani M, Axelsson AK (2018) Young children's participation and environment measure: swedish cultural adaptation. *Phys Occup Ther Pediatr* **38**: 329–342.

Axelsson AK, Granlund M, Wilder J (2013) Engagement in family activities: a quantitative, comparative study of children with profound intellectual and multiple disabilities and children with typical development. *Child Care Health Dev* **39**: 523–534.

Bagatell N (2016) The routines and occupations of families with adolescents with autism spectrum disorders. *Focus Autism Other Dev Disabl* **31**: 49–59.

Bamm EL, Rosenbaum P (2008) Family-centered theory: origins, development, barriers, and supports to implementation in rehabilitation medicine. *Arch Phys Med Rehabil* **89**: 1618–1624.

Boyd JR, Hunsberger M (1998) Chronically ill children coping with repeated hospitalizations: their perceptions and suggested interventions. *J Pediatr Nurs* **13**: 330–342.

Bult MK, Verschuren O, Gorter JW, Jongmans MJ, Piskur B, Ketelaar M (2010) Cross-cultural validation and psychometric evaluation of the Dutch language version of the Children's Assessment of Participation and Enjoyment (CAPE) in children with and without physical disabilities. *Clin Rehabil* **24**: 843–853.

Carlson E, Bitterman A, Daley T (2010) *Access to Educational and Community Activities for Young Children with Disabilities*. Rockville, MD: Westat.

Choong K, Fraser D, Al-Harbi S et al. (2018) Functional recovery in critically ill children, the "WeeCover" multicenter study. *Pediatr Crit Care Med* **19**(2): 145–154.

Coster W, Khetani MA (2008) Measuring participation of children with disabilities: issues and challenges. *Disabil Rehabil* **30**: 639–648.

Cunningham BJ, Rosenbaum PL (2014) Measure of processes of care: a review of 20 years of research. *Dev Med Child Neurol* **56**: 445–452.

Davey H, Imms C, Fossey E (2015) "Our child's significant disability shapes our lives": experiences of family social participation. *Disabil Rehabil* **37**: 2264–2271.

Di Marino E, Tremblay S, Khetani M, Anaby D (2018) The effect of child, family and environmental factors on the participation of young children with disabilities. *Disabil Health J* **11**: 36–42.

Fiese BH, Tomcho TJ, Douglas M, Josephs K, Poltrock S, Baker T (2002) A review of 50 years of research on naturally occurring family routines and rituals: cause for celebration? *J Fam Psychol* **16**: 381–390.

Freitas TC, Gabbard C, Caçola P, Montebelo MI, Santos DC (2013) Family socioeconomic status and the provision of motor affordances in the home. *Braz J Phys Ther* **17**: 319–327.

Hansen M, Harty M, Bornman J (2016) Exploring sibling attitudes towards participation when the younger sibling has a severe speech and language disability. *SAJCH* **10**: 47–51.

Harkness S, Zylicz PO, Super CM et al. (2011) Children's activities and their meanings for parents: a mixed-methods study in six Western cultures. *J Fam Psychol* **25**: 799–813.

Howard S, Vella S, Cliff D (2018) Children's sports participation and self-regulation: bi-directional longitudinal associations. *Early Child Res Q* **42**: 140–147.

Imms C, Granlund M, Wilson PH, Steenbergen B, Rosenbaum PL, Gordon AM (2017) Participation, both a means and an end: a conceptual analysis of processes and outcomes in childhood disability. *Dev Med Child Neurol* **59**: 16–25.

Jarvis JM, Choong K, Khetani MA (2019) Associations of participation-focused strategies and rehabilitation service use with caregiver stress following pediatric critical illness. *Arch Phys Med Rehabil* **100**: 703–710.

Johnson CP, Kastner TA, American Academy of Pediatrics Committee/Section on Children With Disabilities (2005) Helping families raise children with special health care needs at home. *Pediatrics* **115**: 507–511.

Kellegrew DH (2000) Constructing daily routines: a qualitative examination of mothers with young children with disabilities. *Am J Occup Ther* **54**: 252–259.

Khetani M, Graham JE, Alvord C (2013) Community participation patterns among preschool-aged children who have received Part C early intervention services. *Child Care Health Dev* **39**: 490–499.

Khetani MA, Albrecht EC, Jarvis JM, Pogorzelski D, Cheng E, Choong K (2018a) Determinants of change in home participation among critically ill children. *Dev Med Child Neurol* **60**: 793–800.

Khetani MA, McManus BM, Arestad K et al. (2018b) Technology-based functional assessment in early childhood intervention: a pilot study. *Pilot Feasibility Stud* **4**: 65.

Larson E, Miller-Bishoff T (2014) Family routines within the ecological niche: an analysis of the psychological well-being of U.S. caregivers of children with disabilities. *Front Psychol* **5**: 495.

Law M, Anaby D, Teplicky R, Khetani MA, Coster W, Bedell G (2013) Participation in the home environment among children and youth with and without disabilities. *Br J Occup Ther* **76**: 58–66.

Lawlor K, Mihaylov S, Welsh B, Jarvis S, Colver A (2006) A qualitative study of the physical, social and attitudinal environments influencing the participation of children with cerebral palsy in northeast England. *Pediatr Rehabil* **9**: 219–228.

Nakamura MM, Toomey SL, Zaslavsky AM et al. (2014) Measuring pediatric hospital readmission rates to drive quality improvement. *Acad Pediatr* **14**(Suppl): S39–S46.

Newacheck PW, Halfon N (1998) Prevalence and impact of disabling chronic conditions in childhood. *Am J Public Health* **88**: 610–617.

Pfeiffer B, Coster W, Snethen G, Derstine M, Piller A, Tucker C (2017) Caregivers' perspectives on the sensory environment and participation in daily activities of children with autism spectrum disorder. *Am J Occup Ther* **71**: 1, 9.

Phillips R, Hogan A (2015) Recreational participation and the development of social competence in preschool aged children with disabilities: a cross-sectional study. *Disabil Rehabil* **37**: 981–989.

Raina P, O'Donnell M, Schwellnus H et al. (2004) Caregiving process and caregiver burden: conceptual models to guide research and practice. *BMC Pediatr* **4**: 1.

Ray TD, Henry K (2011) Self-efficacy and physical activity in children with congenital heart disease: is there a relationship? *J Spec Pediatr Nurs* **16**: 105–112.

Roberts T, Stagnitti K, Brown T, Bhopti A (2018) Relationship between sensory processing and pretend play in typically developing children. *Am J Occ Ther* **72**(1): 1–8.

Schaaf RC, Toth-Cohen S, Johnson SL, Outten G, Benevides TW (2011) The everyday routines of families of children with autism: examining the impact of sensory processing difficulties on the family. *Autism* **15**: 373–389.

Skille E, Øterås J (2011) What does sport mean to you? fun and other preferences for adolescents' sport participation. *Crit Public Health* **21**: 359–372.

Sood D, LaVesser P, Schranz C (2014) Influence of home environment on participation in home activities of children with an autism spectrum disorder. *Open J Occup Ther* **2**(3): 2.

Soref B, Ratzon NZ, Rosenberg L, Leitner Y, Jarus T, Bart O (2012) Personal and environmental pathways to participation in young children with and without mild motor disabilities. *Child Care Health Dev* **38**: 561–571.

Trevlas E, Matsouka O, Zachopoulou E (2003) Relationship between playfulness and motor creativity in preschool children. *Early Child Dev Care* **173**: 535–543.

Wehmeyer ML, Palmer SB, Shogren K, Williams-Diehm K, Soukup J (2013) Establishing a causal relationship between intervention to promote self-determination and enhanced student self-determination. *J Spec Educ* **46**: 195–210.

In the following vignette a group of Iranian mothers talk about the opportunities their children with impairments have for participation. Creating or seeing opportunities for participation can be dependent on perceptions of the environment: especially whether a situation or context is available, accessible or accommodating to your child's needs, and if accommodations are acceptable to all.

As you read this vignette you may also see the tensions between acceptance and desire for change, and how perceptions of capacity and expectation influence inclusion and participation. Participation in this vignette might be seen to be about doing what is possible and creating enabling contexts.

The Mothers' Wishes and Dreams (Iran)

Farzaneh Yazdani

Aryana, 4 years old, and Shayan, 5 years old, are both diagnosed with spastic quadriplegia and attend an occupational therapist-led group-intervention each Tuesday. Aryana's mother is 35 with two more children, each younger than Aryana. Shayan is the first child in his family and has a 1-year-old sister. His mother is 28. The occupational therapist has arranged a family-oriented session that includes six children of similar ages and diagnoses. At the end of each session, the mothers have 45 minutes to talk to each other about issues they face in managing their family life.

One day, during the mothers' discussion, Aryana, who is playing with her little teddy, looks at Shayan and asks him 'Have you ever been in a park with your friends? My mum take me there every Friday and it's really fun'. Shayan looks at his mother with confusion as if he has never heard of such a thing. 'There is no park near us that could be suitable for Shayan's situation', Shayan's mum says, and looks at Aryana's mother. 'How can you manage that? I neither have opportunity nor really mood to do so… What is the point? They never get better.' As she says this, she looks down to avoid Shayan's eyes; Shayan is curiously listening to this conversation.

Other mothers join in and they all discuss their wishes and dreams for their children to get well and go to mainstream schools. Aryana's mother, however, does not feel comfortable with this discussion. 'I don't think the point is that our children get well and be like other children, it's about us accepting them the way they are and help them live with their full capacity, happy and satisfied', Aryana's mother says.

One of the mothers seems to be very disappointed and distressed by what Aryana's mother said. 'No one cares about our children, people don't understand what it means to have a child with disability and look what facilities we have in the city to help us to take our children around. You are perhaps very lucky to have access to a park that you are able to take Aryana to', she says. Shayan's mother adds: 'What happiness would they have living with their disability? – no education, no future, no achievement. Have you thought what will happen when we are gone? Is there any organisation whatsoever that you can rely on to support our children?'

Aryana's mum feels upset that some mothers are talking with a great level of frustration in front of their children. 'Well, I agree we don't have many facilities available to our children with special needs but we parents have each other and should think that life is not all about achievements in the sense of university degrees, high status job etc....'

Shayan's mother: 'You didn't tell me how you manage to take Aryana to the park?' Aryana's mother said: 'I know it might appear strange in such a difficult situation and with all the environmental barriers that we have managed to take Aryana to a park. We are a group of mothers who have arranged to meet up in one little garden belonging to one of the neighbours and have put a few items like a slide and swings with some adaptation for Aryana to play there. Aryana is the only one with physical limitations. This is what she calls a park!' Shayan's mother keeps silent for a minute and then looks at Shayan and says, 'So it seems it's all down to us, isn't it?'

Participation and School Space: The Role of Environment in Inclusion

Wesley Imms, Benjamin Cleveland and Chris Bradbeer

This chapter focuses on an important overlap between research in education and applied health; the environmental domain. Specifically, it asks if research into the design and use of learning environments can simultaneously accommodate the improved participation of children with early-onset neurological disabilities in learning?

Health and education are often seen as disparate areas of research, but on this topic significant overlaps are evident. This discursive chapter records some commonalities shared by the education and applied health disciplines: a desire to maximise learning experiences for students with a variety of capacities; a belief that the spaces and places within which participation occurs have an effect on the quality of that participation; and an understanding that the goal is not to fit the child into established structures, processes and practices, but to design and use those elements to enable the child to find her or his optimum forms of participation.

Within education, 'spatial conversations' underpinned by principles of personalised learning are gaining traction, but to what degree are the needs of students with disabilities being accommodated? The chapter reflects on the impact of the design of learning environments on children's educational experiences. It explores the presence, or relative absence, of the child with neurological and other disabilities, considering both participation attendance and involvement through brief examination of a sample of actual practices – including some 'applied realities' of inclusion policies – and finishes by hypothesising the potential gains that could result from stronger alliances between research in education, design and allied health.

EDUCATION'S RESEARCH INTO THE EFFECT OF LEARNING ENVIRONMENTS ON STUDENT EXPERIENCE

Ministries of education around the world have been reimagining the physical design of schools and learning spaces. Traditional 30-odd student cellular classrooms with desks facing a front-and-centre teacher (Fig. 6.1) are being replaced by flexible, agile learning environments. Characterised in Figure 6.2, these innovative learning environments (ILEs) allow for an array of learning space sizes (large groups to one-on-one encounters), multiple furniture types and arrangements, and ubiquitous technology. These spaces

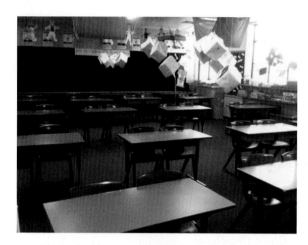

Figure 6.1 A 'traditional' primary school class-room. Photograph: T. Byers, with permission. A colour version of this figure can be seen in the plate section.

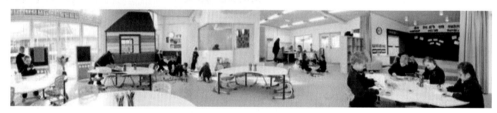

Figure 6.2 An innovative learning environment. Architect: Ken Woodman, No. 42 Architects. Photographer: Erin David-Hartwig, Beechworth Photographers with permission. A colour version of this figure can be seen in the plate section.

may be quickly adapted to alter the teaching/learning situation via reconfigurable walls and dynamic interior elements. The changes are not just physical, however. They are an educational response to significant policy mandates such as the Plowden Report (1967) and in Australia, the more recent Melbourne Declaration (MCEETYA 2008). In essence, these policies argue for differentiated curriculum to replace the tradition of predominately teacher-centred, didactic approaches.

Differentiated curriculum, defined as the delivery of curriculum that is highly flexible to meet the knowledge base, skills, interests and learning needs of individuals (Pendergast and Bahr 2005), has its roots in centuries of educational development. These approaches have re-emerged in recent years under the guise of developing students' so-called 21st century learning skills: communication, collaboration, creativity and critical thinking. These are the attributes demanded of graduates who must work in increasingly dynamic, people-focused employment and social environments (Imms 2018). Such agendas also accept that education must balance contemporary skills development with the transmission of knowledge via texts, lectures and examinations through a blend of progressive and traditional curricula, pedagogies and assessment practices. Of interest for participation of children with disabilities is the interaction between classroom design and the teaching style as well as the impact of design and teaching on inclusion and participation of children with disabilities. The argument is that the design of traditional teaching spaces, with desks facing the front and a teacher occupying the 'fireplace', dictates a pedagogic style that limits students engaging with each other, prevents them from pursuing individual approaches to learning, and privileges a 'hear it and test it' mode of education (McGregor 2004). More concerned with discipline and adherence to a singular curriculum, these teaching spaces dictate a knowledge transfer mechanism that assumes a homogeneous student cohort; it fails to acknowledge the individual, let alone a child with disability. Using a reversal of that logic, ILEs intend to address individualised learning and, with specific relevance to this book, the capacity to facilitate an educational experience that heightens participation for all.

This has not been an easy transition for education to make. The hegemony of the cellular classroom was challenged briefly during the 1960s and 1970s through open-plan classroom designs; schools owned huge spaces where a hundred or more students commonly mingled with peers and teachers. Intended to foster collaborative teaching approaches, individualised learning and stage-not-age progression, open-plan strategies had lofty aspirations, yet failed to account for the wholesale reimagining of teaching and the organisational structures required to make such dynamic educational environments work (Brogden 2007).

The current reimagining of learning space design in education has learned from such mistakes. Evident in the designs themselves, the most effective school facilities (Fig. 6.3 types C–E) offer teachers and students variety in the spaces they can use for particular activities (Imms et al. 2016). The concept of 'spatial typologies' breaks the polarising effect of an 'open-plan versus traditional space' dichotomy – the relative openness of learning spaces extends across a continuum (Fig. 6.3). Pedagogic typologies accept that a range of teaching and learning approaches is what is required, not an 'either-or' approach (Fig. 6.4).

Only when working together – innovative practices in combination with innovative spaces – do we arrive at an innovative learning environment (Mahat et al. 2018).

These environments are now providing some measure of success through evidence showing ILEs can facilitate improved student learning outcomes (Barrett et al. 2015; Byers et al. 2018). More importantly, when compared to traditional classrooms the flexible and adaptive learning spaces of ILEs correlate to high-impact teaching strategies and to increased student deep-thinking skills that is, deep engagement (Imms et al. 2017). These are qualities that promote participation. Hattie's (2009) synthesis of educational meta-analyses that focused on student learning, provides a set of 'teacher mind-frames' that correlate with improved student achievement. Importantly, these mind-frames stress teachers' role as 'change agents' in students' lives,

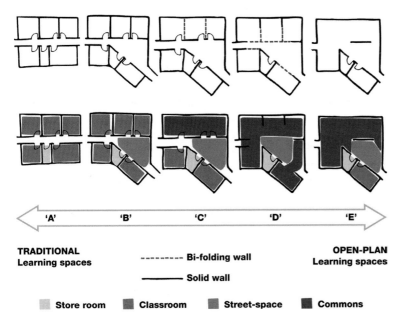

‘A’   ‘B’   ‘C’   ‘D’   ‘E’

TRADITIONAL
Learning spaces

-------- **Bi-folding wall**

———— **Solid wall**

OPEN-PLAN
Learning spaces

Store room   Classroom   Street-space   Commons

Figure 6.3 Spatial design typology. Dovey and Fisher (2014), adapted in Imms (2016). A colour version of this figure can be seen in the plate section.

Typology 1:
Teacher facilitated presentation,
direct instruction or
large group discussion.

Typology 2:
Teacher facilitated small
group discussion
or instruction.

Figure 6.4 Pedagogic typology. Figure used with permission (Imms et al. 2017).

Typology 3:
Team teacher facilitated
presentation, direct instruction
or large group discussion.

Typology 4:
Collaborative/shared learning,
supported by teachers
as needed.

Typology 5:
One-on-one instruction.

Typology 6:
Individual learning.

debunking the assumption they are predominately imparters of knowledge. In terms of learning, across a continuum spanning superficial (learning to pass exams) to deep learning (learning to apply knowledge), 'favourable' curriculum covers not only the basics, but supports the development of students' life-long skills linked with learning how to learn, how to place what is being learned within a personal context, and how to view learning as the individual placing themselves in the wider world (Biggs 1978).

Within ILEs the combination of these two qualities – teachers as change agents and teaching that seeks deep learning skills – appears to impact favourably the ways that students engage and participate in the whole educative experience. There exists some evidence that ILEs assist improved student-centred pedagogies, helping students develop knowledge relevant to their individual needs, interests and capabilities (Imms et al. 2017). Logically, the child with disabilities must benefit from the advent of well-designed and used ILEs. This casts a light onto the existence – or non-existence – of effective educational policies and practices that utilise the potential of ILEs to positively support the participation of students with neurological disorders to achieve desired life-long learning skills.

WHERE AND HOW ARE DISABILITIES RECOGNISED AND ADDRESSED IN THE ENVIRONMENTAL DOMAIN?

Academic literature on students with special educational needs is extensive. Yet, attention to the spatial implications associated with supporting students with disabilities is generally poor. Nevertheless, cross-disciplinary research is developing some progressive concepts of participation that may lead to a more sophisticated understanding of inclusion in schools. This research might be seen to follow five themes of inquiry.

The first theme recognises that *physical spaces mediate and are mediated by the activities that occur within them*. Naraian (2016) encourages the re-conceptualisation of place-based inclusive teaching and learning practices. She suggests that teachers' work with students who require additional support should not be fixed to particular learning spaces but actually occurs across spatially fluid networks of people and experiences that are dynamic and continually changing. Learning spaces need to offer flexibility in curricular and instructional approaches that are applicable to all students (reflected in Figures 6.3 and 6.4), not just those with special educational needs, removing the need to delineate spaces for particular cohorts or individuals.

Similarly, Gibson et al. (2017) promote a dynamic analysis of how dis/abilities are enacted across 'geo-temporal spaces' (p. 497). They suggest researchers should move from 'a reductive focus on evaluating the accessibility of static environmental features' (p. 497) to capture 'the constantly shifting connectivities between heterogeneous elements, including but not limited to bodies, social meanings, places and technologies' (p. 498). Their study of activity–setting–participation of young people with complex communication and/or mobility impairment at home and in the community explores the co-constituting relationship – that is the transactional relationship – between activity and setting. They adopt the perspective that 'settings are particular places that are shaped by people within them and the activities undertaken' (p. 498).

Criticising historic practices that allocate disabled students to 'dedicated environments' and 'special units' (p. 532), D'Alessio (2012) suggests that power relations associated with the use of space and place in schools may contribute to the reproduction of forms of micro-exclusion – even within purposively designed inclusive educational environments. She highlights that inclusive policy and practice does not guarantee exclusion will not be experienced in integrative settings and advocates for creation of new 'hybrid places' that celebrate diversity.

A second emerging theme is the recognition that *spaces transmit meanings and carry implications* for those who occupy them. Again, this applies to all students, but has significant ramifications for those with special educational needs. For example, Pluquailec (2018) challenges historic attention given to the pathology or psychology of individual students with disabilities and their associated behaviour. She suggests that improved understanding of socio-spatial contexts that mediate emotions and behaviour are required and challenges the value placed on students being seated and still. She promotes the provision of spatial variety and choice, or a less prescriptive environment, that accepts the expression of emotion as 'legitimate'. Hoping to open new avenues to discuss the emotional expression of students with autism, she calls for 're-orientating our gaze' towards students' emotions as being socio-spatially mediated, rather than simply perceived as markers or symptoms of disorder.

A third theme highlights that *deeply-informed briefing processes are required to achieve inclusive learning space designs and patterns of occupation*. For example, McAllister and Maguire (2012) developed the Autism Spectrum Disorder Classroom Design Kit, arguing that autism spectrum disorder (ASD) policy guidelines are too general to be useful as a basis for design. They suggest that detailed co-design processes are needed to provide ASD-friendly learning environments, with teachers 'clearly and effectively impart[ing] their knowledge and requirements to architects' (p. 201) through physical models rather than drawing-centric dialogue. Similarly, Durak (2010) argues co-design allows for inclusion: 'an ongoing process during which students develop their capacities with the provision of equal opportunities of access to educational resources, supportive services, teachers, professionals and effective education environments' (p. v). Finally,

> *A deeply informed co-design approach is needed to achieve inclusive learning spaces.*

Cullis (2010) suggests failures at the design briefing stage lead to poor inclusive design due to lack of understanding about how students interact with educational settings.

The fourth theme is the need for *monitoring (evaluation) of the effect of spatialised strategies on students' experiences.* Mostafa (2018) reports on the application of the Autism ASPECTSS™ Design Index in the postoccupancy evaluation of existing school spaces involving seven design criteria: acoustics, spatial sequencing, escape spaces, compartmentalisation, transition zones, sensory zoning and safety. She suggests the ASPECTSS™ outputs offer a 'framework for design thinking as opposed to a prescriptive set of recommendations' (p. 309).

And finally, the fifth theme highlights *the imperative of whole-school approaches to participation and inclusion.* Sanahuja-Gavaldà et al. (2016) highlight the importance of whole-school approaches to collaboration and pedagogy. They suggest the concept of 'support' is evolving from focusing on deficits in students to a focus on the whole school, using an integrative and collaborative approach. Space is required for teacher collaboration to enable them to support students with special educational needs.

The five themes illustrate that spaces both control and react to the activities that occur within; that engagement within learning spaces carry implications and ramifications for those using the spaces; that past 'inclusion' strategies have often restricted, not improved the lot of students with disability; and importantly, the need exists to monitor more closely the impact of policies on actual experience.

INCLUSION AND THE REALITIES OF HOW DISABILITY IS ADDRESSED IN SCHOOLS: ACCOMMODATION, OR MAXIMISING POTENTIAL?

One school located in a reasonably high socio-economic city in New Zealand offers a 'real life' example of how ILEs operate. Its roll of approximately 700 students reveals that about 20% require specific support. Among these are students with special needs related to autism, attention deficit, eyesight, hearing, speech, anxiety, behaviour, dyslexia, dyspraxia, brain injuries, mental health, developmental delays, and the list goes on. Depending on the nature and level of need, short or long-term interventions are developed and implemented at a teacher, team or wider level. The latter regularly draws on collective expertise from external agencies that support learning, health, welfare and family.

The school is a New Zealand pioneer in the development of ILEs. Criticisms of ILEs (they are noisy, students easily 'fall through the cracks' and students with special needs are ignored) are not lost on staff and serve as reminders to consistently monitor how principles of inclusion and participation are enacted in learning space design, spatialised pedagogic practice and students' learning activities. The school demonstrates approaches related to two key principles: *adaptation* and *inclusion*. These are realised as functions of *pedagogy* or *inbuilt-design*. To explain this further, explicit pedagogical adaptation refers to an intervention or modification for a particular student, or sub-set of students. It encompasses how learning is engaged with, activated, accessed, assessed and displayed. This may involve adaptation to communication, curriculum, materials, or the use of assistive technology. For example, students with hearing difficulties benefit from a personal frequency-modulation system, enabling them to hear an individual voice directly to earphones. Students needing to reduce tension can find 'wobbly stools' that encourage movement. Those with auditory processing disorder may utilise noise-reducing headphones. For those with attention-deficit–hyperactivity disorder (ADHD) the use of visual timetables helps to know what to expect, checklists help break tasks into smaller components, and task timers can help in reducing stress. Similarly, opportunities to clamber on playground equipment outside signifies a brief break in their learning, a chance to move before refocusing.

Implicit *pedagogical inclusion* relates to the way an approach and an environment is embraced for all learners, illustrating sensitivity to individual differences and preferences, and a desire to recognise potential barriers to learning and participation. For example, instructions are presented in varied ways, settings within the physical environment are labelled (pictorially and in text) to highlight particular affordances for learning, and routines are reinforced with visual references. Spatially, the variety of furnishings provided across the school enables not only the development of multiple learning settings, but also opportunity to exercise student preference and agency. Differentiated heights and layouts of furniture offer choice and the exercise of free movement.

The addition of calm spaces enables withdrawal and acoustic separation. The classification of breakout spaces for quiet, individual learning are common around the school, often accompanied by student-prepared guidelines on expectations and suitable activities. Acoustic treatments to reduce reverberation time, intended to support English as second language learners and students with auditory processing disorder, benefit all occupants. Additionally, during break times, areas are set aside throughout the school for those not wanting to be outside. So-called 'nurture rooms' are popular destinations where students engage in construction, board games, drawing, writing, reading and conversation. In keeping with Universal Design principles, while their use may originally have been aimed at specific students' needs, they are available to all.

In some cases, it is not only to learning that adaptation is required, but also to the broader environment of the school. One challenge is access, particularly if wheelchairs are needed for mobility. To get inside requires sliding a glass door, not always an easy task for the younger students. The reception area front desk is designed with this in mind; low enough to see across. A lift provides easy access to upper floors. Outside, the gradients of pathways and ramps do not exceed the recommended 1:20 gradient, but do mean that routes are more circuitous than logical, and do not always follow naturally created 'desire lines'. Travel in a wheelchair also reveals a small step across some thresholds to negotiate; although not specified in the architectural drawings, cost clearly played a role in the subsequent decision-making regarding aluminium joinery.

WHERE TO FROM HERE?

The ILE concept brings new possibilities for inclusion and participation, timely indeed considering the challenges that are to be faced. However, the brief description of one school's professional attempts to accommodate all students with special needs is sobering. It illustrates the practical reality of this issue. Teachers have as their primary work output the task of actual teaching. Increasingly, they do so while also attending to a staggering array of secondary demands regarding student needs. These include the requirement to provide for each individual student's physical environment, learning environment, social environment and wellbeing environment. It is no small wonder equitable participation, while unquestionably desired, remains an ephemeral phenomenon.

SUMMARY OF KEY IDEAS

- Addressing the challenge for equitable participation of children with disabilities must be a priority for research into the design and use of innovative learning spaces.
- The goal is not to fit the child into established structures, processes and practices, but to design and use those elements to enable the child to find her or his optimum forms of participation.

- Research must be cross-disciplinary – participation of students with disability is not by any extent an exclusive educational issue.
- A shared inter-disciplinary meaning of terminologies, concepts and theories must be developed.
- Holistic approaches to participation and inclusion, as opposed to isolated interventions, are required.
- Space as a 'pedagogic tool' must be explored by teachers and allied health practitioners to develop differentiated curricula that meet the needs of every child.
- Good cross-disciplinary spatial-use evaluation strategies must be developed. These must focus on closing the gap the between 'inclusive' educational policies and students' and teachers' actual experiences in schools.

REFERENCES

Barrett P, Zhang Y, Davies F, Barrett L (2015) *Clever Classrooms: Summary Report of the HEAD Project.* Salford: University of Salford. Available at https://www.salford.ac.uk/cleverclassrooms/1503-Salford-Uni-Report-DIGITAL.pdf [Accessed 20 August 2019].

Biggs JB (1978) Individual and group differences in study processes. *Br J Educ Psychol* **48**: 266–279.

Brogden M (2007) Plowden and primary school buildings: A story of innovation without change. *Forum* **49**: 55–64.

Byers T, Imms W, Hartnell-Young E (2018) Comparative analysis of the impact of traditional versus innovative learning environment on student attitudes and learning outcomes. *Stud Educ Eval* **58**: 167–177.

Cullis RI (2010) *Children's Relationship with Their Physical School: Considerations of Primary School Architecture and Furniture Design in a Social and Cultural Context.* PhD thesis. London: Brunel University.

D'Alessio S (2012) Integrazione scolastica and the development of inclusion in Italy: does space matter? *Int J Incl Educ* **16**: 519–534.

Durak S (2010) *Searching for a Common Framework for Education and Architecture Through Reconsideration of Universal Design Principles for Promoting Inclusive Education in Primary Schools.* PhD thesis. Ankara: Middle East Technical University.

Gibson BE, King G, Teachman G, Mistry B, Hamdani Y (2017) Assembling activity/setting participation with disabled young people. *Sociol Health Illn* **39**: 497–512.

Hattie J (2009) *Visible Learning: A Synthesis of Over 800 Meta-Analyses Relating to Achievement.* Routledge: Abingdon-on-Thames.

Imms W, Cleveland B, Fisher K (Eds) (2016) *Evaluating Learning Environments: Snapshots of Emerging Issues, Methods and Knowledge.* Rotterdam: Sense Publishers.

Imms W, Mahat M, Murphy D, Byers T (2017) *Type and Use of Innovative Learning Environments in Australasian Schools – ILETC Survey. Technical Report 1/2017.* Melbourne: University of Melbourne. Available at http://www.iletc.com.au/wp-content/uploads/2017/07/TechnicalReport_Web.pdf [Accessed 20 August 2019].

Imms W (2018) Innovative learning spaces: Catalysts/agents for change, or "just another fad". In: Alterator S, Deed C (Eds) *School Space and Its Occupation: The Conceptualisation and Evaluation of New Generation Learning Spaces.* Amsterdam: Sense Publishing, pp. 107–118.

Mahat M, Bradbeer C, Byers T, Imms W (2018) *Innovative Learning Environments and Teacher Change: Defining Key Concepts.* Melbourne: University of Melbourne. Available at http://www.iletc.com.au/wp-content/uploads/2018/07/TR3_Web.pdf [Accessed 5 September 2019].

McAllister K, Maguire B (2012) A design model: The Autism Spectrum Disorder Classroom Design Kit. *Br J Spec Educ* **39**: 201–208.

McGregor J (2004) Spatiality and the place of the material in schools. *Pedagogy Cult Soc* **12**: 347–372.

Ministerial Council on Education, Employment, Training and Youth Affairs (MCEETYA) (2008) *Melbourne Declaration on Educational Goals for Young Australians.* Melbourne: Ministerial Council on Education, Employment, Training and Youth Affairs.

Mostafa M (2018) Designing for autism: an ASPECTSS™ post-occupancy evaluation of learning environments. *Archnet-IJAR* **12**: 308–324.

Naraian S (2016) Spatializing student learning to reimagine the "place" of inclusion. *Teach Coll Rec* **118**: 1–46.

Pendergast D, Bahr N (2005) *Teaching Middle Years: Rethinking Curriculum, Pedagogy and Assessment*. Crows Nest, NSW: Allen & Unwin.

Plowden Report (1967) *Children and Their Primary Schools: A Report of the Central Advisory Council for Education (England)*. London: Her Majesty's Stationery Office.

Pluquailec J (2018) Affective economies, autism, and "challenging behaviour": socio-spatial emotions in disabled children's education. *Emot Space Soc* **29**: 9–14.

Sanahuja-Gavaldà JM, Olmos-Rueda P, Morón-Velasco M (2016) Collaborative support for inclusion. *J Res Spec Educ Needs* **16**: 303–307.

Social Contexts: Communication, Leisure and Recreation

Beata Batorowicz and Martine Smith

A developing child needs meaningful social experiences to develop competencies, skills, self-efficacy and self-determination, a sense of belonging and friendships. Having friends, spending time together, sharing activities and conversations, seeking and providing help or emotional support to others, are of significant importance to development, health and well-being. Researchers have linked positive developmental outcomes to involvement in play, communication, and social interactions with peers, freedom of expression, and the opportunity to develop a sense of social belonging (Petrenchik et al. 2011). Thus, opportunities for experiences that have meaning are at the heart of the developmental process.

When Lund and Light (2007) studied long-term outcomes of seven young men with cerebral palsy who had severe motor and communication impairments, they found that, despite relatively strong language and communication skills, the young men had few meaningful relationships beyond immediate family members. Indeed, an emerging body of research points to social isolation and loneliness of children and young people with complex disabilities (e.g. Wickenden 2011). According to Lund and Light (2007), the factors that best supported positive outcomes for their participants were social, especially relationships that provided physical and emotional support, nurturing and assistance. The authors suggested that social interaction might be a stronger predictor than language skills for real-life participation outcomes of children with communication impairments.

In this chapter we give particular attention to communication and social relationships within the context of leisure and recreational activities. The examples provided concern children with severe motor and communication disabilities that use augmentative and alternative communication (AAC); however, many of the points raised in this chapter are relevant to all children and young adults with disabilities. The parent quotes are drawn from an international study of children acquiring language using communication aids [see von Tetzchner (2018a) for full description]. The term AAC is used here to refer to non-speech modes of communication, including gestures, facial expressions, communication boards and high-tech communication aids, all of which are used in contexts where an individual has little or no functional speech that can be understood by others, even highly familiar family members.

First, we discuss the conceptualisation of the social context of participation. Next, we highlight leisure and recreation as contexts of social participation and consider communication as related to children and young people with disabilities. Finally, we raise some issues related to practice and enabling social interaction and participation of children with complex disabilities.

SOCIAL CONTEXT

The Integrated Model of Social Environment and Context suggests that opportunities for meaningful reciprocal child–environment interactions are created on the level of *social context* and it is at that level that service providers need to work with children (Batorowicz et al. 2016a). Children are embedded in specific environments where they 'meet' and experience places, people, activities and objects – in time. Furthermore, children's subjective experiences with other people matter, as do the patterns of activities, the social roles and interpersonal experiences that arise from interactions between children and their immediate surroundings over time.

Children experience their world as an environment of relationships. Relationships engage children in ways that help them define who they are and how and why they are important to others. Relationships emerge over time in daily interactions. Therefore, considering relationships requires careful attention to the nature and extent of the opportunities, resources and supports that are available to children to engage in meaningful ways in activity settings. Furthermore, how these opportunities are experienced by a child will depend on the qualities of the places, people, objects and activities as well as a child's personal factors (e.g. preferences, interests), and how both transact over time.

Social context is dynamic and changes over time as individuals engage with others in their daily lives. Therefore, variations in life experiences are unique to each child. Experiences can be developmentally supportive or inhibiting; they can shape and reinforce interests, choices and creative expression, and may nurture interpersonal relationships. Positive experiences may erase negative ones as new meanings develop (Seligman and Csikszentmihalyi 2000).

SOCIAL CONTEXT AND PARTICIPATION OF CHILDREN WITH MOTOR AND COMMUNICATION IMPAIRMENTS

The impact of combined motor and communication impairments on a child's participation, life and development is weighty. These children typically have very limited ability to exert physical control on their environment as well as very limited functional speech, making it hard for them to express their desires, needs and thoughts. The environment can mitigate some of these challenges and provide opportunities for meaningful participation through the knowledge and skills of other individuals. Evidence to date overwhelmingly suggests that many children with motor and communication impairments have limited interaction opportunities and sparse and restricted social networks. They tend to participate in activities close to home, have restricted locations for activity engagement compared to children with typical development; have reduced scope for activity participation, especially with peers, and profoundly limited social networks (Batorowicz et al. 2014; Smith 2014). There is a strong connection between social network patterns and social participation and multiple studies indicate that children using AAC interact most frequently with close family members, adults with close ties to the family and professionals (e.g. Thirumanickam et al. 2011).

LINK TO VIGNETTE 7.1
'Gift and the Snake that Wouldn't Go to Sleep', p. 76.

In sum, the profound challenge for children with motor and communication impairments is to be active and in control, both of which are key not only to daily functioning but also to development (von Tetzchner 2018b). Given the nature of their motor impairments, effective communication skills present a crucial support for active engagement and control. Research points to the need to create more opportunities to (1) support autonomous and genuine communication; (2) be involved together with peers with and without disabilities; and (3) support relationship-building through participation in activities with the same peers over time, thus allowing deeper connections to develop. Adults using

AAC have identified building and maintaining friendships as a key priority of AAC research (O'Keefe et al. 2007).

LEISURE AND RECREATION AS CONTEXT OF INTERACTION

Play, leisure and recreational activities offer particularly important opportunities to children for genuine connections with others. In leisure activity
settings children get involved together, argue, have fun, and create and derive
meaning. Participation is based on interests, choice and preferences. Children

LINK TO VIGNETTE 7.2
*'In the Shadow of
Rockets', p. 78.*

with and without disabilities may try different activities before forming preferences. Therefore, providing
opportunities for activities is not sufficient: variety is also important. Children often choose different
leisure activities than their parents or teachers (Kulis and Batorowicz 2016); their views are important as
motivation and personal preference has been linked to meaningful engagement (King et al. 2006).

In a study involving children with cerebral palsy, Kramer and Hammel (2011) found that doing lots
of things was important to the participants. In another study of more than 600 children with disabilities
(Eriksson and Granlund 2004), this positive experience of control (i.e. in charge in an activity) was perceived as key to supporting participation.

Children with disabilities are at risk of limited opportunities to engage meaningfully in leisure and
recreational activities. They may be welcome to attend and may be present in settings where activities are
held; however, engaging children with disabilities in what is going on, and involving them in meaningful
ways, usually requires not only careful physical planning, but also individualised supports and resources.
Describing her experience in collecting her young son who uses AAC from her local preschool, one
mother recalled:

> So Brian wasn't at the little table, not at the big table … only at the middle so she [the personal
> assistant] was at the big table and she was able to feed him while he was in the middle, he was at
> neither table … you know … and that broke my heart.

Given the experience of being physically but not socially present in group activities, individuals with
complex impairments may seek out solitary activities. For example, when asked about what her 10-year-
old son typically does after school, one mother stated:

> He likes to be by himself and work on his computer and look up information. He searches the
> Internet for different movies and different characters, or … he does his homework on there.

Relationships develop in the context of social activities and friendship and
lasting social connections are created in shared activities. The provision of
opportunities to meet within the context of leisure activities and to be with
peers is only the first step. What is needed to develop lasting interpersonal
connection is engagement and shared meaning. In particular, repeated

LINK TO VIGNETTE 7.3
*'Reveal the Abilities',
p. 80.*

encounters and shared experiences, lead to familiarity and provide an opportunity to form strong and
more intimate relationships (Milner and Kelly 2009). Relationships are bound to opportunities to be
with people meaningfully – doing things together and communicating. However, outside of school and
home, children with disabilities may only have access either to programmes specifically for children with
disabilities, or inclusive programmes that have therapeutic goals, or seasonal programmes, like summer
camps (Batorowicz et al. 2014).

The advent of social media platforms offers new opportunities for overcoming some of the practical
barriers to being 'together' with others, such as geographic distance, physical accessibility of locations and

even the challenge of time. Messages can be expressed in real time without revealing the preparation time that can make co-present interactions challenging. Having access to social media platforms has been identified as motivating and powerful both for youth (Hynan et al. 2015) and adults (Caron and Light 2016) who use AAC. However, there are significant language, literacy and physical access barriers to effective use of social media for many individuals who use AAC, significantly constraining the extent to which these platforms are used by the majority of children and youth who use AAC. Furthermore, such platforms may complement, but do not replace in-person interactions with peers in shared, natural contexts. A key question, therefore, is whether children with disabilities have opportunities to be with their classmates and neighbourhood friends in the same leisure and recreational activities (e.g. dancing, talking or just hanging out together), thereby building networks of relationships that are embedded in their communities (Smith 2014).

Leisure services are often not funded and seem to be considered less important than school work or home participation. Preliminary research suggests that awareness of the burden of the cost (financial, time and/or physical) of leisure activities for families is a factor that influences leisure activity choices of young adults with motor and communication impairments (Hajjar et al. 2016), potentially nudging individuals towards solitary activities, rather than activities together with neighbourhood peers.

PARTICIPATION THROUGH COMMUNICATION: RECIPROCITY

Authentic communication implies reciprocity and a shared responsibility on all those involved in an interaction, although the balance of responsibility shifts developmentally. The human drive to engage in meaning-making is evident even in the earliest interactions between adults and babies. Although very young children are usually dependent on the willingness of others to engage in interactions, these interactions provide the context in which they develop language, communication and interaction skills to enable them to express themselves, assert their personalities, and determine their desired communication partners. Effective communication skills link to social competence, peer acceptance and psychosocial adjustment (Berk 2003) and are pivotal to the social experiences of children (Marshall and Goldbart 2008) and adults who use AAC (Trembath et al. 2010). Through communication, children learn to control and understand their world. Consequently, communication skills have profound importance for all aspects of life – doing, choice, being in control and decision making. Choice and control are instrumental to children's wellness and quality of life (Prilleltensky et al. 2001). Adults using AAC have reported that autonomous communication is a key factor enabling successful social participation (Trembath et al. 2010). Language and AAC provide a mechanism for children to be active in the world and to develop autonomy, particularly if individuals have severe motor impairments (Batorowicz et al. 2016b).

To enable genuine reciprocity in interaction, children need access to people to talk to and interesting things to talk about. Therefore, they need experiences that extend beyond the predictable and routine contexts of home and school. They require resources and supports to enable genuine communicative exchange (e.g. time, knowledgeable partners, accessible places, motivation, interests), as well as a means of expressing themselves. The importance of having access to an independent means of expression is captured in the following quote from a mother of 12-year-old boy:

> I remember the first conversation we ever had, so … It'll make me cry. I was invited to the school for, I think it was Mother's Day. And he said 'Hi Mom' [using his new communication device] when I walked in the classroom. And I'm like 'Alex, is that you?' And yeah, it was him. Yeah, that was a milestone.

Time represents a major barrier to successful social interactions for children who use AAC. The slow pace of communication using AAC has often been attributed to a child's abilities or limitations of technology (e.g. Fager et al. 2012). More recently, the focus has shifted to the extent to which communication partners allow sufficient time to support successful interactions with children (Batorowicz et al. 2014) or adults (Trembath et al. 2010) who use AAC.

Interaction experiences over time with people in activity settings lead to particular outcomes. If a child meets people who are not willing to 'listen' and take time to have a meaningful interaction, the child may become 'passive', as there is no gain or worth in trying to communicate. Moreover, if a child is treated as immature or having cognitive delays, when the child is functioning cognitively at their peer's level, the child may be frustrated (Batorowicz et al. 2014). The reported notion of passivity and lack of initiation in children may reflect the reaction of children to specific people, based on prior experiences.

Genuine reciprocity is at the heart of successful interactions as captured by a mother of a 14-year-old, 'Sometimes she says [to others] "I'm not a baby, I'm a normal teenager, so talk to me like one"'. Real-life interactions, in children's typical activity settings, such as local stores, theatres, or libraries may lead to changes in children as their experiences grow and as other people become familiar with the use of AAC. A parent of a 10-year-old girl noted:

> It's just a matter of getting it out there. If there's more than just my kid at the mall using her talker …, we have a better chance of people going to them and asking them questions and initiating conversations.

In sum, social interactions are context bound; they happen within activity settings. Participation in leisure and play activities over time with the same people provides unique opportunities to develop bonds with others. Social interactions are the foundations for forming connections and potentially more deep and intimate relationships.

COMMUNICATION PARTNERS

Although individuals with motor and communication impairments may engage disproportionately in solitary activities, given a choice, they opt for activities with others (Batorowicz et al. 2014). They also express preferences for activity settings based on the people present there, rather than the activities themselves (King et al. 2014). Therefore, patterns of participation understood as attendance may depend not only on place or activity, but also on the people present, who represent potential interaction partners.

Robust social networks are populated by a diverse range of potential interaction partners, ranging from intimate and highly familiar to unfamiliar or passing acquaintances and context-specific individuals, such as the serving staff in a local coffee shop. Children with severe motor and communication impairments have expressed desires to be social, to be with peers, to interact with unfamiliar people, and to interact with people with and without disability, but have also reported that they lacked opportunities to demonstrate their abilities (e.g. Batorowicz et al. 2014). Of special concern is a general lack of peers in the child's social context, often despite parents' efforts to arrange time to be together with peers (e.g. Wickenden 2011). One father of a 6-year-old girl reflected:

> All of her friends are adults – all of our adult friends. She relates very well to adults … and she struggles with her peer group. Outside of her sister, no. There's no-one she hangs out with.

Concerns about limited opportunities for peer interaction are not new and even within interactions with peers, peers have been found to adopt the role of helpers (e.g. Raghavendra et al. 2012), rather than equal

> *Methods and strategies are needed to engage children meaningfully in activity contexts with their peers, with expectations of shared distribution of control and responsibility.*

participants. Further, while children who use AAC may have more interactions with adults in comparison to children without disabilities, lower levels of meaningful engagement may still occur (King et al. 2014). A mother of 12-year-old boy captured the power of this reciprocity:

> Then … later, I heard him talk to his friends, like … with friends that are verbal, they actually have conversations, like somebody told me the other day they were talking about girlfriends, and that was just like … 'are you kidding me?' But yeah, he's 12.

Siblings may play a special role in creating these equal relationships. As one mother of a 10-year-old boy commented:

> With his brother … they play the Wii together. … They're good … they can fight, they're just like regular brothers. They pick on each other constantly – they're just … they're brothers. You wouldn't know that Jack has a communication problem.

A QUANTUM LEAP FOR SERVICES

Acknowledging Different Perspectives

Professionals may not be supported to take time to interact directly with a child who uses AAC (noted also in relation to adults; Smith and Murray 2011); instead, they may talk to parents or educational assistants about the child. Consequently, their knowledge about the child's social context may be limited. Parents and therapists may have different perspectives on what is most important as a focus of intervention. This is not surprising, given that therapists may be biased towards performance and attainment of functional goals, with an associated pressure for competence, outcomes and *doing* things. They may prioritise the development of physical independence, activity and skill learning, all of which are valuable aspirations. For parents, a focus on social interaction and simply *being* may be equally important. For example, the mother of one 8-year-old who used AAC said, 'There's no place where he can just, have a break, be himself, just, be himself and just you know, just do what he can do and that's enough'. Parental priorities may be informed by an understanding of social networks as a key to healthy living and by a focus on future contexts and a desire to ensure their children do not find themselves alone.

Addressing Social Environmental Influences

Social influences on participation concern opportunities, resources and supports that are present in a particular activity setting. Meaningful participation is most likely to occur where there are communication partners who expect participation, who are willing to talk, who have the skills to interact with a child using AAC, and who can offer the time needed for interaction using AAC. Such opportunities have lasting value if they occur in accessible community settings where children with communication and motor impairments can attend on an equal footing with peers, where the play and leisure activities allow them to be meaningfully involved, and where there are objects (e.g. adapted books, communication aids) that support their autonomy and engagement.

Building Natural Interaction Opportunities

Exploiting social contexts requires the availability of programmes and activities welcoming all children, formal activities as well as places for informal play (e.g. playgrounds), activities that are accessible, interesting, age appropriate, inviting, and that offer natural interaction opportunities (in contrast to therapeutic and respite care programmes). There is a need to provide choices for children and to involve them in decision making about their preferred activities. For example, because of safety concerns and school policies a child who used a wheelchair and

Being involved includes providing opportunities for self-advocacy and decision making.

a communication device was not allowed to walk from home with her peers, a context that would otherwise offer rich opportunities for informal social interactions and for building friendships. Her mother reported:

> She advocated for herself to be able to walk home from school, and at first she wasn't able to walk home from school until they approved it through the board, and she wrote her own letter, she was really upset at first that the initial … answer was no, … so she now can walk home with her friends, and she does a lot of talking while she walks home.

Emphasising Participation

There seems to be a discrepancy between accepted social models of practice and actual practice. Perhaps because of the operational demands of many communication aids, clinical work may focus on technology more than on social interaction and social context (Light and McNaughton 2013), leaving little time to focus on supporting a child's actual participation in different social settings, especially outside of school (Batorowicz et al. 2006). Professionals may rely on discussions with parents, teachers and other healthcare professionals to gain an insight into a child's participation opportunities, offering only partial information. However, a review of qualitative research with children and youth with disabilities showed that children had meaningful participation experiences when services were individualised to their unique needs and strengths within their various life circumstances (Kramer et al. 2012).

For services to support the emergence of inclusive places, attention must be paid to ensuring:

- *multiple opportunities* for welcoming activity settings offered in a child's own neighbourhood, out of home and with peers;
- *supportive people* who know how to engage and involve the child with opportunities to engage and adapt an activity as needed;
- *places* that naturally encourage peer interactions, tools/technology to support interaction, communication and choice within those interactions;
- *resources* to support meaningful activity participation;
- *time:* opportunities for children to attend activity settings with the same peers over time to develop lasting connections and friendships.

In sum, such inclusive leisure activity settings create opportunities for children to be engaged in collective experiences, particularly in meaningful peer interactions in activities with other children, where experiences are child-directed, natural and genuinely reciprocal. Services need to be re-oriented to focus on meaningful real-world participation opportunities. While the measurement of performance and functioning in areas of self-care and productivity continue to be relevant, the focus needs to expand to incorporate social participation in context of leisure and direct services focusing on supporting children's interactions with others. The need for such a transformation is best captured by a father of a 5-year-old girl:

> I think it needs to become more real time for these kids. I think this part of therapy needs to make a quantum leap forward because these kids are going to be left behind when they get involved in the real world.

In conclusion, family and client-centred practice points to the importance of supporting the active participation of children within their families and communities in accordance with their own interests and goals. Children need opportunities to choose the activity settings, to meaningfully engage in typical childhood activities in their neighbourhoods and have a say in things that are important to them. Interventions must address the contextual elements needed to support an *active* child, recognising that being active need not always involve *doing*.

SUMMARY OF KEY IDEAS

- It is a profound challenge for children with motor and communication impairments to be in control.
- Genuine reciprocity in children's interactions is needed within leisure activity settings.
- Children need a variety of communication partners, and especially opportunities to participate with peers.
- *Being* is as least as important as *doing*.
- We need to take a quantum leap – to reorient services to meaningful, in real-world, participation opportunities.

REFERENCES

Batorowicz B, Campbell F, von Tetzchner S, King G, Missiuna C (2014) Social participation of school-aged children who use communication aids: the views of children and parents. *Augment Altern Commun* **30**: 237–251.

Batorowicz B, King G, Mishra L, Missiuna C (2016a) An integrated model of social environment and social context for pediatric rehabilitation. *Disabil Rehabil* **38**: 1204–1215.

Batorowicz B, Stadskleiv K, von Tetzchner S, Missiuna C (2016b) Children who use communication aids instruct peer and adult partners during play-based activity. *Augment Altern Commun* **32**: 105–119.

Batorowicz B, McDougall S, Shepherd TA (2006) AAC and community partnerships: the participation path to community inclusion. *Augment Altern Commun* **22**: 178–195.

Berk LE (2003) *Child Development*. Boston, MA: Allyn and Bacon.

Caron J, Light J (2016) "Social media has opened a world of 'open communication'": Experiences of adults with cerebral palsy who use augmentative and alternative communication and social media. *Augment Altern Commun* **32**: 25–40.

Eriksson L, Granlund M (2004) Conceptions of participation in students with disabilities and persons in their close environment. *J Dev Phys Disabil* **16**: 229–245.

Fager S, Bardach L, Russell S, Higginbotham J (2012) Access to augmentative and alternative communication: new technologies and clinical decision-making. *J Pediatr Rehabil Med* **5**: 53–61.

Hajjar DJ, McCarthy JW, Benigno JP, Chabot J (2016) "You get more than you give": Experiences of community partners in facilitating active recreation with individuals who have complex communication needs. *Augment Altern Commun* **32**: 131–142.

Hynan A, Goldbart J, Murray J (2015) A grounded theory of internet and social media use by young people who use augmentative and alternative communication (AAC). *Disabil Rehabil* **37**: 1559–1575.

King G, Law M, Hanna S et al. (2006) Predictors of the leisure and recreation participation of children with physical disabilities: A structural equation modeling. *Child Health Care* **35**: 209–234.

King G, Batorowicz B, Rigby P, Pinto M, Thompson L, Goh F (2014) The leisure activity settings and experiences of youth with severe disabilities. *Dev Neurorehabil* **17**: 259–269.

Kulis A, Batorowicz B (2016) *Views of Children and Parents on Choosing Extracurricular Activities*. 1st COTEC-ENOTHE Congress, Galway, Ireland.

Kramer JM, Hammel J (2011) "I do lots of things": Children with cerebral palsy's competence for everyday activities. *Int J Disabil Dev Educ* **58**: 121–136.

Kramer JM, Olsen S, Mermelstein M, Balcells A, Liljenquist K (2012) Youth with disabilities' perspectives of the environment and participation: a qualitative meta-synthesis. *Child Care Health Dev* **38**: 763–777.

Light J, McNaughton D (2013) Putting people first: re-thinking the role of technology in augmentative and alternative communication intervention. *Augment Altern Commun* **29**: 299–309.

Lund SK, Light J (2007) Long-term outcomes for individuals who use augmentative and alternative communication: part III – contributing factors. *Augment Altern Commun* **23**: 323–335.

Marshall J, Goldbart J (2008) "Communication is everything I think." Parenting a child who needs augmentative and alternative communication (AAC). *Int J Lang Commun Disord* **43**: 77–98.

Milner P, Kelly B (2009) Community participation and inclusion: people with disabilities defining their place. *Disabil Soc* **24**: 47–62.

O'Keefe BM, Kozak NB, Schuller R (2007) Research priorities in augmentative and alternative communication as identified by people who use AAC and their facilitators. *Augment Altern Commun* **23**: 89–96.

Petrenchik TM, King GA, Batorowicz B (2011) Children and youth with disabilities: Enhancing mental health through positive experiences of doing and belonging. In: Bazyk S (Ed) *Mental Health Promotion, Prevention, and Intervention in Children and Youth: A Guiding Framework for Occupational Therapy*. Bethesda, MD: American Occupational Therapy Association, pp. 189–205.

Prilleltensky I, Nelson G, Peirson L (2001) The role of power and control in children's lives: an ecological analysis of pathways towards wellness, resilience and problems. *J Community Appl Soc* **11**: 143–158.

Raghavendra P, Olsson C, Sampson J, McInerney R, Connell T (2012) School participation and social networks of children with complex communication needs, physical disabilities, and typically developing peers. *Augment Altern Commun* **28**: 33–43.

Seligman ME, Csikszentmihalyi M (2000) Positive psychology. An introduction. *Am Psychol* **55**: 5–14.

Smith MM, Murray J (2011) Parachute without a ripcord: the skydive of communication interaction. *Augment Altern Commun* **27**: 292–303.

Smith M (2014) Adolescence and AAC: intervention challenges and possible solutions. *Comm Disord Q* **36**: 112–118.

Thirumanickam A, Raghavendra P, Olsson C (2011) Participation and social networks of school-age children with complex communication needs: a descriptive study. *Augment Altern Commun* **27**: 195–204.

Trembath D, Balandin S, Stancliffe RJ, Togher L (2010) "Communication is everything:" The experiences of volunteers who use AAC. *Augment Altern Commun* **26**: 75–86.

von Tetzchner S (2018a). Introduction to the special issue on aided language processes, development, and use: an international perspective. *Augment Altern Commun* **34**: 1–15.

von Tetzchner S (2018b). *Child and Adolescent Psychology: Typical and Atypical Development*. New York: Routledge. doi:10.4324/9781315742113.

Wickenden M (2011) Talking to teenagers: using anthropological methods to explore identity and the lifeworlds of young people who use AAC. *Comm Disord Q* **32**: 151–163.

In the following vignette, participation can be seen as connecting with communities through communication. Although we may focus on the importance of enabling the child's communication (and that is important), in this vignette the importance of really listening to parents and carefully observing children in context is also highlighted. As you read this vignette, consider the impact on parents when their children feel or are 'invisible' or misunderstood.

Gift and the Snake that Wouldn't Go to Sleep (South Africa)

Juan Bornman

'You shouldn't worry so much that your son is not talking. He is a boy. Every day we see that boys are slow talkers. They don't start talking when they are young – they are not like the girls.' Mrs Serudu (not her real name) knew that the doctor was trying to comfort her, but the uneasiness she felt about her 5-year-old son, Gift, who had not yet started talking, would not leave her.

This uneasiness was like a snake in her tummy and the snake was angry. The more fear she felt, the angrier the snake became. Mrs Serudu knew that at home her husband would be angry for wasting a whole day travelling to the city to go to the hospital to hear what the doctors thought was wrong with Gift. There would not be a plate of hot food waiting for him when they returned home, and on top of it all, the taxi trip to the hospital had cost the equivalent of a week's salary. Mr Serudu was also of the opinion that his wife should just leave Gift alone, he would talk when he wanted to talk. After all there was already enough noise in their tiny two-roomed house with four other children.

Gift was attending a crèche in their little rural village. The teacher was not a qualified teacher, but a grandmother who looked after a group of preschool children to allow their mothers to work in the city. The 'teacher' said that Gift was doing well at school. He was well behaved and she experienced no problems with him. However, one day when Mrs Serudu arrived early to pick up Gift, she noticed that he was sitting in the back of the class, all by himself rocking forwards and backwards while humming. Suddenly the snake started stirring in her tummy again. She had never seen Gift do this before. He looked as if he was not even aware of her presence. 'You see, Mama', the old teacher triumphantly said, 'He is happy and he is well behaved. We have no problems with Gift'. The snake was very angry now. How could Gift be happy if he was in a school with so many other children who ignored him? When his teacher thought that he was well behaved because he sat humming all by himself in the back of the classroom? How can so many people see him, but at the same time not see him? If only Gift would talk.

Mrs Serudu knew that Gift never looked her, or anybody else in the eye. She knew that he preferred playing by himself – if you could call it playing. He liked putting things in neat rows – from stones to teaspoons, everything he could lay his hands on. She knew that even though Gift did not speak, he understood things that she said to him, and if she made a sign with her hand, like waving, he seemed to understand her even better. She knew that he has strong preferences for certain foods, and that he requests 'more' food by smacking his lips in a specific way. She knew that Gift showed her when he was 'finished' with something, because that is when he closed his eyes and turned his head away. She knew so many things about her 'Gift', he was truly a gift to her, and the stories spilled out as she explained them to the pastor at her church. He listened patiently, nodding his head to encourage her. Eventually he spoke and said that he heard about a young girl, they called her a speech therapist, who had recently started working at the hospital. Mrs Serudu and Gift would be welcome to go to the hospital on Wednesday with the church taxi.

With the speech therapist listening closely, Gift's story spilled out of Mrs Serudu. Not once did the speech therapist interrupt, until she said, 'We can help Gift to start communicating. We can give him therapy, using pictures and signs and maybe even a talking machine. It will not be easy and it will not be a quick fix – but everyone can and every one does communicate. We just have to find the right way of communicating for Gift'. And so, for the first time in many years, Mrs Serudu felt as if the snake finally went to sleep.

VIGNETTE

7.2

This vignette highlights the challenges for children growing up under chronic life-threatening situations; where 'normal' activities and contexts in the community are seemingly impossible, and in which participation is itself a coping mechanism. As you read this vignette reflect on those children whose vulnerabilities further restrict opportunities for participation, the role of resilience and the need for creativity in finding solutions.

In the Shadow of Rockets (Israel)

Orit Bart and Limor Rosenberg

Rachel is a healthy, intelligent, 5-year-old girl. Dan is her 7-year-old brother; he has developmental coordination disorder. They live in the south of Israel, in a quiet little town surrounded by green fields. Yet for the last couple of decades, the citizens of this town have been living with constant threat of rocket attacks. Rachel and Dan were born into this reality.

Like other children their age, Rachel and Dan participate in the routine activities of daily life. Every morning they brush their teeth and get dressed. Rachel fixes her ponytail independently, while Dan needs help tying his shoelaces. When Rachel goes to the toilet she prefers to have her mother nearby. They both like attending school and play with siblings and friends. Rachel enjoys doing arts and crafts and spending time outdoors at the playground.

Dan, however, refuses to play outdoors despite all the protective measures taken. Dan is afraid he will not be able to reach the secure area quickly enough. In the context of ongoing exposure to life-threatening situations, Dan's developmental disabilities are having a worsening impact on his daily routines and involvement.

At bedtime, Rachel and Dan like listening to their parents read them stories. Often, they are afraid at night and crawl into bed with their parents.

Without any notice, at any time day or night, the Red Alert siren can go off, warning residents of an incoming rocket attack. When this happens, Rachel and Dan have only 15 seconds to seek shelter before the rocket hits. This short warning does not enable people to reach a safety place if they are in the shower, for example, or driving their children in the car.

Because of this situation, increasing numbers of children like Rachel and Dan are being diagnosed with post-traumatic stress. They may experience anxiety, sleep disturbance, night wetting and may react aggressively.

How can children maintain their daily routines and continue to function normally under these circumstances? In our study, we found that mothers also exhibit a high level of stress and post-traumatic symptoms. Nevertheless, they allow their children to participate in their daily activities and normal routines. Their behaviour may be explained by mothers' resilience (ability to adapt well to adversity, trauma,

78

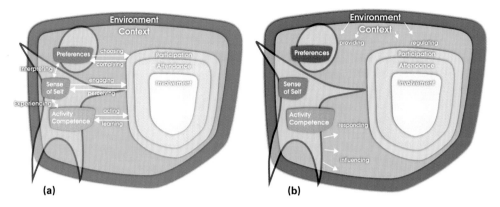

Figure 1.2 The family of participation related constructs: **(a)** person-focused processes, **(b)** environment-focused processes (Imms et al. 2017)

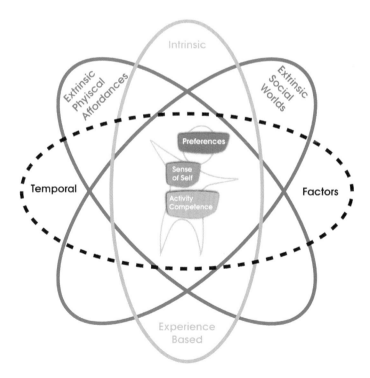

Figure 4.1 Transactional influences of the family of participation related constructs over time. Figure adapted from the fPRC, Imms et al. (2017), with permission.

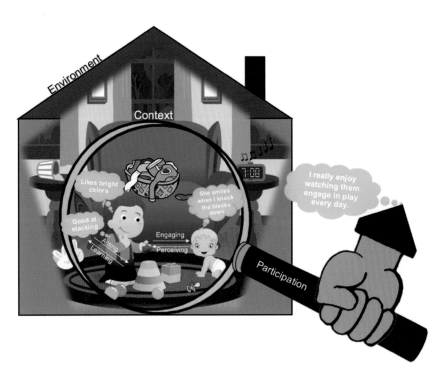

Figure 5.1 Participation-related constructs specific to indoor play and games.

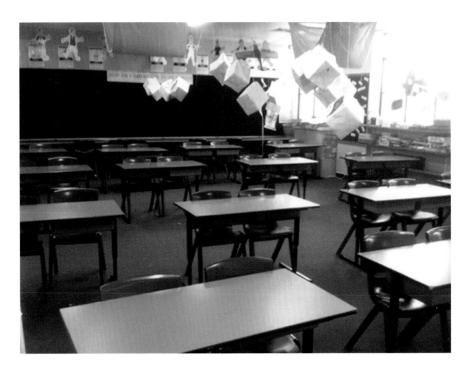

Figure 6.1 A "traditional" primary school classroom. Photograph: T. Byers with permission.

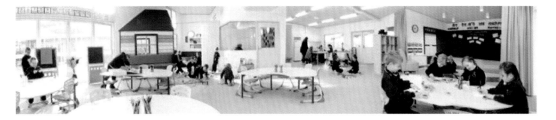

Figure 6.2 An innovative learning environment. Architect: Ken Woodman, No. 42 Architects; Photographer: Erin David-Hartwig, Beechworth Photographers.

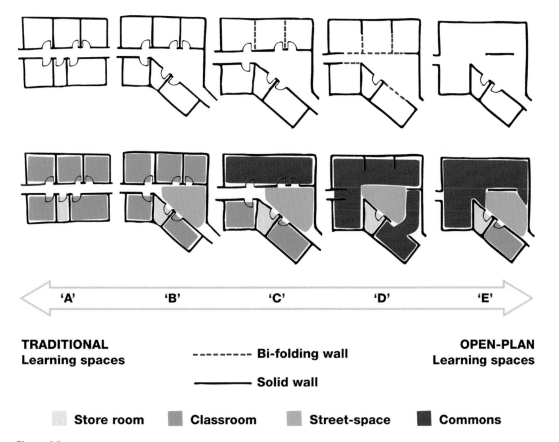

Figure 6.3 Spatial design typology. Dovey and Fisher (2014), adapted in Imms (2016).

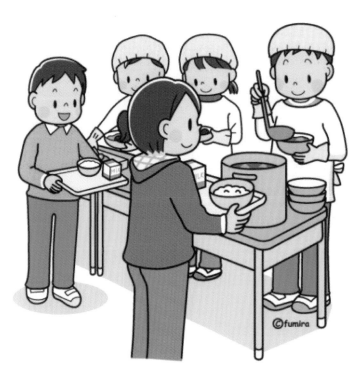

Figure V17.1 Compulsory school lunch (reprinted with permission © fumira).

Figure V17.2 The school lunch (reprinted with permission © fumira).

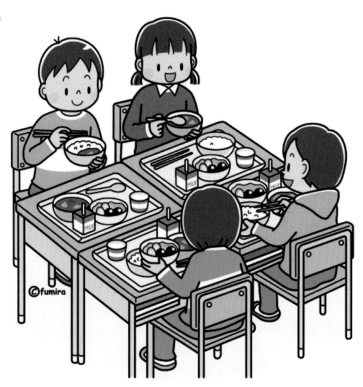

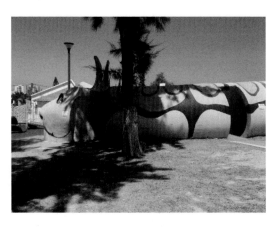

Figure V7.2 Specially designed playground shelter.

tragedy or threats). We found that higher levels of maternal resilience were associated with higher levels of children's independence and enjoyment while participating in their routine activities.

Rachel, Dan and the family are part of a supportive community, which allocates many resources to enhance the physical safety and mental health of its citizens. For example, a special school curriculum was developed. When the Red Alert siren is sounded, the children routinely sing a reworded familiar nursery rhyme to help them hurry into the secure area, manage their stress and relax (see https://www.youtube. com/watch?v=e7fFqeofXfU).

Colour red! Colour red! Hurry up hurry up to a safe area…

My heart is beating Boom, Boom, Boom.

My body is shaking Doom, Doom, Doom.

But I am overcoming because I am a little different …

Shake your hands, loosen your legs,

Breath in deep, breath out far, we can laugh.

This creative activity aims to help teachers and children maintain their daily routine at school. Special shelters were built and cement walls were constructed around bus stops. Special playgrounds were designed to enable children to play outdoors, with the playground apparatus adjusted to provide a secure space while maintaining a playful atmosphere (Fig. V7.2).

Across the globe, political issues are threatening to hamper children's participation in daily life activities. Nevertheless, human and environmental factors can mediate the negative impact, thus enabling children to participate and live their lives despite the security threat.

Cultural expectations for behaviour may be implicit or explicit; influencing actions as well as aspirations for both parents and children with disabilities. When reading this vignette, reflect on the story of a father who risks alienation to enhance opportunities for participation in education and employment for his son. We can take inspiration from the positives that arise when focusing on strengths and building on preferences.

Reveal the Abilities (Vietnam)

Yen-Thanh Mac

In Vietnam, men have 'low participation' in childcare overall, with about 30% spending just less than 1 hour/day with their children (Jennings 2017). The practices and norms of the Vietnamese society still engender male dominance with Confucian ethics deeply affecting Vietnamese culture. Although there have been laws, regulations and women's rights movements recently, the concept of male superiority over women remains; the man (father) as breadwinner with absolute authority in the household. The woman becomes the housewife and mother; expected to be the caregiver, more likely to bathe, feed and mind the children. Consequently, when there is a child with a neurodevelopmental disorder, mothers experience more stress than fathers; they are the main caregivers and financially dependent on their husbands. In addition, there

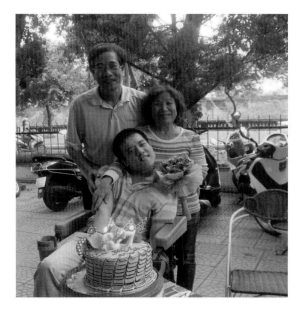

Figure V7.3 Mr Van, his wife and Hong. Hue, Vietnam.

is stigma attached to the mothers. Their husbands' family, and even their husbands blame them: 'She did something wrong in her past life, she did not know how to be pregnant and delivery the baby well.' This stigma directly affects the activities and participation of those children. Higher levels of parenting participation by fathers have been associated with lower levels of parenting stress in mothers (D'Antonio and Shin 2009). That in turn, affects the participation of their children. Therefore, enhancing the parenting role of fathers of children with neurodevelopment disorders is crucial to maximising outcomes.

I am going to tell you the story of Mr Van, the father and the main caregiver of a young man named Hong. This is a success story. Hong has cerebral palsy with severe physical limitations and lives in Hue, Vietnam. Hong is an English teacher, an inspirational writer and speaker. Hong did not go to any formal school – he was self-taught with support from friends. Hong calls himself 'a happy man who has more experience than others'.

There are many wonderful things to say about Mr Van, but I am going to focus on four aspects: *playing*, *encouraging risk*, *protecting* and *disciplining*.

To support playing, Mr Van developed shared hobbies between him and Hong to provide a unique place for connection, fun and memory. While most parents in Vietnam do not allow their children to play video games, Mr Van believed allowing and monitoring was better than prohibiting. He not only helped Hong buy video games but also learned about them for shared fun. These things helped Hong to participate in peers' conversations and entertainment, equally and happily.

Mr Van has not sacrificed his own interests while maximising Hong's ability. He taught Hong to write 'Đường Poem' (a traditional Chinese style poem, requiring good language, perception and creativity), as he loves this art. Hong has become an active and outstanding member of the 'Đường Poem' writers' group in Vietnam and overseas.

Mr Van also encouraged risk. Hong has speech difficulty. Mr Van's plan was for Hong to learn to become a computer teacher, but Hong has a passion for teaching English. Although Mr Van was aware that teaching a language would be almost impossible for someone like Hong, he encouraged Hong to follow his dream. Hong worked hard to find a native speaking teacher online. Fascinatingly, it is much easier for Hong to speak English than Vietnamese. Now, Hong earns money designing curricula for an English language centre.

Mr Van lets Hong be as independent as possible. Hong has an electric wheelchair but the streets in Hue are not easy. His father guides him about safety and lets him go out on his own but the wheelchair stops working when it (frequently) rains. When this happens Mr Van must escort Hong and the wheelchair back home without the electrical support, enjoying the adventure. Certainly, Hong does not think his physical disability should stop him doing anything he likes.

When Hong was a small child, his heaviest punishment was not receiving gifts from Santa Claus in his socks every night. Mr Van encouraged Hong by having a gift for him when he made the effort to learn each day. That acknowledged Hong's efforts and helped him keep trying; building confidence that he is a good and useful person in society.

It's difficult to believe that this is a story of a father who, 27 years ago, was told by his best friend, a paediatrician: 'You should have another child, Hong has 'brain failure', he will not have any cognition or perception'!

REFERENCES

D'Antonio E, Shin JY (2009) Families of children with intellectual disabilities in Vietnam: Emerging themes. *Int Rev Res Mental Retard* **38**: 93–123.

Jenings R (2017) From Vietnam to Taiwan, Why Asian fathers are caring more for their children. *Forbes, June 15.* Available at: https://www.forbes.com/sites/ralphjennings/2017/06/15/fathers-day-asia-why-asian-fathers-are-caring-more-for-their-children/#4030ddbf6660 [Accessed 20 August 2019].

Societal Influences on Participation

Dido Green and Bengt Westerberg

> *I only have cerebral palsy now and again*
> – Teenager with cerebral palsy (Jahnsen et al. 2017)

In this chapter we explore societal influences, attitudinal and institutional, and potential impacts on participation of individuals living with disability, their families and their communities. We begin by highlighting different constructs of disability and discuss how language influences the ways societies respond to, and support, people with disabilities. We then consider the impact of legislation to facilitate access and inclusion. We reflect on how institutional and socio-political landscapes provide a foundation for attitudes and policies that shape expectations and define opportunities. We end with discussion of the challenges to forming inclusive societies.

DISABILITY – WHAT DOES THIS MEAN IN THE CONTEXT OF PARTICIPATION?

Differing perspectives of human behaviour can help us think about why societies operate the way they do. Four main models for conceptualising the nature of disability have been identified in disability literature (Berghs et al. 2016). Different understandings of impairment and disability are evident; from a focus on individual impairment (and functional variability) in the medical model, the accessibility of society in critical disability studies, or an interaction between the two in a biopsychosocial model. A fourth, human rights model, focuses on the fundamental rights of individuals with disability, thus, is technically not a model of disability (Berghs et al. 2016). These models have their critics, particularly from individuals with disability, not only in view of the perspectives of disability defined from those without, but also with respect to the limitations of the models in accounting for the dynamic interactions among physical and emotional experiences in multiple and changing environments (Abrams 2016; Shakespeare 2013). Nonetheless, these models influence the frameworks for care practices and legislative policies adopted by different cultures (e.g. Toro-Martínez 2015). Whether practices and policies take a caring, restorative or emancipative perspective, can be seen to reflect as well as shape societies' attitudes towards those individuals defined as having disabilities.

The International Classification of Functioning, Disability and Health (ICF) and the Child and Youth version (ICF-CY) have made major contributions to shifting perspectives of health and function away from participation restrictions purely residing in the individual, to considering environmental and societal impacts (WHO 2001). Nevertheless, from the perspective of those with disability, the embodied experience of ability or disability is not realised in the ICF model and 'disability' is viewed as negative or problematic; the antithesis of an 'able' or desired form of human existence (Abrams 2016). Notably, the ICF fails to define Personal Factors beyond a mix of features; for example, sex, age, education, social background and 'other factors that influence how disability is experienced by the individual' (WHO 2001, p. 11). Or in the words of an 8-year-old with cerebral palsy: 'It's cool because you're different …. I like being different, so I like having hemiplegia, because you're different, you're not the same. You're different in your own way' (Green 2015). Abrams (2016) argues that notions (and hence definitions) of disability, ability or other human attributes are not simply structures of human existence but reflect instead complex interactions that unfold over time and which then define meaningful interactions. In illustration of this, we may see attributes of an individual with autism, such as lack of distraction for social interactions and persistence in attention to detail, as disadvantaging in one environment but advantageous in another. Westerberg (in press) highlights the difficulty in defining a person as 'disabled' when considering functional variability; one individual can simultaneously have certain exceptionally well-developed abilities alongside considerable weaknesses. Nevertheless, there is often an economic impact for individuals who require different levels of physical, educational or social supports to access mainstream facilities.

The perspective of an individual is fundamental to participatory experiences. Abrams (2016) incorporates the work of the philosopher Martin Heidegger to redefine constructs of 'disability' and consider the 'politics of disablement' to encompass the subjective essence of human experience. This phenomenological approach to understanding disability is consistent with the transactional influences between participation constructs of 'being' and 'being involved while being there' (Imms et al. 2016); focusing on embodiment in the personal experience and the cultural concepts of disability (Abrams 2016). These are essential tenets on which we consider 'participation' as incorporating the physical state of 'being' (attendance) alongside the personal experience of 'being there' (involvement). Policy decisions to promote participation for individuals with disabilities arise from perspectives and models of disability within differing societies as well as economic capacity (Stevens 2013). The next section explores political impacts on the cultural and institutional organisation of 'disability' within society.

PARTICIPATION – A POLITICAL PERSPECTIVE FROM SWEDEN

How legislation and policies impact on individuals, families and communities is pertinent to understanding macro (societal) contexts for participation opportunities and experiences. In this section we discuss participation from a political perspective, and use Swedish and North American experiences as cases representing high resource countries before discussing challenges in low-resource countries.

Political decisions influence legislation supporting advocacy and inclusion. Inclusion may mean different things in different contexts.

The Swedish constitution emphasises that public organisations shall work for all individuals to obtain participation and equality in society, to safeguard the rights of children and to prohibit all kinds of discrimination including disability. Participation is seen as a comprehensive goal for the United Nations (UN) Convention on Rights for Persons with Disabilities (CRPD; UN 2006), and also for Swedish disability policy.

The wordings of relevant Swedish documents emphasise that people with disabilities shall be citizens with the same conditions and rights as others and that a person with a disability must never be regarded as an object of measures, but always seen as an individual with rights. This mode of thought has been echoed in other contexts and reflected in the writings of Abrams (2016), Shakespeare (2013) and others.

Participation in One's Own Life and in Social Activities

The World Health Organization defines participation as engagement in a life situation (WHO 2001). It can be understood in at least two respects: on the one hand, as participation in decisions about one's own life, and, on the other, as participation in individual meaningful activities or social activities of different kinds. In this chapter we focus on societal influences on 'social' participation.

When looking at the outcome of participation in social activities one can talk about different degrees of participation, from mere attendance to deeply felt experiences of involvement. Ultimately, only the individual can estimate his or her own engagement. Politically determined goals for legislation are mainly about creating prerequisites for participation.

Goals of Procedure and Outcome Influencing Participation

In this field, one of the most important Swedish national laws is the Act Concerning Support and Service for Persons with Certain Functional Impairments (LSS), which aims to provide services to people in need of substantial support. Goals are set in the law which can roughly be related to procedure or outcome:

- Procedural goals concern how support is provided; giving regard to the integrity and individual needs of the beneficiary in order to guarantee his or her influence, co- and self-determination.
- Outcome goals concern the results that the measures aim for, such as full participation in social life, good living conditions, opportunities for an independent life and living as others do.

Self-determination of a beneficiary is not obvious. He/she is often, to a larger degree than people without disabilities, dependent upon the views of others. Others might be municipal administrators having opinions about which support should be provided, in what way, when and by whom, or the personnel tasked to give services.

The right to influence support and services and self-determination is thus emphasised in the LSS (and other laws), with positive impacts on daily life evident. However, many beneficiaries indicate that in practice, there is a tendency towards a Big Brother (over-controlling) attitude from agencies and agency personnel. These practices risk limiting choice and over-riding the experiences of participation of the individual.

Decision makers and service providers need to offer opportunities for participation, and consider these from perspectives of beneficiaries, rather than assume they 'know best'.

Regarding social activities in which participation is important, the CRPD (UN 2006) calls attention to five areas:

- education;
- health, habilitation and rehabilitation;
- work and employment;
- political and public life;
- culture, recreation, leisure activities and sports.

These areas are addressed in Swedish disability policy, and evident also in other societies in which the UN Convention and a social model of disability have informed legislation (see, e.g. impact on Argentinian legislation in Toro-Martínez 2015).

Differences in Participation

The CRPD claims that people with disabilities, in spite of many measures taken, continue to meet obstacles to their participation as equal citizens. This is true also in Sweden; illustrated with a few examples from a report on participation, reflecting the situation in 2015:

- There is a gap in educational level between people with disabilities and people without disabilities, that is, the proportions of people with disabilities completing postsecondary school education is 32% compared to 44% in the general population.
- There is a similar gap in the regular labour market; the rate of employment is 62% in contrast to 81% respectively.
- Of people with disabilities, 49% visited a cinema or a theatre compared to 64% of the general population. People with disabilities also have lower frequency and variation of social participation (34%) than the general population (15%); seldom participating in activities such as study circles, demonstrations or private parties.

Studies of Western societies over the past decade have consistently highlighted the reduced participation, in both frequency of attendance and diversity of activities in leisure/recreation and physical activities of young people with disabilities reflecting discrepancies similar to those above (King et al. 2013).

Removing Restrictions/Differences to Participation

Removing restrictions to participation is an important goal of the CRPD as well as of Swedish disability policy. In 2017, the Swedish Parliament decided upon new national goals within disability policy. The overall goal is to reach equality in living conditions and equal opportunities for participation in society (including making choices and access) for people with disabilities (Westerberg in press).

Accessibility and Individual Support

From a political perspective, restrictions of participation are mainly of two (related) types; deficient accessibility in environments and lack of provision of support to compensate for individual impairments. With improved accessibility, the frequency of impairments impacting on participation is reduced. Improved accessibility may decrease need for individual support; but conversely may also increase it. For example, if cultural or sport arenas are made more accessible, the need for some people with disabilities to obtain personal assistance to get there, and be involved while there, may increase. It should be underscored that accessibility is not limited to physical accessibility, including also, for example, accessibility to media (e.g. use of symbols for communication).

Children's Right to Participation

Children are always more or less dependent upon their parents. However, if they have the capacity to have opinions of their own, according to the UN Convention on the Rights of the Child (CRoC; UN 1989), they shall be secured the right to freely express their opinions on all issues affecting them, and those opinions shall be valued in relation to their age and maturity. In CRoC, as well as in the CRPD, it is emphasised that this is also valid for children with disabilities.

Levels of participation of children can be described on a scale from 1 to 5 (Shier et al. 2014):

1. Children are listened to.
2. Children get support to express their opinions and views.
3. Children's opinions and views are taken into consideration.
4. Children are involved in the processes of decision making.
5. Children share the influence and responsibility for decision making.

To live up to the CRoC's requirement for participation, actions to support levels 1 to 3 are required, which means that children's opinions and views are at least taken into consideration.

In Swedish studies mapping children's participation and restrictions of participation children have been asked for example (Socialstyrelsen 2017, pp. 53–55):

- how often they participate in various activities;
- how important the various activities are for them;
- if they can carry out the activities by themselves or need support from others;
- if they want support to be able to execute the activities.

Respondents have claimed that many activities were important for them, but infrequently carried out, like getting in touch with new friends, going on holidays, washing their own clothes, participating in sport activities, going to the cinema, visiting grandparents, playing with others or going to restaurants/cafés. Thus, while having access to a range of important activities, participation was less frequent.

Participation in School

School is an arena of particular interest for the participation of children. Szönyi and Söderqvist Dunkers (2012) outlined a model for analysing participation illustrating six aspects of it applied on three different cultural elements prevailing in school: education, caring and friendships. In Table 8.1 we expand on this model to consider the roles and functions across participation constructs in the school environment. Good accessibility can be regarded as a key factor for all other aspects of participation.

Belonging and acting together concern the interplay with peers: an individual needs to feel affiliated to the group, be able to participate in group activities on the same basis as others, and be respected by his/her class mates. Engagement and autonomy relate to self-experienced participation and prospects for influence

Table 8.1   Cultures of education for special needs in Sweden and participation related constructs

Aspects of participation	Cultures of participation		
	Education	Caring	Friendship
Accessibility	Overcoming physical, sensory and learning barriers	Attitudes	Opportunities
Belonging	Including	Enabling	Relating
Acting together	Learning	Supporting	Doing
Recognition	Acknowledgement	Respect	Equality
Engagement	Experience	Involvement	Interacting
Autonomy	Self-determination	Inter-dependence	Influence

and self-determination. These reflect the degree of involvement, not only attendance, in line with self-determination theory's ideas of relatedness, competence and autonomy (see Chapter 2).

School is an important arena requiring a balance between accessibility of the environment and individual support. Problems in school can be attributed to the children or to the school environment. Historically in Sweden, the problem has been placed 'inside the children' in line with the more traditional medical model perspective (Hjörne 2016). Problems have often, within a culture of diagnostics, been explained by a diagnosis, such as attention-deficit–hyperactivity disorder, autism spectrum disorders or post-traumatic stress disorder, with these children often placed in special educational groups or resource schools. While justification for specialist provision can never be excluded as a possibility in certain circumstances, there is risk that the consequence will be less participation. Developmental work carried out in schools in Sweden has tried to turn the perspective around, in line with the ICF biopsychosocial model; placing the onus of solving problems on the school environment and not the individual. The experience shows more pupils in regular classes, which is in accordance with the political intentions expressed in the School Law (Hjörne 2016).

Participation in Working Life

To have a job contributes to economic independence, and also to structure life and provide a social network. The political goal is that as many persons with disabilities as possible have a job in the regular labour market. Through the Law on Discrimination (and other laws) a certain pressure is put on employers to accommodate people with disabilities. The Swedish Public Employment Service may pay wage subsidies for persons, who, because of a disability, are less productive. Those who cannot find a job in the regular market can be provided a form of social employment, organised by municipalities (or private firms on behalf of municipalities).

> *Participation in working life is a particularly important aspect of participation in social life.*

Research on careers for young people with reduced mobility showed that choices of education and profession are affected by many circumstances, such as accessibility of the universities, albeit with risk of over-protection by surrounding world of adults (Söderberg 2014). Adults with a low belief in a young person's capability, may not encourage expectations and may accept less ambitious goals. Another problem might be that adults, including teachers, assistants or employers, may give more support than needed because of low beliefs in the young person's capabilities, resulting perhaps in 'learned helplessness' and/or leading to more limited participation.

PARTICIPATION – INFLUENCE OF ATTITUDES AND PERCEPTIONS

Children with disabilities are protected by the CRoC, and CRPD. In the previous section we considered how treaties and legislation coming from these treaties may influence practice and support participation of children and young people with disabilities, using Sweden as a case example. A relatively recent review of public policy and health interventions, showed that most of these conceptualised disability, and relative cost to the general public, in relation to individual dependency and 'deservingness' (Berghs et al. 2016, p. 92).

Promoting equal physical access for opportunities is possibly easier than shifting attitudes to reframe 'disability'. Even subtly expressed negative attitudes may contribute to parental dis-beliefs, less hope and low expectations that may impact upon opportunities conceived of, and or made available for their child. Encounters with other families, including parents of non-disabled children and members of the community as well as positive behaviours of professionals (health, education and public service) may all go to reinforce the beliefs that shape expectation and give rise to experience [see the Disability Matters programme (Brokenbrow et al. 2016) and Chapter 7]. A positive, empowering attitude from professionals, especially during early encounters with families, has been shown to be a vital component contributing to equality of access and also to supporting long-lasting belief systems of parents (Brokenbrow et al. 2016).

A systematic review of non-disabled children's contact with people with disabilities shows a general, if not universal, association between greater exposure and reporting of more positive attitudes towards disability (MacMillan et al. 2014). Ensuring these encounters contribute to positive interactions to build respect and inter-dependency is more difficult to enshrine in policy. The positive imagery projected by the photographer Rick Guidotti of individuals with genetic, physical, intellectual or other conditions may help shift societal attitudes towards difference (see https://positiveexposure.org/).

Lessons learned from Nicaragua highlight the importance of respect and belief in co-production, when defining objectives and priorities, as preconditions to enable children to influence policy (Shier et al. 2014, pp. 7–8). Including children and young people with disabilities in decisions that will have a life-long impact on their opportunities is vital and is enshrined in the quote: 'Nothing about us without us' (Loring 2016).

PARTICIPATION – SOCIO-POLITICAL CHALLENGES

Access to equal opportunities for participation (with freedom of choice), is an overall goal for the Swedish policy for persons with disabilities. By the 1990s, it was noticed that general principles are not enough to reach the goal of accessibility. In 2000, the Swedish Parliament decided on a plan of action with more tangible goals for various social areas and a clearer responsibility for different public agencies to reach them. This first plan was adapted for 2001–2010, followed by a second plan for 2011–2016. An evaluation in 2016 showed progress, but only 40% of goals set in 2011 were achieved. In 2015 more stringent rules were introduced in the Swedish Law on Discrimination. Insufficient accessibility from that date is regarded as discrimination if a person with a disability in any environment is disadvantaged compared to a person without disability.

However, even in the most accessible environment, one cannot eliminate the consequences of all impairments and compensatory measures are required. In Sweden, individual support has developed gradually. One of the measures of LSS (promulgated by the Swedish Parliament in 1993) provides for personal assistance. Personal assistants are at the disposal of the beneficiary who can decide on activities that he/she will carry out. Even though most of the assisted hours are spent on activities such as personal hygiene, eating and dressing/undressing, the assistance is also available for participation in social activities.

Co- and self-determination are important when designing individual packages of support; a particular challenge arises when the support is provided for those with limited autonomy where decisions are based on other people's judgements and interpretations of their wishes. When the beneficiaries are children it is usually up to parents or guardians to make these assessments. This raises legal issues as well as other challenges in identifying solutions in the best interest of the child.

There are further challenges in defining (understanding) mental capacity and addressing 'advocacy'. There is a balance between advocating individual choice and decision making for children and providing support for their choices, while not exposing them to harm. While the CRoC stipulates the rights of children to freely express their opinions on all issues affecting them and have their opinions valued, the appropriate attitudes of those listening, are more difficult to enshrine in legislation.

Challenges for Inclusion – Beyond Sweden

Inclusive education is similarly beset with problems of 'equal participation'. In many Western societies, children with disabilities are *integrated* into regular education classes with provision of an untrained teacher aide (learning support assistant). Ostensibly to enable access to the curriculum and school activities, these individuals may equally hinder true participation (Rutherford 2012). Providing just the right balance of support without singling out a student as different, or getting in the way of friendships, while allowing 'risk taking' and independent problem solving, requires considerable skill in school environments. A meta-analysis of inclusive physical education, showed that some aides/physical education teachers removed students with disabilities from their peers to complete one-on-one instruction in the belief that this would encourage 'participation and a positive experience for all students' (Pocock and Miyahara 2018, p. 761). Obtaining the balance between inclusion in 'essential activities' (e.g. physical fitness exercises) and participation in physical education, is not easy to implement in practice. Provision of personal or teaching assistants, whether at school, home or community, may facilitate access to particular environments and opportunities. However, this provision may have unintended effects; limiting aspirations and contributing to an imbalanced dependency or inadvertent segregation. Implementing policies to provide assistance and access to curricula may inadvertently isolate or create barriers to some peer activities and friendship opportunities.

In the United States the perception of inclusion of people with disabilities is often considered through the lens of legislation for people with disabilities, notably the Americans with Disabilities Act (ADA) of 1990 and the Individuals with Disabilities Education Act (IDEA) of 1975. Both legislations are exceptional models for creating an inclusive society. Indeed, the CRPD is an international treaty modelled after the ADA; designed to promote international legislation and policies that embrace the rights and dignity of all people with disabilities. But despite these notable disability rights laws, the experience of raising a child in the United States can be fraught with ongoing struggles to ensure participation and inclusion in local communities and beyond, as evidenced in the vignette 'Legislation is Not Enough'.

LINK TO VIGNETTE 8.1
'Legislation is Not Enough', p. 93.

What is the disconnect in the United States between these legislative models of inclusion and disability rights and the actual experience of people with disabilities and their families? One of the biggest issues is that there is no regular enforcement mechanism for most disability rights legislation. This means that individuals with disabilities and their family members must advocate for adherence to these principles by bringing forth civil rights violations themselves. This is done either by directly addressing the appropriate leadership, by filing complaints with the Department of Justice, or by filing lawsuits against entities that refuse to comply. This kind of assertive action requires courage, energy and knowledge of existing laws and financial resources, along with being able to afford the time required to undertake these actions. Issues surrounding physical access and inclusion can happen so frequently within the individual's own community and when they attempt to travel, that advocacy for one family member could be a full-time job. Additionally, taking action against a local business or government agency can lead to further isolation and stigma in one's own community – the very thing the individual or family is fighting against. But, unless a lawsuit threat is in the forefront of the city planner's, architect's, business owner's or landlord's mind, or unless these individuals are personally motivated to create inclusive spaces and programming, physical access and inclusion may be sacrificed in the name of economics or for the sake of simplifying the programme execution.

Challenges Ahead

Our chapter has focused on describing societal influences on policies and impact on individuals with disabilities in resource rich countries like Sweden and the United States. These are echoed to some extent by policies and practice in other 'Western' cultures. Within these contexts, it is evident that while legislation is behind policies to support full integration and inclusion of individuals with disabilities within society, a number of challenges in translating policy to everyday practice exist. These challenges in low-resource countries, or those with even less emancipated views of disability, may be much greater. If financial incentives are required to instigate action, let alone sustain it, in resource rich countries, how can policies for inclusion and participation be facilitated in areas where basic health and social care are extremely limited and the rights to 'be' and live free from persecution are more pressing? However, at another level, provision of personal assistance (and other personnel-intensive services) may be more affordable options in low-middle income countries where wage costs are lower.

LINK TO VIGNETTE 4.1
'I Will Not Kill My Child'.
p. 46.

Similarly, as we map progress of young people with neurodisabilities into adulthood to ensure opportunities for employment, how can we support participation in productive or valued activities where no 'social employment' support is available?

These examples reflect Western models of ability (health) and disability in which social welfare may be provided by the 'State' and supported through legislation and policies. However, other cultures may not have such divergent views of 'ability' and 'disability'. This is illustrated in the vignette of an Aboriginal child, which describes a more seamless integration of individuals of all 'abilities' included in Aboriginal society, where participation is seen as taking on roles that match your capacity – without reference to 'disability'. Western cultures of disability and social care, 'caring for', may not necessarily equate to 'enabling' and or providing (safe) opportunities for risk taking.

LINK TO VIGNETTE 8.2
'Starting School', p. 95.

CONCLUDING THOUGHTS

Legislative policies may go some way towards supporting attendance in life situations, but it is more challenging to use legislation to support the experiences of 'being involved while being there' because involvement is influenced by multiple factors, including attitudinal. Many organisations may claim they support and even implement a social model yet translation to practice is less evident than the rhetoric, even in societies with more progressive legislation. Professionals in health and education arenas in particular, may find it more rewarding to help an individual (a medical model approach) rather than spend time changing the system (a social model approach). Designing policies that enable equal opportunities and allow for individual choices for participation requires creativity as well as financing. Shifting (some) societal attitudes underpinning legislation is more difficult. It is essential to include individuals with disability and their families and advocates in public discourse and debate and involving them in policy making and research (see Chapter 10) is a necessary step in the right direction.

SUMMARY OF KEY IDEAS

- The way societies operate and approach people with disabilities emerges through a very complex and diverse set of systems and people interacting together in uncountable combinations.
- Legislation may play an important role in providing for physical and financial support to promote participation; but on its own may not be enough for implementation of the 'spirit' of the law.
- Inclusive policy design requires creativity and financing, shifting (some) societal attitudes behind legislation is a greater challenge.

REFERENCES

Abrams T (2016) *Heidegger and the Politics of Disablement.* Toronto: Palgrave Macmillan.

Berghs MJ, Atkin KM, Graham HM, Hatton C, Thomas C (2016) Implications for public health research of models and theories of disability: a scoping study and evidence synthesis. *Pub Health Res* **4**: 1–166.

Brokenbrow L, Horridge K, Stair H (2016) *Disability Matters in Britain 2016: Enablers and Challenges to Inclusion for Disabled Children, Young People and Their Families.* London: Royal College of Paediatrics and Child Health.

Green D (2015) HOPE: Expectations for therapy and relationship to confidence and competence in intervention outcomes for children with unilateral cerebral palsy. Paper presented at Beit Issie Shapiro International Conference on Disabilities Unity and Diversity in Action. Tel Aviv Israel.

Hjörne E (2016) The narrative of special education in Sweden: History and trends in policy and practice. *Discourse: Studies in the Cultural Politics of Education* **37**(4): 540–552.

Imms C, Adair B, Keen D, Ullenhag A, Rosenbaum P, Granlund M (2016) "Participation": a systematic review of language, definitions, and constructs used in intervention research with children with disabilities. *Dev Med Child Neurol* **58**: 29–38.

Jahnsen R, Hollung SJ, Elkjær S et al. (2017) "I only have cerebral palsy now and then" – a study on children and youth with an "invisible" disability. Poster. Unpublished Conference Proceedings, *29th European Academy of Childhood Disability Conference* 17–20 May, Amsterdam.

King G, Imms C, Palisano R et al. (2013) Geographical patterns in the recreation and leisure participation of children and youth with cerebral palsy: a CAPE international collaborative network study. *Dev Neurorehabil* **16**: 196–206.

Loring A (2016) Nothing about us without us. *Dev Med Child Neurol* **58**: 787–787.

MacMillan M, Tarrant M, Abraham C, Morris C (2014) The association between children's contact with people with disabilities and their attitudes towards disability: a systematic review. *Dev Med Child Neurol* **56**: 529–546.

Pocock T, Miyahara M (2018) Inclusion of students with disability in physical education: a qualitative meta-analysis. *Int J Incl Educ* **22**: 751–766.

Rutherford G (2012) In, out or somewhere in between? Disabled students' and teacher aides' experiences of school. *Int J Incl Edu* **16**(8): 757–774.

Shakespeare T (2013) *Disability Rights and Wrongs Revisited.* London: Routledge.

Shier H, Méndez MH, Centeno M, Arróliga I, González M (2014) How children and young people influence policymakers: lessons from Nicaragua. *Child Soc* **28**: 1–14.

Socialstyrelsen (The National Board of Health and Welfare) (2017) Vägar till ökad delaktighet Kunskapsstöd för socialtjänsten om arbete med stöd och service enligt LSS [Ways to increased participation. Knowledge support for social services on work with support and service according to LSS]. Stockholml Socialstyrelsen.

Szönyi K, Söderqvist Dunkers T (Eds) (2012) *Där man söker får man svar.* Delaktighet i teorin och praktik för elever med funktionsnedsättning [Where you search you find answers. Participation in theory and practice for pupils with disabilities]. Stockholm: Specialpedagogiska skolmyndigheten (SPSM) (The National Agency for Special Needs Education and Schools).

Söderberg E (2014) *Grynnor och farleder i karriärvalsprocessen.* Unga med rörelsehinder och deras handlingsutrymme [Reefs and Fairways in the Career-Selection Process. Young adults with mobility impairments and margins for manoeuvres]. PhD thesis, Stockholm University. ISBN: 9789176490327.

Stevens CS (2013) *Disability in Japan.* London: Routledge.

Toro-Martínez E (2015) [The social model of disability in Argentina: paradigm of decision-making support and safeguards in the new Argentine Civil Code]. *Vertex* **26**: 284–291.

UN General Assembly (1989) Convention on the Rights of the Child. *United Nations. Treaty Ser* **1577**: 3.

UN General Assembly (2006) *Convention on the Rights of Persons with Disabilities (A/61/106).* Paris: UN General Assembly.

Westerberg B (in press) *Funktionshinder och samhällsstöd* [Disabilities and Socal Support]. In: Kilman L, Andin J, Hua H, Rönnberg J (Eds) *Leva som andra. Bio-psyko-sociala perspektiv på funktionsnedsättning och funktionshinder (To live as others. Bio-psycho-social perspectives on impairment and disability).* Lund: Studentlitteratur.

WHO (2001) *International Classification of Functioning, Disability and Health: Short Version.* Geneva: World Health Organization.

In this vignette, a mother shares a common experience of difficulty gaining access. She talks about the struggle to ensure that her child can attend varied community settings despite legislation and community rhetoric that should enable both attendance and involvement. As you read this account, consider how legislation and policies are applied from a practical perspective – what actions and behaviours need to be part of day-to-day practice to enable access and involvement?

Legislation is Not Enough (USA)

Michele Shusterman

When my daughter was 2.5 years old we moved to a new city in the southeastern United States. Shortly thereafter, I approached a popular recreation centre about having our daughter (who has cerebral palsy and epilepsy) participate in their children's summer programme of story time and crafts. I was very excited since it would give her a chance to socialise with her peers. On her application I candidly described the extra support she needed and stated that we would provide the staff or other resources necessary for her to participate safely and comfortably. I asked for the programme director to contact me to discuss her accommodations further. After 6 weeks of having my follow-up calls ignored, their central office finally told me that they did want to have my daughter attend their camp. I was sad, angry and shocked, particularly because this was a place that seemed to pride themselves on the principles of inclusion. Unfortunately, their inclusivity didn't include my child.

I arranged a meeting between the Executive Director, several of the organisation's board members and myself. I will never forget when the Executive Director turned to me during the meeting and said, 'If I welcome your daughter to our camp then I cannot uphold the religious mission of our organisation which includes physical activity'. Wow, I thought to myself, did this man really just say this out loud and did he hear himself? He also went on to defend his organisation by pointing out their programming for kids with intellectual disabilities, thereby illustrating their commitment to inclusion. I told him that although those programmes were important, organisations cannot selectively exclude people solely on the basis of the kind of disability they have. What's more, I was asking for my daughter to be included in story time and crafts which was clearly not incompatible with his mission concerns. I did my best during this meeting to educate the individuals about how they mishandled this situation from both a values perspective and from a civil rights standpoint.

Determining whether a programme is appropriate for a particular child should be a thoughtful process. These discussions should begin by searching for solutions that meet that child's particular needs, rather than immediately turning them away. After two meetings and more phone calls, they asked for me to give them another chance. I was satisfied that my concerns were taken seriously and that there would be systematic changes in how this centre approached families with children who have disabilities, but I never wanted to send my daughter to one of their programmes. Although I succeeded in changing the way this group of leaders thought about their obligations to uphold my daughter's civil rights, I was not sure they could provide a welcoming and warm environment for her.

All of our experiences in fighting for our daughter to have physical access to a building or a bathroom, or to be thoughtfully included in a programme, go well beyond legislation – the barriers are rooted in the values and perspectives of the people in society. If people are motivated to include my child in their programme, we can overcome most obstacles and the practical details often come together easily. But, most of the time people have not been very motivated to include her. They are afraid of her needs and they often over-analyse how to make it work. Other people cite economic barriers that they perceive as insurmountable. And, sometimes, people just skip past their excuses and say that they do not want to include children who are different.

Even though the United States has some of the best disability rights laws in the world, inclusion doesn't happen unless people fundamentally believe in its importance. If only the adults in charge would take their cues from children. Without interference from adults, my daughter's peers and older children often naturally include her in their interactions and play, offering the most beautiful and graceful examples of how it can and should be done. I believe because children often act instinctively from their hearts, they make room for more creative solutions to emerge.

Transition to school opens opportunities across multiple contexts in which children from varied backgrounds and educators may come together to create learning spaces, establish relationships and build skills. School is mandated in Australia; however for Indigenous peoples, perceptions of accessibility and evidence of accommodations are influenced by an overt welcome (e.g. art work). The visible presence of cultural connections can be critical to developing a sense of safety and acceptance. As you read the following vignette, consider the people, place, objects, activities and time needed to support Brandon's involvement. In this vignette, cultural understandings of disability are also described in which participation in Indigenous communities is seen as taking on roles that match your capacity.

Starting School (Australia)

Loretta Sheppard and Nicole Cassar

Brandon is a 5-year-old Aboriginal boy living in metropolitan Melbourne with his maternal grandmother. He has just started school but the shift from his preschool setting to primary school is presenting some challenges. For the last 2 years, Brandon attended a preschool local to his home where there was a strong Aboriginal presence with several Aboriginal families providing a network of support and sense of community which was both welcoming and culturally familiar. Since starting school, Brandon and his grandmother are finding they are cut off from this cultural support. The school where most of Brandon's friends went to is too far for Brandon and his grandmother to access by taxi, and Brandon's grandmother's health is such that she is unable to use public transport.

At the school Brandon is attending he is increasingly sitting alone in class and playing by himself in the playground. He tells his grandmother the other kids tease him and won't let him play with them and is indicating he does not feel safe at school. Four weeks into the school year, Brandon is reluctant to get ready each morning and is refusing to participate in class activities when at school.

Brandon has a diagnosis of autism and there are multiple factors impacting his participation at school. He is currently *attending*, but he is not yet *involved* at school, and whilst it might be usual for children with autism to take longer to settle in a new setting than their peers, there are cultural perspectives to consider too. For example, disability is not as heavily accentuated in many Australian Aboriginal cultures – disability is part of life and people with disability are included naturally in community, taking on roles that match their capability. 'No one is expected to "do everything"; everyone does what they are capable of' and contributes in their own way to the community. This contrasts with a view of disability commonly found in Western cultures where disability might be seen as belonging with the individual and interventions focus on changing or improving the individual rather than matching abilities to roles and activities, or altering the environment.

It is important for all children to feel safe at school, but this need may be heightened for Aboriginal children and their families because of the impact of past history and events. Brandon's grandmother was part of the Stolen Generations so was taken from her family at a young age; she is worried that Brandon may be taken from her by welfare and anxious that he fits into school and behaves well. She does not want to speak to the teachers at the school about Brandon's experiences in the playground and classroom in case this reflects on her parenting. She feels isolated from the school community because there are no visible signs of inclusiveness of Aboriginal people and no indicators of who she could approach to get cultural support; yet this support and sense of belonging to community is integral to her being able to participate in Brandon's education. She is missing the network she had at Brandon's preschool, yet cannot afford the transport needed to get to the school where his preschool friends are because of the impact of generational disadvantage.

Sustained school attendance and involvement are impacted negatively for many Indigenous Australian students but Brandon's grandmother is extraordinarily resilient and committed to ensuring he can attend school despite poor health, financial disadvantage, and in full knowledge that the education her grandson will receive is unlikely to affirm his cultural identity. Facilitating Brandon's participation at school requires attention to things that will support the involvement of his grandmother too. Involvement at school will require adjustments to the environment to acknowledge it may appear strange and unwelcoming without visible Aboriginal signs and symbols, as well as active linking with other Aboriginal families to garner a sense of belonging.

Therapy as a Life Situation

Christine Imms

The family of participation related constructs (fPRC) framework is neutral about the activity or setting in which participation is considered (Imms et al. 2017). Life situations of children are, however, commonly described and investigated within three key environments: home, preschool or school, and community. In this chapter, consideration is given to therapy as a life situation.

If therapy is a life situation in which children and families (along with us, as health professionals) participate, then we need to consider carefully aspects of attendance and involvement including barriers and facilitators of both aspects. Therapy is defined here as situations or events that comprise therapeutic interventions. A therapeutic intervention is defined variously as the 'act of intervening, interfering or interceding with the intent of modifying the outcome'; or an 'effort made by individuals or groups to improve wellbeing'; or 'medicine or surgery to treat or cure' a condition (Dictionary.com 2018). In childhood onset neurodisability, therapeutic interventions might involve occupational therapy, physiotherapy, speech therapy, equipment prescription and or orthopaedic surgery among many others. In this chapter, the focus is on therapy from the perspective of participation; focusing on attendance and involvement in therapeutic interventions as a mechanism for continuing to improve both *what* therapy is provided and *how* therapy is delivered, with the goal of enhancing the quality of therapeutic transactions and outcomes.

ATTENDING THERAPY

When we think about participation attendance we seek to understand and optimise the frequency, time spent, or diversity of activities in which people take part (see Chapter 1). Although we often measure attendance in activities as discrete items, we are really interested in understanding and optimising the patterns of attendance in home, school and community across the life course. Most participation research to date has focused on showing changes in 'how much' attendance has occurred following an intervention (Adair et al. 2015; Reedman et al. 2017). It is more complex, but arguably more important, to understand what a desirable pattern of attendance might be.

> *If therapy is a life situation, we need to ask: how much is enough, and what is a desirable pattern of attendance across the lifespan?*

'How much is enough?' is a common therapeutic question, but to date, research has not directly addressed this question about participation-focused interventions. Research that addresses the question of what might constitute a desirable pattern of attendance in therapy across the life course for those with childhood onset neurodisability has not to date been undertaken. What should this research look like, and for what outcomes? If we think about all therapeutic interventions that a child and family may experience as a gestalt, our goal will surely be wellness, wellbeing, participation and quality of life. How do we get there? How do we ensure that provision is sufficient but is not too much? Too much attendance may result in participation in therapy as a way of life, rather than a means to live your life.

In therapy, attendance has often been equated with a client and/or family's response to following regimes and adhering to recommendations or advice with the goal of achieving a therapeutic dose or effect (Jansen et al. 2003). Unfortunately these requirements can be met with the parent's lament 'I don't want to be my child's therapist' and for some parents increased stress and reduced wellbeing (Jansen et al. 2003). Collaborative team approaches (Nijhuis et al. 2007) and family centred care principles (King et al. 2004) aim to address these issues, by coordinating health professional efforts and placing the child and family at the centre. Assessments such as the Measures of Processes of Care (Cunningham and Rosenbaum 2014) provide insight for organisations and therapists about how well they are doing in this regard. In addition, new knowledge about effective methods to train skills and enhance early development has helped to reduce traditional attendance in never-ending weekly therapy, as may have been experienced some decades ago.

INVOLVEMENT IN THERAPY

One element of the therapeutic 'package' that may influence the amount of attendance needed, is the extent to which children and families are involved while attending. Involvement in the fPRC is defined as the experience while attending which might include engagement, persistence, affect and perhaps social connection (Imms et al. 2017). In healthcare literature the term 'engagement' in therapy is used more commonly than 'involvement'. Engagement in healthcare has been defined as a 'co-constructed process and state. It incorporates a process of gradually connecting with each other and/or a therapeutic programme, which enables the individual to become an active, committed and invested collaborator in healthcare' (Bright et al. 2015, p. 650).

Engaging in Therapy

Engagement in therapy has been described as a 'patient state', defined as the 'internal experience expressed by observable behaviours' (Bright et al. 2015, p. 649). This state of 'engaging in' has been further described as 'being with what you are doing … participating … beyond talk', contributing, persisting, being deliberate, intentional and effortful (Bright et al. 2015, p. 650). Engaging in therapy can, therefore, be seen as a multifaceted state of affective, behavioural and cognitive investment in therapy (D'Arrigo et al. 2017). Affective investment might be observed in clients' emotional connection, positive affect, excitement, enthusiasm joy, interest, energy or alertness. Behavioural engagement might be recognised by the asking of questions, sharing thoughts, positive body language and uptake of recommendations, and cognitive engagement might be visible in the effort, readiness for change and perceived need for intervention by the client (D'Arrigo et al. 2017).

When these very positive attributes of engagement in therapy are present, clients (children, families and others) are primed and ready to respond and use clinician knowledge to inform their goals and actions. When conditions are not right, and engagement is low, there may be reduced effects of intervention, and/or increased time (attendance) required to reach desired therapy goals, or disengagement, lack of attendance or abandonment of therapy.

Engagement with Therapy

While 'engaging in' describes a client's state, *'engagement with* therapy' is defined as a process of connection between the client and practitioner or service. 'Engagement with' is relational, involving collaboration,

Table 9.1 Conditions for engagement	
Therapist	**Client**
• Persistence	• Persistence
• Caring attitude	• Positive stance to intervention
• Active listening	• Collaborative stance
• Client-centred approach	• Appointment keeping
• Making information and activities meaningful	• Perceived usefulness of intervention
• Understanding the client's perspective	• Being open to communication
• Co-established priorities	• Initiation of activity
• Ability to create a climate of engagement	• Respect and appreciation
• Empathy	• Commitment
• Trust	• Effort
	• Willingness
	• Trust

Adapted from Bright et al. (2015)

a client-centred approach to care and co-established priorities (see Table 9.1). D'Arrigo et al. (2017) described supporting 'engagement with' by applying self-determination theory, whereby autonomy can be supported through collaborative goal setting and providing opportunities for choice; relatedness by attending to the quality of the therapeutic relationship and building rapport; and competence by the careful observation and noting of changes, providing opportunity for challenge and mastery through therapy.

When engagement with and in therapy are high, therapists and children and families together create transactional contexts in which learning and other positive client outcomes are facilitated through the availability of opportunities, fostering of positive experiences and provision of supports and resources for success (King et al. 2016, 2018). When conditions for engagement are not met, then children and families and clinicians may become disconnected from (or never connect to) the therapeutic alliance, parents may act to protect their child from experiences viewed as harmful to their child's identity, children and families may become passive recipients of, rather than collaborators in the rehabilitation or healthcare encounter (O'Connor et al. 2019). Although some medical procedures can be provided to an individual as a passive recipient, there are few therapeutic interventions in which the quality and effectiveness will not be impacted by the level of engagement of the child and family.

Strategies to Support Engagement in Therapy

Strategies to support engagement in/with therapy are well known from literature related to family centred practices and therapeutic relationships (King and Ziviani 2015; Carman et al. 2013). It is no secret that the therapeutic alliance is a critical element of any successful therapeutic outcome. Recent research investigating how youth with physical disabilities can be supported to engage in therapy supports prior findings, but also helps us see the connection between ideas of *engagement in* as an affective, cognitive and behavioural state (Smart et al. 2017).

Smart et al. (2017) undertook a series of repeated semi-structured interviews with youth with physical disabilities to explore the strategies used to support therapeutic engagement. Affective strategies included building a relationship based on familiarity and reciprocity, and guiding the programme using the youths' preferences and strengths. These strategies can be visualised within the transactional exchanges between context (which includes the therapist) and individual as described in the fPRC (Imms et al. 2017). Strategies to support behavioural engagement included: ensuring youth had access to resources, providing youth with multiple opportunities to make decisions and enabling them to showcase their capabilities. Cognitive strategies were described as assisting youth to envisage meaningful change, using youths' learning styles and promoting youths' awareness of their goal progress (Smart et al. 2017). These cognitive strategies can be seen to support the interpretation of the experiences in therapy of the youth as they progress from setting goals to achieving them.

Barriers to either attendance or involvement in therapy may occur for many reasons. These may include socio-economic factors (e.g. financial and/or geographic access; see Chapter 21), attitudes and beliefs in general or in relation to particular therapeutic approaches, or unsatisfactory transactions among the child, family and therapist (Bright et al. 2015). Understanding potential barriers will be important to optimise therapeutic time and experience.

LINK TO VIGNETTE 9.1
'Therapy Means Work, Not Play', p. 103.

Where and How Should Therapy Happen?

In child development research and practice we have traditionally focused on providing interventions with the aim of seeing children develop increasingly complex behaviours – understood to be synonymous with developing activity competence (fPRC) – typically seen as following a normative process. But if we focus on children meeting developmental norms, we risk losing sight of diversity and disenfranchise those whose bodies work differently or whose level of interdependence is greater than others. In addition, if we focus on development of skills or activity competences out of context, then we risk missing the idea that learning for life is done by living your life and find ourselves focusing on the constructs (blobs/shapes) in the fPRC instead of the transactions (the arrows). The fPRC aims to bring into focus the transactions at play in varying activity settings or life situations (Imms et al. 2017). Because transactions involve person-in-context, they bring into focus both 'where' therapy occurs and 'how' it occurs.

Learning for life is done by living your life.

One example of focusing on transactions comes from a study (Heesh 2018) of the completion of daily living routines when children with cerebral palsy are classified at level IV or V of the Gross Motor Function Classification System (Palisano et al. 2008). In Heesh (2018), parent–child dyads collected a video record of the completion of a daily routine that was important to them but difficult to achieve – such as getting dressed, or mealtime. The video was subsequently watched by the parent, child and therapist-researcher and an interview conducted to elicit how the child–parent dyad worked together to complete these routines. Both video and interview were collected in the child's usual setting: at home. What emerged from these thoughtful interviews and the subsequent analyses was a description of the complex but successful negotiation that occurs daily to achieve the routines. How routines were achieved varied across days and times, but the routines were achieved. The children required the assistance of the parent/carer to achieve the routine, and would always do so, but they also contributed to the completion of the task in various ways. This process of careful observation of the transactions among the child, parent, and other elements of the real-world context (such as equipment, hallway, rooms and beds) allowed generation of knowledge about *when* and *how* child and parent engagement in learning could be supported. This study provides a window into the varied daily life transactions of these dyads: that is, involvement in the moment, day-after-day, that over time leads to both skill development and future participation.

If therapy is situated in real life contexts, like daily routines at home, or playing with your friends in the park, then engagement will be in other life situations, not 'therapy'. When therapy is situated in real life contexts, then therapy will be about seeking opportunity and experiences to support participation attendance and involvement, that is focused on naturally occurring transactions and supporting in-context experiences and capacity development in situ. The practitioner's roles will be as advocates, knowledge brokers, collaborators, facilitators, educators and coaches – not experts doing to.

CONCLUSION

Engagement should be given special consideration in therapeutic interventions. It will shape how the child and family and practitioner experience the intervention. If therapy is the life situation, participation attendance and involvement must be the means to other outcomes than continuing to come to therapy. If therapy is a special life situation, then maximising outcomes in the minimum time might be imperative.

The extent to which we can measure and understand what constitutes sufficient therapy attendance for any one child over the years is probably not known at this time. I would argue though, that this is important to understand, even though it is likely to be an evolving and shifting target as we discover and deliver more effective interventions, in hopefully shorter time periods.

If involvement is defined as engagement, persistence, affect and perhaps social connection, then current literature suggests that *engagement in therapy* can be supported as both as a process and a state, and the state of engagement includes persistence and affect (which can be further described as affective, cognitive, behavioural engagement) and that social connection is a critical component of the therapeutic relationship.

Transactional frameworks focus on shifting rehabilitation to 'real-world' contexts where participation and environment are in focus more than body function and activity (King et al. 2018). With this shift in focus comes a change to the outcomes of interest which will relate to enabling participation in day-to-day life over time. To achieve that shift requires a broader/deeper awareness of the lives of children and families and of the transactional processes of change over the life course. It might also require a complete re-conceptualisation of how we deliver health and community services.

SUMMARY OF KEY IDEAS

If therapy is a life situation in which children and families along with health professionals participate, then we need to consider carefully aspects of attendance and involvement.

- We need to know that the amount of therapy provided is sufficient but not too much: too much attendance may result in participation in therapy as a way of life, rather than a means to live your life.
- When engagement with and in therapy are high, therapists and children and families create transactional contexts in which learning and other positive client outcomes are facilitated.
- Because transactions involve person-in-context, they bring into focus both 'where' therapy occurs and 'how' it occurs – the actions and reactions of the practitioner are as much in focus as those of the client.

REFERENCES

Adair B, Ullenhag A, Keen D, Granlund M, Imms C (2015) The effect of interventions aimed at improving participation outcomes for children with disabilities: a systematic review. *Dev Med Child Neurol* **57**: 1093–1104.

Bright FA, Kayes NM, Worrall L, McPherson KM (2015) A conceptual review of engagement in healthcare and rehabilitation. *Disabil Rehabil* **37**: 643–654.

Carman KL, Dardess P, Maurer M et al. (2013) Patient and family engagement: a framework for understanding the elements and developing interventions and policies. *Health Aff (Millwood)* **32**: 223–231.

Cunningham BJ, Rosenbaum PL (2014) Measure of processes of care: a review of 20 years of research. *Dev Med Child Neurol* **56**: 445–452.

D'Arrigo R, Ziviani J, Poulsen AA, Copley J, King G (2017) Child and parent engagement in therapy: what is the key? *Aust Occup Ther J* **64**: 340–343.

Dictionary.com (2018) Therapeutic intervention. *Dictionary.com* [Online]. Available: www.dictionary.com [Accessed 7 December 2018].

Heesh R (2018) *Daily Living Transactions.* Master of Health Science Research (Occupational Therapy). Australian Catholic University.

Imms C, Granlund M, Wilson PH, Steenbergen B, Rosenbaum PL, Gordon AM (2017) Participation, both a means and an end: a conceptual analysis of processes and outcomes in childhood disability. *Dev Med Child Neurol* **59**: 16–25.

Jansen LM, Ketelaar M, Vermeer A (2003) Parental experience of participation in physical therapy for children with physical disabilities. *Dev Med Child Neurol* **45**: 58–69.

King GA, Ziviani J (2015) What does engagement look like? Goal-directed behaviour in therapy. In: Poulson AA, Ziviani J, Cuskelly M (Eds) *Goal Setting and Motivation in Therapy.* London: Jessica Kingsley Publishers.

King S, Teplicky R, King G, Rosenbaum P (2004) Family-centered service for children with cerebral palsy and their families: a review of the literature. *Semin Pediatr Neurol* **11**: 78–86.

King G, Kingsnorth S, McPherson A et al. (2016) Residential immersive life skills programs for youth with physical disabilities: A pilot study of program opportunities, intervention strategies, and youth experiences. *Res Dev Disabil* **55**: 242–255.

King G, Imms C, Stewart D, Freeman M, Nguyen T (2018) A transactional framework for pediatric rehabilitation: shifting the focus to situated contexts, transactional processes, and adaptive developmental outcomes. *Disabil Rehabil* **40**: 1829–1841.

Nijhuis BJ, Reinders-Messelink HA, de Blécourt AC et al. (2007) A review of salient elements defining team collaboration in paediatric rehabilitation. *Clin Rehabil* **21**: 195–211.

O'Connor B, Kerr C, Shields N, Adair B, Imms C (2019) Steering towards collaborative assessment: a qualitative study of parents' experiences of evidence-based assessment practices for their child with cerebral palsy. *Disabil Rehabil* **23**: 1–10.

Palisano RJ, Rosenbaum P, Bartlett D, Livingston MH (2008) Content validity of the expanded and revised gross motor function classification system. *Dev Med Child Neurol* **50**: 744–750.

Reedman S, Boyd RN, Sakzewski L (2017) The efficacy of interventions to increase physical activity participation of children with cerebral palsy: a systematic review and meta-analysis. *Dev Med Child Neurol* **59**: 1011–1018.

Smart E, Aulakh A, McDougall C, Rigby P, King G (2017) Optimizing engagement in goal pursuit with youth with physical disabilities attending life skills and transition programs: an exploratory study. *Disabil Rehabil* **39**: 2029–2038.

Marcel's story shows that shifting priorities for therapy can present challenging contexts for parents, children and therapists. Therapists in Romania who desire a focus on participation in play and self-care, may have difficulty harmonising this with traditional expectations of parents (and others) who are focused on academic skill development and settings where independence is required for attendance. As you read this vignette, consider how we can transition to focusing on participation in situations in which all of children's activities are viewed as opportunities for learning for life.

Therapy Means Work, Not Play (Romania)

Liana Nagy and Stefania Bibolar

Marcel is a 6-year-old boy, who presents with significant developmental delay and visual difficulties; diagnosed with agenesis of corpus callosum before birth. Marcel attends occupational therapy, physiotherapy, speech therapy, massage and hydrotherapy. At present, Marcel can stand for approximately 2 minutes with minimal support and can walk if held by one hand. He drinks from a cup and feeds himself pureed food using a teaspoon. Marcel matches geometrical shapes with some support although lacks consistency. He points to main body parts on another person and plays with toys for short periods before losing interest.

The focus within the paediatric therapy environment in Romania is often driven by parents' values. One of the most valued aspects for parents is the child's ability to do well in school. Doing well in school is related to reading, writing and completing classroom tasks at similar levels to typically developing children. The typically developing child is a point of reference for day-to-day participation and activity engagement. Because performing well in school activities comes first, the importance of dressing, washing, eating independently or playing with other children is commonly overlooked. There is often a lengthy debate between the therapist and the family to help the family see the importance of independence with self-care.

Play, in particular, is not valued. This might be why many therapeutic interventions lack playfulness: going to therapy is sometimes a chore for the child. Parenting in Romania doesn't involve the degree of children's choice we see in the western world, or much playfulness. Therapists are familiar with the attitude 'My child didn't come to therapy to play, but to learn'. This is a cultural perspective within Romania, and perhaps other eastern countries, where playfulness might be perceived an unnecessary feature of therapy. Although attitudes are changing, we have not yet caught up with all the evidence on play. With most of research published in English we might experience delays in encouraging participation in play for children with disabilities.

Marcel's family were keen for him to attend nursery school. Their application was rejected though, because Marcel was not independent with mobility and feeding. Marcel's main goals were established in agreement with the occupational therapist and physiotherapist; goals focused on improving lower limb and core muscle tone with the aim of improving self-care abilities. This focus on body function goals as opposed to activity performance and participation is common in Romania.

Marcel's family have been dissatisfied with the cumbersome access to health and social services and felt that it has delayed rehabilitation. Financial pressures are often a barrier for accessing therapy in Romania as not all therapy services are freely available. Marcel's family fund therapy from their own resources along with fundraising, to obtain the amount required for a year of therapy. Others who cannot do this, access fewer services. Cultural perspectives and parent self-funding of therapies may contribute to challenges in working towards a more participation-focused approach in therapy.

Involvement of Young People and Families in All Stages of Research: What, Why and How?

Marjolijn Ketelaar, Dirk-Wouter Smits, Karen van Meeteren, Martijn Klem and Mattijs Alsem

INTRODUCTION

If you want to go fast, go alone. If you want to go far, go together
– African proverb

We have illustrated this chapter with the journey that we, researchers, clinicians and parents, embarked upon in our quest for meaningful collaboration in research. It shows our struggles and pitfalls, the stretches where we could only progress because of our different backgrounds, and our discussions and expectations about our goal and direction.

START OF OUR JOURNEY

Our journey started a number of years ago when some of us, a group of scientists in the field of child-hood disabilities, aimed to develop research on the needs of families of children with disabilities, and on development of participation of young people with cerebral palsy.

In earlier projects our research group collaborated with patient organisations, but – to be honest – mainly focusing on the initial stage of funding, and on the last stages of a project. It was only when we had the scientific results, that we started to discuss ideas for knowledge translation with patient organisations and families. These discussions were inspiring and mostly resulted in products aiming to increase knowledge, such as factsheets and infographics. We all realised that building on each other's expertise from the beginning would greatly enrich our studies by combining research expertise with experience-based expertise. We all felt the potential value of meaningful collaboration in all stages and all aspects of research, and we decided to start our next journey together.

In our journey we learned from other examples; from colleagues, discussions, articles from around the world, but we also learned by 'just doing'. Travelling together through new, beautiful and sometimes challenging landscapes, careful listening to each other, and not being afraid to take unknown roads. Sometimes taking directions or shortcuts that turned out to be not the most fertile areas, sometimes taking parallel tracks that merged later, and sometimes discovering beautiful tracks we never thought would be possible.

In this chapter we discuss involvement of families and other 'end-users' in research, based on literature and our own experiences during our journey. 'End-user' in this chapter refers to patients, people/children with disabilities, and their carers, parents and families. We will use 'young people and families' most of the time, while referring to end-users broadly. We discuss various aspects of involvement of young people and families in research, including benefits and challenges. Roles and preferences for involvement in research as well as examples and suggestions for meaningful involvement in research will be presented. With this chapter we aim to inspire researchers, clinicians, patients and families, and to increase the effects of meaningful collaborations.

FROM FAMILY-CENTRED SERVICES TO FAMILY INVOLVEMENT IN RESEARCH

The family-centred approach to services of children with disabilities is widely accepted as *the* foundational approach to service delivery in paediatric healthcare (King and Chiarello 2014). The core of a family-centred approach contains some general principles: recognition of the family as central in a child's life, recognition of the family as expert, partnership between family and service providers, and the importance of supporting the family's role in decision making. Increasingly, the value of these principles is being acknowledged not only in healthcare, but also in research (Domecq et al. 2014). More and more questions are being asked, such as: To what extent are research questions grounded in knowledge of the priorities of children and families? Are interventions acceptable and feasible? What is the likelihood that findings will be meaningful to children and families in their daily lives? (Palisano 2016).

Overall there is growing consensus about the crucial role of end-user involvement in research, and initiatives and publications on this topic are increasing rapidly (Domecq et al. 2014). This shift is also illustrated by the focus of leading journals such as BMJ (Richards and Godlee 2014; Crowe and Giles 2016) and the establishment of new journals; for example, *Research Involvement and Engagement*.

Many arguments for end-user involvement come down to three key premises, summarised by Morris et al. (2011), and described more elaborately by van der Scheer et al. (2017). First, from a philosophical perspective, patients and families should be involved in deciding the research that concerns them and those in similar life circumstances. These arguments often refer to the slogan 'Nothing about us without us' (Chu et al. 2016). People have the right to participate in decisions that will (eventually) affect their lives (UN 2007). Second, from a quality perspective, active involvement concerns the contribution of experiential knowledge. Patients and families possess unique knowledge and specific experiences, have ideas about relevant research questions, ideas about research designs and research procedures that are acceptable to them, and provide another perspective on findings and their interpretation. Third, from a societal perspective, involving end-users is more frequently becoming mandatory when applying for government-sponsored funding streams. This is predicated on the fact that it is the end-user's taxes which are used to subsidise the research, and therefore they have a democratic right to influence what is supported.

YOUNG PEOPLE AND FAMILY INVOLVEMENT IN RESEARCH

There is no uniform terminology for end-user involvement and participation in research; sometimes also referred to as patient and public involvement (PPI). First, there is no uniformity in the use of the terms 'participation' or 'involvement'. In the Netherlands the active role of end-users in research is called 'participation', in North America it is called 'engagement', and in the United Kingdom 'involvement' is used to refer to active involvement in research projects and research organisations (Liabo et al. 2018). In this chapter we use the terminology of INVOLVE (see Box 10.2), one of the most influential organisations supporting active public involvement in research. INVOLVE defines public involvement in research as 'research being carried out "with" or "by" members of the public rather than "to", "about" or "for" them' (http://www.invo.org.uk/find-out-more/what-is-public-involvement-in-research-2/). When using the term 'public', INVOLVE means to include patients, potential patients, carers and people who use health and social care services, as well as people from organisations that represent people who use services.

INVOLVE uses the following terms to distinguish between different activities: involvement, engagement and participation. 'Involvement' refers to activities where end-users are actively involved in research projects and in research organisations. Examples include: involvement in identifying research priorities, as members of a project advisory or steering group, commenting and developing patient information leaflets or other research materials, undertaking interviews with research participants, and patients and/or carer researchers carrying out the research. 'Engagement' refers to activities where information and knowledge about research is provided and disseminated, particularly to end-users. 'Participation' refers to activities where people take part in a research study, for example completing a questionnaire or participating in a focus group as part of a research study, i.e. being a participant in a study.

In the family of Participation-Related Constructs (fPRC), participation has two essential components: 'attendance', defined as 'being there' and measured as frequency of attending, and/or the range or diversity of activities; and 'involvement', the experience of participation while attending. Involvement might include elements of engagement, motivation, persistence, social connection and level of affect (Imms et al. 2017). Although the terminology differs, in both the INVOLVE and the fPRC terminology the term 'involvement' refers to an active role, including elements such as motivation and affect, as distinguished from other, more passive concepts.

In this chapter we use 'end-user involvement' and 'PPI' to refer the active roles of young people and families in all aspects of research; including developing ideas, priority setting, designing studies, finding funding, carrying out the research, interpreting results and disseminating results (Fig. 10.1).

WHAT THE LITERATURE TELLS US

The impact, value and challenges of PPI, including family and young people involvement, in research has been systematically described and evaluated (e.g. Bailey et al. 2015; Camden et al. 2015; Shen et al. 2017). Reviews demonstrate that robust evidence for the impact of family and young people's involvement in research is lacking, with most findings about impact and challenges being descriptions of experiences. However, some general patterns can be found in this young field.

Benefits of Involving End-Users in Research

Reported benefits for the research itself include:

- prioritisation of research questions that are relevant and important to families and young people;
- more meaningful and culturally socio-economically appropriate research;

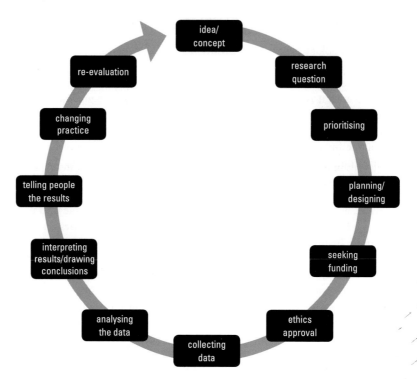

Figure 10.1   Stages of the research cycle; www.pencru.org. © PenCRU, used with permission.

- identification of issues and details that researchers may not be aware of, for example, focus on outcomes that matter for the individuals concerned;
- study protocols and interventions that are more acceptable and sustainable;
- more age-appropriate and accessible recruitment and advertising materials;
- greater credibility and interest in studies, among families and young people as well as professionals;
- positive contribution to data collection;
- enrichment of perspectives in data analyses and interpretation;
- improved dissemination to the extent that reporting was more meaningful and understandable for participants; and
- increased reach of dissemination (summarised from Bailey et al. 2015; Camden et al. 2015; Shen et al. 2017).

Moreover, there is some evidence of the impact of patient involvement on rates of enrolment and retention in clinical trials (Crocker et al. 2018). People are more likely to take part in studies that address their own priorities, and that fit their lives and family situations.

Patient and public reviewers provide valuable perspectives that complement those provided by academic reviewers.

In the process of publication of findings, some journals have established patient and public reviews alongside the scientific peer review process. Editors report that patient and public reviewers provide valuable perspectives that complement those provided by academic reviewers. These include insights into the wider impact of illness – biological, psychological and social, the 'burden' of treatment, how people self-manage conditions, and whether interventions are practicable (Hickey et al. 2018).

The benefits for families and young people that have been reported include: empowerment, with increased confidence, self-esteem, enhanced knowledge, skills and access to decision making; increased awareness of health issues and sense of control over health service involvement; greater responsibility and independence, and increased likelihood of being involved in community programmes after completion. Aspects of involvement related to these benefits include the opportunity to socialise with peers, the opportunity to share frustrations and appreciations, knowing that their views and opinions are respected and valued, knowing that they can make a difference, and knowing that their efforts may help others (summarised from Bailey et al. 2015; Shen et al. 2017).

Benefits for the researchers have been reported too and include increased awareness of patients' perspectives; increased skills in relating to end-users and enhancing data collection; increased motivation, and increased satisfaction (Vale et al. 2012; Dudley et al. 2015).

Challenges When Involving End-Users in Research

While most reports indicate mainly positive effects of involvement, it is also clear that the positive effects of involvement are not always easy to attain. We will summarise most important challenges based on several studies (Domecq et al. 2014; Bailey et al. 2015; Camden et al. 2015; Shen et al. 2017, de Wit et al. 2018; Phoenix et al. 2018).

First, challenges included the need for greater resources to involve end-users, and extra time necessary for building relationships, and to incorporate ideas and feedback. From the perspective of families and young people the issue of time (constraints) and (in)flexibility due to personal circumstances has often been reported.

A second group of challenges was more relational in character and included power imbalance, potential conflicts, and disagreement about roles and foci of interest. Researchers were perceived to be driven by literature gaps and funding agency directives, not always aligning with the concerns of the end-users. Moreover, it can be difficult for researchers to truly share power when universities are often the main recipients of research grants and academics are ultimately accountable for how the money is spent (Hickey et al. 2018). From the perspectives of families and young people, differences in educational levels and research expertise could result in disappointment, frustration and powerlessness.

A third cluster of challenges in involving end-users in research is the issue of tokenism, with only symbolic efforts to involve end-users, without 'true' openness to the ideas of others. Finally, a common finding is the inconsistency of involvement in the various stages of the research process. End-users are most often involved in the early stages and in the final stages of research.

Currently, the setting of research priorities is undergoing a major shift in thinking; increasingly end-users are being recognised as the key stakeholders in defining research agendas and research priorities (Morris et al. 2015; Gross et al. 2018). The James Lind Alliance (JLA) plays an important role in end-user involvement in agenda setting. JLA is a non-profit initiative, bringing patients, carers and clinicians together to identify and prioritise uncertainties, or unanswered questions. The methods developed by JLA are now being used widely in various areas. This is an important development that has great impact on decisions about which research is being funded. This is a crucial step in recognising the importance of the voice of the end-user, the real challenge for the future, however, is to have true involvement in all stages of the research cycle (Fig. 10.1).

We found that challenges in research involvement may be overcome when researchers and end-users make potential roles more explicit for various stages in the research cycle.

OUR JOURNEY — STAGE 1

During our journey we aimed for close collaboration between researchers, patient organisations and parents in all stages and all aspects of research. Various perspectives clearly enriched the projects. However, we think we learned most from our struggles; in some phases we travelled at different speeds, or even on different routes. Researchers and parents noticed an imbalance in activities and duties; for researchers doing research was their main job, but for the parents it wasn't. Moreover, it became clear that continuity and routines are not self-evident. Unexpected events in the lives of the families almost always showed how difficult it can be to combine working and private life for a parent of a child with a disability. Combining these caring roles with involvement in research puts even more pressure on this fragile balance.

Despite all our good intentions and shared ambitions, we learned that is of utmost importance to talk about and agree upon tasks, roles, expectations and responsibilities. Not only those of parents, but also those of researchers, and not only at the start of the project, but repeatedly: after and before each new phase. Moreover, we more and more realised that involvement requires a lot of flexibility from all parties. Prioritising and planning research tasks flexibly was needed to fit the schedules of all individuals. From these experiences we learned to prospectively plan and discuss expectations, roles, tasks and deadlines. Respect, good relations and flexibility have enabled us to move forward.

Roles of Families and Young People in Research

Different expectations about roles and responsibilities can disrupt even the most promising end-user involvement in research. To facilitate collaboration, we believe the distinction between involvement in research and participation in research (Liabo et al. 2018) is not enough. We believe there needs to be a further distinction of individuals' roles.

Arnstein's ladder of citizen participation (Arnstein 1969) is often used as a basis for describing and discussing patient involvement in research projects. The implicit assumption in this model is that involvement in decision making is hierarchical in nature (Stewart and Liabo 2012). This assumption does not always align with individuals' reasons for engaging in decision-making processes (Morris et al. 2011; de Wit et al. 2018).

During our journey we acknowledged the need for a non-hierarchical description of roles families can play. We decided to use roles instead of levels to facilitate our discussions about collaboration. We have adopted a five-role framework, including the following roles: *Listener* (is given information, either verbally, visually or in writing; e.g. the project leader gives the parent the project plan to read);

> *Consider the roles collaborators might assume: Listener, co-thinker, advisor, partner, decision maker*

Co-thinker (is asked to give his/her opinion; e.g. parents are requested to give their opinions about an information letter for study participants); *Advisor* (gives solicited or unsolicited advice; e.g. parents propose improvements to the content of questionnaires); *Partner* (works as an equal partner; e.g. parent and researcher write an implementation plan together), and *Decision maker* (takes the initiative and/or makes the necessary decisions; e.g. parents develop and maintain a website to share information coming from the project).

Involvement, Roles and Preferences

In thinking about involvement and roles in the research process, the fPRC framework (Imms et al. 2017) is helpful in that it describes personal factors that contribute to, and that are being developed from participation and involvement experiences. These personal attributes include activity competence, sense of self and preferences. Mostly roles of end-users in the research process are rather implicit, while if roles are being discussed explicitly and are based on preferences, notions like motivation and affect are likely to become important, and people thus become more involved. Distinguishing the various roles in research involvement facilitates the discussion of individual preferences. In our experience the discussion of preferred involvement in various stages of a research project not only increases commitment, it also clarifies mutual expectations.

OUR JOURNEY – STAGE 2

An interesting insight was gained during our journey through one of the projects in which parents and researchers collaborated. Halfway through the project we together realised the importance of distinguishing the various roles described above, and we decided to take a step aside and look back to the roles taken. When we (parents and researchers) discussed the roles of individuals in the project we found, to our surprise, we had totally different views on, for example, the role of a mother in the project so far. These views varied from Listener and Co-thinker, from the perspective of the mother, to Partner, from the perspective of the Researcher. We realised that, if the preferred and expected role in each stage had been discussed in advance, the mother might have behaved differently. She might have felt more freedom to give feedback and be stronger in her opinions earlier in the project.

At that moment, it showed how important it was to be really open and honest with each other in order to have a true partnership. Although it was not easy to disagree with each other, we acknowledged the need and shared a willingness to find common ground. This created a new, stronger foundation for future collaboration. The conclusion was that discussing the role of the parent (and researchers) beforehand and on a regular basis might prevent misunderstandings and make it clear for everybody what everyone expects from one another.

Involvement, Roles and Preferences – Current Debates

While the focus in this chapter lies on experiences in applied research, there are two additional topics currently being debated. First, there is some critical discussion about patient involvement in the field of basic research, such as science that takes place in laboratories. Most important arguments refer to the complexity of the issues and necessary expertise, and the long and mostly unknown distance and relationship between basic research and practice. On the other hand, others are proponents of the benefits of patient involvement in this kind of research, advising that to ensure a more effective movement from basic science to relevant and useful clinical applications, involvement of patients is critical (e.g. van der Scheer et al. 2017). There is some scepticism about 'true partnership' in the middle stages of research; in the design, conduct and analysis of the research. In this debate, the discussion focuses on the risk of tokenism because of inequality between researchers and 'lay persons' in their research skills and expertise (e.g. Ives Damery and Redwod 2013).

We agree that there is always a risk of tokenism in PPI. However, we do not agree that this is inherent to inequality in research skills and expertise. The power of bringing skills and expertise of both researchers and end-users together is that they complement each other. An open discussion about each other's roles in various stages, and more specifically in various activities, is key to avoiding tokenism (Bailey et al. 2015).

YOUNG PEOPLE AND FAMILY INVOLVEMENT IN RESEARCH: HOW?

The field of PPI is developing rapidly. There are so many differences in (research) contexts, end-users and researchers, that make it impossible and not helpful to aim for an extensive overview of instruments, tools or advice on how to involve young people and families in research. Currently, there is still a lack of clear

Box 10.1 Recommendations for involving families and young people (end-users) in research	
Timing and planning	• Involve end-users as early as possible • Involve end-users in all stages of the research process • Share ideas and plan activities well in advance of deadlines • Plan for unpredictability; be flexible about project plans, timings, etc.
Roles	• Discuss (preferred) roles openly and honestly before each stage, and be clear on expectations • Be clear that roles can differ for different stages of the research, based on individual preferences • Evaluate involvement and roles regularly during the entire process
Communication and attitude	• Make agreements on roles explicit • Invest in building relationships • Recognise end-users as experts and equals • Avoid using complicated and technical language • Take into account any differences in educational levels and research expertise • Be responsive to individual lifestyles • Be aware of the busy home lives individuals have • Explicitly ask end-users for their opinion; e.g. if they think the research is feasible and relevant in their daily lives • Provide encouragement to end-users for their contributions • Discuss how end-users prefer to be valued for their contributions • Be flexible; accommodate to each other's knowledge, skills and attitudes • Make the research process transparent and ensure end-users are aware of everything from the start, including the inherent unpredictability of research
Organisation	• Let end-users be part of the research group and meetings • Provide relevant training to end-users • Provide relevant training to researchers • Have a trusting and positive work environment • Provide structural supports, e.g. meet in convenient places, provide incentives/reimbursements, provide food and childcare • Create group guidelines • Develop conflict resolution strategies • Provide support, and recognition to end-users for their contributions

guidance about methods for engaging patients in research (Camden et al. 2015; Phoenix et al. 2018). The current state-of-the-art is experience based: there is no empirical evidence about what works and what does not in end-user engagement. We can learn however from each other. We will illustrate some 'lessons learned' with examples from the field of childhood disability, as food for inspiration, including concrete recommendations in Box 10.1 and examples of organisations, tools and websites in Box 10.2.

Early 'lessons learned' suggest the benefits of establishing meaningful partnerships at an organisational level, including the importance of in-person contact for relationship building (Forsythe et al. 2016). A first inspiring example includes a web-based research advisory community, connecting a group of parents of special needs children with researchers at CanChild, Centre for Childhood Disability Research. This group started as a Facebook group run by two parents who worked in consultation with CanChild. In a couple of years this group became an established community of parents and researchers with active engagement and knowledge exchange in all phases of research (Russell et al. 2016).

A second example is the research vision and organisation of PenCRU (www.pencru.org), a partnership between researchers, families and healthcare professionals. The ethos of the unit is to involve families affected by childhood disability in all aspects of research and related activities. This is organised around their Family Faculty, comprising families and carers of children with neurodisability. The handbook

Box 10.2	Organisations, tools and websites
INVOLVE (UK) www.invo.org.uk	INVOLVE is an advisory group to the National Institute for Health Research (NIHR), charged with supporting active public involvement in the national health system, public health and social care research.
	Example: Briefing notes for researchers
	http://www.invo.org.uk/resource-centre/resource-for-researchers/
James Lind Alliance (JLA) (UK) www.jla.nihr.ac.uk	The James Lind Alliance brings patients, carers and clinicians together in Priority Setting Partnerships to identify and prioritise unanswered questions about the effects of treatments that are important to all groups. The aim is to make sure that health research funders are aware of the issues that matter most to patients and clinicians.
	Example: Guidebook providing step-by-step guidance to establish Priority Setting Partnerships
	http://www.jlaguidebook.org/
Patient-Centered Outcomes Research Institute (PCORI) (US) www.pcori.org	The Patient-Centered Outcomes Research Institute (PCORI) was established in 2010 to fund research that can help patients and those who care for them make better-informed decisions about the healthcare choices they face every day, guided by those who will use that information. This is achieved by engaging patients, caregivers and all other stakeholders in the entire research process.
	Example: Engagement Plan
	https://www.pcori.org/about-us/our-programs/engagement/engagement-resources
PenCRU www.pencru.org	PenCRU (Peninsula Cerebra Research Unit) is a childhood disability research team. They are a partnership between researchers, families and healthcare professionals.
	Example: Handbook Family Faculty. The handbook was created with members of the Family Faculty to explain who PenCRU and the Family Faculty are, and to provide a clear statement about how they work together.
	http://www.pencru.org/getinvolved/handbook/
	Example: Tips to involve young people as partners in health research
	http://www.pencru.org/media/universityofexeter/medicalschool/subsites/pencru/pdfs/Review_of_involving_DCYP_Plain_english_summary_FINAL.pdf
Research Involvement and Engagement (journal) https://researchinvolvement.biomedcentral.com/	*Research Involvement and Engagement* is an interdisciplinary, health and social care journal focusing on patient and wider involvement and engagement in research, at all stages. The journal is co-produced by all key stakeholders, including patients, academics, policy makers and service users.
GRIPP reporting checklists http://www.equator-network.org/reporting-guidelines/gripp2-reporting-checklists-tools-to-improve-reporting-of-patient-and-public-involvement-in-research/	Tools to improve reporting of patient and public involvement in research.

(Continued on next page)

Box 10.2   (Continued)

Involvement Matrix: www.kcrutrecht.nl/involvement-matrix	The Involvement Matrix was developed, by the Center of Excellence for Rehabilitation Medicine and BOSK, to facilitate end-user involvement in research, by discussing individual preferences in various stages and activities of a research project.
Feedback from researchers to PPI Contributors: Guidance for Researchers https://www.clahrc-eoe.nihr.ac.uk/wp-content/uploads/2016/05/Guidance-for-Researchers-PPI-Feedback_2018.pdf	This guidance for researchers provides practical tips on Who?, Why?, When?, What? and How? researchers could improve their feedback to PPI contributors. Developed by the Center for Research in Public Health and Community Care (CRiPACC).

---

explaining how PenCRU and the Family Faculty work together is an inspiring tool for researchers and families. Experiences support the role of family coordinator as critical to the team for building relationships and in-person contact.

Finally, the importance of clearly defining roles and expectations in the various stages and activities of a project, and adapting to needs and preferences, is a major lesson we have learned from our own experiences. During our journey together we became increasingly aware of the importance of discussing individual preferences in various stages and activities. With the aim of facilitating this discussion, we developed the Involvement Matrix which brings together the roles and stages in research (Fig. 10.2). Roles are not fixed; they can, and often do, change in the course of a project, depending on individual needs and preferences in relation to activities that are most central in a specific stage.

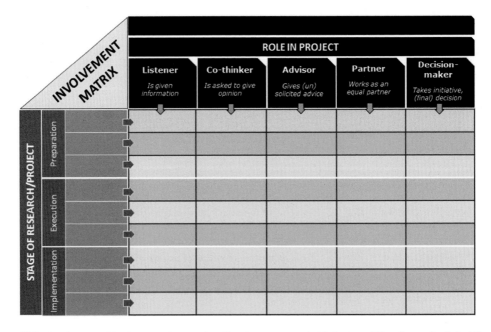

Figure 10.2   Involvement Matrix; www.kcrutrecht.nl/involvement-matrix. © Center of Excellence for Rehabilitation Medicine Utrecht, used with permission.

NEXT STEPS

The benefits and challenges of PPI in research are increasingly recognised. The field is developing rapidly, and major steps have been taken recently. However, there are still many issues to resolve, such as questions related to potential bias in the groups involved in research; for example, the involvement of people with intellectual disabilities, young children, and 'difficult to reach' groups. Moreover, there are still many steps to be taken in the development and evaluation of strategies for meaningful involvement. Family and young person involvement in research asks for major changes in the mind-set and routines of individuals. The recommendations in Box 10.1 make clear that more flexibility, changes in resources, and new skills are required to facilitate involvement. In our journey we have experienced that both parties were forced to step out of their comfort zone. Not easy, but with high impact!

Next steps should focus on the 'how'; which strategies have the greatest positive impact on research quality and usefulness to end-users of the research, including careful evaluation of barriers and facilitators. Some influential organisations (Box 10.2), at the level of research funding, research publication and patient interests, are progressing the development of this field, aiming to make research more relevant and useful.

Finally, the field would benefit much from sharing and reporting on experiences (Fergusson et al. 2018). Recently international evidence based, consensus informed guidelines have been published for reporting PPI in research (Guidance for Reporting Involvement of Patients and the Public; GRIPP) (Staniszewska et al. 2017). These guidelines aim to improve the quality, transparency and consistency of the international PPI evidence base, to ensure PPI practice is based on the best evidence. By sharing experiences in a systematic way, we can learn from each others' journeys in many ways!

> *Share experiences and report on it so we can move this new field forward.*

OUR JOURNEY — REFLECTION

We started this journey together with a shared goal to make research more relevant and to make a difference in research for children and young people with disabilities and their families. Travelling together through new, beautiful and sometimes challenging landscapes, careful listening to each other, and not afraid to take unknown roads. We shared a goal, respected each other's position and expertise, and we valued the different perspectives that were brought in, that would otherwise not have emerged. We have learned a lot and we are certain our research projects would be completely different and of less relevance and quality without our close collaboration. In our bumpy journey we learned that good intentions, mutual respect, clarity about roles, a lot of time and flexibility, and above all, passion, sense of humour and creativity can lead to beautiful vistas and a drive to explore new areas.

SUMMARY OF KEY IDEAS

- People have the right to participate in decisions that will (eventually) affect their lives.
- Active involvement concerns the contribution of experiential knowledge. Patients and families have ideas about relevant research questions, about research designs and research procedures that are acceptable to them, and provide another perspective on findings and their interpretation.
- Involvement of patients in research benefits the research, but also the patients and researchers themselves.
- Respect, good relations and flexibility are key.
- Discussion of (preferred) roles increases commitment, and clarifies mutual expectations.

ACKNOWLEDGEMENTS

Our journey and this chapter would not have been possible without the great, inspiring, and very open discussions with many people; patients, individuals with disabilities, researchers, parents and carers, including BOSK, OuderInzicht, the teenager ambassadors of Participation in Perspective, and the youth panel of ZéP FNO. The development of the Involvement Matrix has been supported financially by FNO, the Netherlands. A reflection on our journey from the perspective of the two parents in our group, Karen van Meeteren and Martijn Klem, has been included in the PhD-thesis of Mattijs Alsem (van Meeteren and Klem 2018).

REFERENCES

Arnstein SR (1969) A ladder of citizen participation. *J Am Inst Plann* **35**: 216–224.

Bailey S, Boddy K, Briscoe S, Morris C (2015) Involving disabled children and young people as partners in research: a systematic review. *Child Care Health Dev* **41**: 505–514.

Camden C, Shikako-Thomas K, Nguyen T et al. (2015) Engaging stakeholders in rehabilitation research: a scoping review of strategies used in partnerships and evaluation of impacts. *Disabil Rehabil* **37**: 1390–1400.

Chu LF, Utengen A, Kadry B et al. (2016) "Nothing about us without us" – patient partnership in medical conferences. *BMJ* **354**: i3883.

Crocker JC, Ricci-Cabello I, Parker A et al. (2018) Impact of patient and public involvement on enrolment and retention in clinical trials: systematic review and meta-analysis. *BMJ* **363**: k4738.

Crowe S, Giles C (2016) Making patient relevant clinical research a reality. *BMJ* **355**: i6627.

de Wit M, Beurskens A, Piškur B, Stoffers E, Moser A (2018) Preparing researchers for patient and public involvement in scientific research: development of a hands-on learning approach through action research. *Health Expect* **21**: 752–763.

Domecq JP, Prutsky G, Elraiyah T et al. (2014) Patient engagement in research: a systematic review. *BMC Health Serv Res* **14**: 89.

Dudley L, Gamble C, Preston J et al. (2015) What difference does patient and public involvement make and what are its pathways to impact? Qualitative study of patients and researchers from a cohort of randomised clinical trials. *PLoS One* **10**: e0128817.

Fergusson D, Monfaredi Z, Pussegoda K et al. (2018) The prevalence of patient engagement in published trials: a systematic review. *Res Involv Engagem* **4**: 17.

Forsythe LP, Ellis LE, Edmundson L et al. (2016) Patient and stakeholder engagement in the PCORI pilot projects: Description and lessons learned. *J Gen Intern Med* **31**: 13–21.

Gross PH, Bailes AF, Horn SD et al. (2018) Setting a patient-centered research agenda for cerebral palsy: a participatory action research initiative. *Dev Med Child Neurol* **60**: 1278–1284.

Hickey G, Richards T, Sheehy J (2018) Co-production from proposal to paper. *Nature* **562**: 29–31.

Imms C, Granlund M, Wilson PH, Steenbergen B, Rosenbaum PL, Gordon AM (2017) Participation, both a means and an end: a conceptual analysis of processes and outcomes in childhood disability. *Dev Med Child Neurol* **59**: 16–25.

Ives J, Damery S, Redwod S (2013) PPI, paradoxes and Plato: Who's sailing the ship? *J Med Ethics* **39**: 181–185.

King G, Chiarello L (2014) Family-centered care for children with cerebral palsy: conceptual and practical considerations to advance care and practice. *J Child Neurol* **29**: 1046–1054.

Liabo K, Boddy K, Burchmore H, Cockcroft E, Britten N (2018) Clarifying the roles of patients in research. *BMJ* **361**: k1463.

Morris C, Shilling V, McHugh C, Wyatt K (2011) Why it is crucial to involve families in all stages of childhood disability research. *Dev Med Child Neurol* **53**: 769–771.

Morris C, Simkiss D, Busk M et al. (2015) Setting research priorities to improve the health of children and young people with neurodisability: a British Academy of Childhood Disability-James Lind Alliance Research Priority Setting Partnership. *BMJ Open* **5**: e006233.

Palisano RJ (2016) Bringing the family's voice to research. *Phys Occup Ther Pediatr* **36**: 229–231.

Phoenix M, Nguyen T, Gentles SJ, VanderKaay S, Cross A, Nguyen L (2018) Using qualitative research perspectives to inform patient engagement in research. *Res Involv Engagem* **4**: 20.

Richards T, Godlee F (2014) The BMJ's own patient journey. *BMJ* 348: g3726.

Russell DJ, Sprung J, McCauley D et al. (2016) Knowledge exchange and discovery in the age of social media: the journey from inception to establishment of a parent-led web-based research advisory community for childhood disability. *J Med Internet Res* **18**: e293.

Shen S, Doyle-Thomas KAR, Beesley L et al. (2017) How and why should we engage parents as co-researchers in health research? A scoping review of current practices. *Health Expect* **20**: 543–554.

Shippee ND, Domecq Garces JP, Prutsky Lopez GJ et al. (2015) Patient and service user engagement in research: a systematic review and synthesized framework. *Health Expect* **18**: 1151–1166.

Staniszewska S, Brett J, Simera I et al. (2017) GRIPP2 reporting checklists: tools to improve reporting of patient and public involvement in research. *Res Involv Engagem* **3**: 13.

Stewart R, Liabo K (2012) Involvement in research without compromising research quality. *J Health Serv Res Policy* **17**: 248–251.

UN (2007) Convention on the Rights of Persons with Disabilities. *Eur J Health Law* **14**: 281–298.

Vale CL, Thompson LC, Murphy C, Forcat S, Hanley B (2012) Involvement of consumers in studies run by the Medical Research Council Clinical Trials Unit: results of a survey. *Trials* **13**: 9.

van der Scheer L, Garcia E, van der Laan AL, van der Burg S, Boenink M (2017) The benefits of patient involvement for translational research. *Health Care Anal* **25**: 225–241.

van Meeteren K, Klem M (2018) Parental involvement: a critical reflection. In: Alsem MW (Ed) *Family Needs and the Role of Information in Paediatric Rehabilitation Care*. Utrecht: Utrecht University, pp. 199–215.

PART III

Measuring Participation

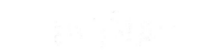

An Overview of Measurement Issues Related to Participation

Christine Imms

This chapter provides an overview of measurement principles and poses questions and challenges to measuring participation, which will be further addressed in subsequent chapters. I do not intend to provide a detailed account of measurement or psychometric research, but rather highlight key issues, especially where participation measurement may require additional thought.

WHY MEASURE PARTICIPATION?

Measurement can be undertaken for a variety of reasons:

- to describe patterns of participation in a group or population;
- to determine or describe the current participation attendance and involvement of an individual as a baseline;
- to determine if an individual or community or societal level intervention would be desirable;
- to determine if change occurs following an intervention, thus providing evidence of its effectiveness; or
- to capture 'natural' history or longitudinal patterns of participation.

Measuring participation is consistent with best practice in healthcare, where careful observation of relevant phenomena supports professional decision making. Development and validation of measures takes considerable time, as constructing tools that will capture the phenomenon of interest – especially personal, subjective constructs – and then gathering data to confirm the validity and reliability of the tool requires a series of interrelated research activities (Fawcett 2007; Mokkink et al. 2006; Terwee et al. 2017).

While early methods of participation data gathering may be informal or begin as checklists that become validated and substantiated over time, every measure or assessment must have a clear definition of the construct of interest. The definition of participation, published in the International Classification of Functioning, Disability and Health (ICF) in 2001 'involvement in a life situation' (WHO 2001) has been used as the basis for development of measures in health sciences. In addition, the fields of psychology and education have had a long-standing interest in 'engagement in learning' and also have a range of measures of this construct (Fredricks et al. 2004; Harcourt and Keen 2012). In these fields, engagement has been defined in terms of behavioural engagement (the 'doing' element, often further defined as doing it correctly or as expected), emotional engagement (positive and negative values and feelings) and cognitive engagement (motivation, effort and application of cognitive strategies for learning) (Zyngier 2008). In health sciences, the term engagement has more commonly been explored in relation to 'engagement in healthcare' and defined as either a process of collaboration (engagement with) or an internal state (engagement in) (Bright et al. 2015).

The WHO definition of participation has led to diverging practices in participation measurement (Adair et al. 2015; Imms et al. 2016). A systematic review of participation measures, referenced since publication of the ICF in 2001, found 118 published measures, 61 measures that were designed specifically for the reported study without further evidence of psychometric properties, and 130 measures that counted a variety of behaviours deemed by their authors to be related to participation (Adair et al. 2018). This proliferation of potential measures means that it is possible that researchers and practitioners will be able to select a valid measure for use. However, the caveat must be that the measure chosen must focus on the construct of interest (not a related construct) and be valid, reliable and useful.

CORE PRINCIPLES FOR SELECTING MEASURES

General principles associated with selecting measures for use in practice and research include making decisions based on the evidence about validity, reliability and utility of available measures. The overarching goal is to select a measure that captures what you want to know (e.g. it captures the participation construct) about the individuals you wish to know it (i.e. it is valid for your population of interest in terms of age, condition and/or situation), and information is collected from the most relevant source (e.g. the individual themselves, a proxy respondent or direct observation) (De Vet et al. 2011). The COnsensus-based Standards for selection of health Measurement Instruments (COSMIN; www.cosmin.nl) (Mokkink et al. 2012) provides a detailed overview of the methods that are most appropriate to evaluate the validity of a measure. Table 11.1 provides a summary of definitions of the core constructs that have been described as necessary properties of measures.

Validity is not an 'all or none' construct. Evidence of validity of a measure is built over time through research that specifically tests assumptions about validity. One of the challenges to practice is that tools are often selected for use in practice and research because they have been reported in the literature – sometimes with little evidence that the tool is valid and reliable for the current purpose. Thus, a tool becomes popular, but may or may not meet appropriate standards for validly assessing the construct or measuring change over time. This appears to be true in relation to participation measures. Popular tools that have not been rigorously assessed typically have at least some face validity – that is they provide a sense of authenticity regarding capturing the construct. However, if the tool is not valid and reliable, then what is learned is unclear and any reported change over time or differences between respondent groups is unlikely to be valid.

Once a tool has been designed, then the next most important element to establish is the extent to which the measure is reliable. That is, whether the measure delivers consistent scores when no change in the construct is expected. There are several different types of reliability. Internal consistency is closely related to the structural validity of the tool but is typically described as a measure of reliability because it relates to the consistency of responses to like-items. Other forms of reliability are related to determining the level of consistency of scores obtained when different raters assess the performance. In self-report measures, which are commonly used to assess participation, test–retest reliability is important as there can only be one rater.

All measures contain some error. The sources of error are varied, and may include error associated with different raters, with usual variation in day-to-day performances, or difference in equipment used, for example. If the standard error of measurement of a measure is known, then it can be used to describe the 95% confidence interval surrounding the individual's score, thus indicating the likely precision of the score (Streiner and Norman 2003). Large standard errors of measurement indicate lower reliability. Measuring change in participation requires the use of tools that are valid, reliable and responsive. Measures that are reliable and have small measurement error are more likely to be responsive to identifying when change in participation has occurred.

Table 11.1   Definitions of measurement properties

Property	Definition	Sources of information
Validity	The degree to which a tool measures what it is intended to measure	Streiner and Norman (2003)
Content	The degree to which the scale contains all relevant elements and no irrelevant aspects of the domain of interest	Law (2004)
Face	The degree to which the tool appears to measure what it is intended to measure	Portney and Watkins (2000)
Ecological	The extent to which tool results relate to real world, everyday performances	Spooner and Pachana (2006)
Construct	The ability of the tool to measure an abstract idea, assessed by evaluating how scores respond when tested against a range of hypothesised outcomes and relationships among differing constructs. Includes cross-cultural validity which is the extent to which the tool validly captures the same construct in different cultural settings	Mokkink et al. (2012)
Criterion	The correlation of scores between the measure and other criterion standard measures of the same construct	Mokkink et al. (2012)
Responsiveness	The extent to which the measure can show change in scores in the presence of actual change	Fawcett (2007)
Reliability	The extent to which a measure is dependable, consistent and free of error when repeated under ideal conditions	McDowell and Newell (1996)
Internal consistency	The degree of relatedness between items in the same scale	Mokkink et al. (2012)
Test-retest	Stability of the measure when re-taken at a subsequent time when no change is expected	Mokkink et al. (2012); Streiner and Norman (2003)
Intra-rater	Consistency of the measurement scores when the same individual rates the same performance on a repeated occasion/s	Mokkink et al. (2012); Streiner and Norman (2003)
Inter-rater	Consistency of the measurement scores when different individuals apply it to the same performance	Mokkink et al. (2012); Streiner and Norman (2003)
Measurement error	The extent to which differences in scores can be attributed to error in measurement rather than true change	Bland and Altman (1986); Streiner and Norman (2003)
Utility	The extent to which the measure can be readily applied within a setting. Includes elements of cost, time, effort and materials needed, clarity of instructions, acceptability to users and respondents, training required to administer	Fawcett (2007); Law (2004)

Validity and reliability are the primary properties that should influence the decision about whether to use a measure. However, some high-quality tools may be difficult to use in practice. The utility of a measure is influenced by cost, the need for specific materials, equipment or setting for administration, time needed to complete, the requirement for training to administer the measure, and the acceptability of the measure to respondents. Measures that are distressing or burdensome to respondents, or that appear to be irrelevant to the needs of the respondent, are likely to be deemed to have low utility.

HOW DO I USE INFORMATION ABOUT MEASUREMENT PROPERTIES TO CHOOSE A PARTICIPATION MEASURE?

There are four key criteria that need to be met when selecting a measure of participation. First, the tool must define the construct that is being measured in a way that is consistent with the definition of participation, that is, it must be designed to measure 'attendance' or 'involvement' in a life situation. When selecting measures, it is critical to attend to the definition and the operationalising of the definition in the measure. To do this, you need to review three pieces of information:

1. the definition of the construct provided by the author/s of the measure;
2. the content of the item phrasing; and
3. the descriptors assigned to the scale that is scored.

It is these three elements, with an emphasis on the third element, which will ultimately determine what is scored or quantified, by a measure.

Second, there needs to be evidence that the measure is valid in relation to content and construct and it has been validated for the population (age, clinical characteristics) with whom you intend to use it. Third, there needs to be high levels of reliability so that scores can be trusted. Fourth, the utility of the tool must be sufficient that the information gained is of greater benefit than the burden of measurement.

WHO IS THE RESPONDENT AND WHY DOES IT MATTER?

If choosing to measure participation, consideration needs to be given as to who the most relevant reporter or observer is likely to be. Deciding this will depend on the nature of the participatory experience of interest – attendance or involvement; and whose perspective (individual, professional and/or societal) is required to inform decision making. Attendance is often observable and can be measured in terms of frequency (e.g. number of times per day or week), time (e.g. minutes spent per session), pattern (e.g. days of the week), or diversity (e.g. number of activities undertaken, or type of activity undertaken). Because attendance is observable, it is possible to collect data through self- or proxy-report using diaries, or recall surveys or measurement devices such as activity monitors.

Because involvement (while attending) is a subjective experience, it is likely that self-report will be the most valid method of measurement. However, proxy-report is also used in a range of measures (e.g. parent report is used in the Participation and Environment Measure for Children and Youth; PEM-CY) (Coster et al. 2011). Proxy measures are developed on the premise that the level of involvement can be observed by another individual. This may or may not be true. The extent to which differences between a proxy assessment and the individual's actual experiences matter, will depend on the nature of the issue for which participation assessment is required.

It may not be possible to accurately observe the level of involvement.

CAN CHILDREN SELF-REPORT?

One key question in relation to self-report, is the age at which we can ask children to provide an assessment of their own participation. There is evidence that an appropriately constructed scale assessing health-related quality of life can be completed by children as young as 5 years of age (Varni et al. 2007). Other research suggests that 6-year-olds can understand health states and are becoming reliable, and self-report can be used more confidently with those older than 7 years (Riley 2004). In this review, Riley reported that the development of the scale was important – younger children tended to use the extremes of a five-level scale, thus in effect converting it to a three-level scale.

There are several key issues to consider when determining if children can reliably self-rate. It may not be sufficient to simply apply the same assessment procedure for younger children or those with cognitive impairments, as for older children and adults. The work of Kramer and Schwartz has highlighted aspects of assessment tools to attend to, to ensure cognitive accessibility. They highlight three key features, including content, layout and administrative procedures, that need to be carefully considered and purposefully designed to support self-report (Kramer and Schwartz 2017). The more abstract the construct under consideration, the more important it is to ensure the way the item is phrased, and the examples provided, are accessible to the intended rater.

It is not always possible to obtain a valid or reliable self-report; for example, when children are very young, or when individuals have such significant cognitive or communication impairments that they are unable to express and/or hold an opinion about their involvement. Proxy responses from those who know the individual well in these instances are valuable. To obtain these responses though, requires careful consideration of what participation involvement 'looks like'.

> *How do I know if a child has sufficient understanding to be the respondent?*

WHAT ABOUT PARTICIPATION GOAL SETTING?

Paediatric rehabilitation has embraced child- and family-centred goal setting as a key element of evidence-based practice. This has seen widespread use of both the Canadian Occupational Performance Measure (COPM; Law et al. 2005) and the Goal Attainment Scale (GAS; Kiresuk et al. 1994) as valid, reliable tools to set and measure client-centred goals across diagnostic groups and in varied settings. Both measures have been used to set and measure participation-based goals and outcomes. Both the COPM and the GAS have been described as 'empty scales' (Adair et al. 2018) in that the client's issues/goals become the 'items' that are rated. While both tools can be used to set participation goals, it is very important to note that the measurement construct of the COPM is occupational performance, and the scales of measurement are self-perceived 'level of performance' and 'satisfaction with performance'. Often, the performance problems identified by clients using the COPM relate to skill development, rather than participation attendance and involvement. This is also commonly true when the GAS has been used in research. It is possible to establish participation goals using the COPM and the GAS, but if that is the intent, care must be taken to ensure that the goals set are about the participation construct.

WHAT TO DO WHEN YOU CANNOT LOCATE A SUITABLE MEASURE FOR YOUR PURPOSES

This feels like a common experience; however, our systematic review of measures that aim to assess participation identified a total of 309 different measures in use since 2001, many of which had been developed because 'there was nothing suitable available'. It can be tempting to design a new measure or measurement approach specific for your research or practice purposes; however, the journey to develop a tool that demonstrates validity and reliability (and therefore can be used with confidence) typically takes 5–10 years. If there is truly no appropriate measure, consideration should be given to developing a new measure, or to further developing an existing measure, using appropriate measurement development methods, such as those set by COSMIN (Mokkink et al. 2012).

IS THERE SOMETHING SPECIAL ABOUT MEASURING PARTICIPATION?

Not really – it is possible to select measures that validly and reliably assess either attendance or involvement; the following chapters will provide a range of examples. However, our research investigating measures of participation suggests that often participation measures have been designed that conflate multiple constructs (Imms et al. 2016; Adair et al. 2018). For example, a measure may be described as assessing participation, perhaps defined as taking part in activities in the same situation with peers, but the individual's scores are reduced if a support person is required. This example conflates independence (being able to be there on my own) with participation (being there). When more than one construct is included in the score, it is very difficult to know what has been measured.

SUMMARY

This chapter has provided a brief overview of key issues in selecting measures. The following chapters provide examples of measures of participation to support the readers' thinking about what is important to measure in their own situations, and how to think about measurement of the key constructs. Readers will be provided with examples of tools (methods to collect data/information) that could be used as well as a framework to support their rationale for use in practice.

REFERENCES

Adair B, Ullenhag A, Keen D, Granlund M, Imms C (2015) The effect of interventions aimed at improving participation outcomes for children with disabilities: a systematic review. *Dev Med Child Neurol* **57**: 1093–1104.

Adair B, Ullenhag A, Rosenbaum P, Granlund M, Keen D, Imms C (2018) Measures used to quantify participation in childhood disability and their alignment with the family of participation-related constructs: a systematic review. *Dev Med Child Neurol* **60**: 1101–1116.

Bland JM, Altman DG (1986) Statistical methods for assessing agreement between two methods of clinical measurement. *Lancet* **1**: 307–310.

Bright FA, Kayes NM, Worrall L, McPherson KM (2015) A conceptual review of engagement in healthcare and rehabilitation. *Disabil Rehabil* **37**: 643–654.

Coster W, Bedell G, Law M et al. (2011) Psychometric evaluation of the Participation and Environment Measure for Children and Youth. *Dev Med Child Neurol* **53**: 1030–1037.

De Vet HCW, Terwee CB, Mokkink LB, Knol DL (2011) *Measurement in Medicine: A Practical Guide.* New York: Cambridge University Press.

Fawcett AJL (2007) *Principles of Assessment and Outcome Measurement for Occupational Therapists and Physiotherapists: Theory, Skills and Application.* Hoboken, NJ: John Wiley & Sons.

Fredricks JA, Blumenfeld PC, Paris AH (2004) School engagement: potential of the concept, state of the evidence. *Rev Educ Res* **74**: 59–109.

Harcourt D, Keen D (2012) Learner engagement: has the child been lost in translation? *Australas J Early Child* **37**: 71–78.

Imms C, Adair B, Keen D, Ullenhag A, Rosenbaum P, Granlund M (2016) "Participation": a systematic review of language, definitions, and constructs used in intervention research with children with disabilities. *Dev Med Child Neurol* **58**: 29–38.

Kiresuk TJ, Smith A, Cardillo JE (1994) *Goal Attainment Scaling: Applications, Theory and Measurement.* Hillsdale, NJ: L Erlbaum Associates.

Kramer JM, Schwartz A (2017) Reducing barriers to patient-reported outcome measures for people with cognitive impairments. *Arch Phys Med Rehabil* **98**: 1705–1715.

Law M (2004) *Outcome Measures Rating Form Guidelines* [Online]. Hamilton, Ontario CanChild Centre for Disability Research. https://canchild.ca/system/tenon/assets/attachments/000/000/372/original/measrate.pdf [Accessed 4 October 2019].

Law M, Baptiste S, Carswell A, Mccoll M, Polatajko H, Pollock N (2005) *Canadian Occupational Performance Measure*. Ottawa, ON: CAOT Publications ACE.

McDowell I, Newell C (1996) *Measuring Health: A Guide to Rating Scales and Questionnaires*. New York: Oxford University Press.

Mokkink LB, Terwee CB, Knol DL et al. (2006) Protocol of the COSMIN study: COnsensus-based Standards for the selection of health Measurement INstruments. *BMC Med Res Methodol* **6**: 2.

Mokkink LB, Terwee CB, Patrick DL et al. (2012) COSMIN checklist manual. http://fac.ksu.edu.sa/sites/default/files/cosmin_checklist_manual_v9.pdf [Accessed 4 October 2019].

Portney LG, Watkins MP (2000) *Foundations of Clinical Research: Applications to Practice*. Upper Saddle River, NJ: Prentice Hall Health.

Riley AW (2004) Evidence that school-age children can self-report on their health. *Ambul Pediatr* **4**(Suppl): 371–376.

Spooner DM, Pachana NA (2006) Ecological validity in neuropsychological assessment: a case for greater consideration in research with neurologically intact populations. *Arch Clin Neuropsychol* **21**: 327–337.

Streiner DL, Norman GR (2003) *Health Measurement Scales: A Practical Guide to Their Development and Use*. Oxford: Oxford University Press.

Terwee C, Prinsen B, Chiarotto A et al. (2017) COSMIN standards and criteria for evaluating the content validity of health-related patient-reported outcome measures: A Delphi study. *Qual Life Res* **27**: 1159–1170.

Varni JW, Limbers CA, Burwinkle TM (2007) How young can children reliably and validly self-report their health-related quality of life? An analysis of 8,591 children across age subgroups with the PedsQL 4.0 Generic Core Scales. *Health Qual Life Outcomes* **5**: 1.

WHO (2001) *International Classification of Functioning, Disability and Health: Short Version*. Geneva: World Health Organization.

Zyngier D (2008) (Re)conceptualising student engagement: doing education not doing time. *Teach Teach Educ* **24**: 1765–1776.

Measuring Participation as an Outcome: Attendance and Involvement

Brooke Adair, Annette Majnemer and Christine Imms

INTRODUCTION

Everyone with a disability has the right to 'full and effective participation and inclusion in society' according to Article 3 of the Convention on the Rights of Persons with Disabilities and Article 30, which refers to the right to participation in cultural life, recreation, leisure and sport (UN General Assembly 2007). The UN Convention on the Rights of the Child (Article 31) further articulates the right to play and to participate fully in society, with equal opportunities for cultural, artistic, recreational and leisure activity (UN General Assembly 2007). While many of the Articles are concerned with environmental elements that can be legislated about – such as access, opportunity and freedom from discrimination – others are concerned with ensuring people with disabilities can participate fully. We cannot, however, know if we are meeting our participation obligations under the Conventions if we do not measure participation effectively.

When choosing a measure, the primary consideration should always be 'what is the question to be answered' with the information gained from the assessment? The more focused and clear your question, the more likely you will select an appropriate measure and ultimately discover a useful answer. The shift in focus in childhood-onset disability research and practice to understanding participation outcomes, has given rise to a plethora of 'participation' measures; however, the measures have not all captured a clearly defined and distinct construct (Imms et al. 2016; Adair et al. 2018). Often, the measures chosen were originally designed to quantify the capability of an individual, their ability to exercise choice, or their preferences. There are measures available that quantify participation attendance – these can support measurement of whether individuals with disability attend the same activities as others. There are fewer measures of involvement. Measures of involvement will provide information about the extent to which participation actually occurs when an individual attends particular activity settings or life situations.

In this chapter we define the participation constructs of interest and situate measurement choice within key topics that need to be considered when selecting a measure. The chapter will also include examples of measures of participation, described in ways that aim to assist the reader to make reasoned choices when new measures become available, or, if you are a researcher, to consider the measurement gaps that might be filled by the development of a new measure.

This chapter is particularly focused on understanding participation as an outcome – thus the measures of interest are those that tap participation attendance and involvement. We predominantly consider the participation of children; however, most of the topics are also pertinent to adults.

DEFINITION OF THE PARTICIPATION CONSTRUCT

In the International Classification of Functioning, Disability, and Health (ICF), participation is defined as 'involvement in a life situation' (WHO 2001). Although the ICF was instrumental in identifying participation as an important concept for health professionals to understand and promote, the definition lacked clarity, making it difficult to ascertain what constituted participation.

This lack of clarity, combined with the overarching need to optimise participation and address participation restrictions, was the driving force behind the development of the family of participation-related constructs (fPRC) (Imms et al. 2016, 2017). According to the fPRC, participation is a multidimensional construct that has two key components: 'attendance' and 'involvement' (Imms et al. 2016, 2017). In addition, there are three important participation-related concepts ('activity competence', 'sense of self' and 'preferences') that are not synonymous with participation but can influence or be influenced by a person's participation experiences (Imms et al. 2016, 2017).

Many measures have been developed that have focused on a person's ability to complete an activity, quantifying successful participation according to whether a child met specific criteria or performed the activity 'correctly' (Adair et al. 2018). According to the definition provided by the ICF, these measures could be considered to quantify participation because of their focus on 'performance', in particular, their focus on quantifying 'correct' or 'independent' performance in natural settings. Operationalising participation as performance is problematic as it equates ability with participation, and therefore, all individuals with need for special support to complete activities will, by definition, be deemed to experience low levels of participation. Individuals who attend and are involved in activities with equipment or personal support may disagree with this conceptualisation, as do we. Within the fPRC, measures that quantify performance or ability are defined as measures of 'activity competence' (Imms et al. 2016, 2017). In this chapter, we focus on the measurement of participation 'attendance' and 'involvement'.

> It is problematic to operationalise participation as performance as it equates ability with participation.

DEFINITIONS OF ATTENDANCE AND INVOLVEMENT

Attendance is defined as 'being there', or whether a person is physically (or virtually) present in a situation. Attendance is a necessary condition for participation in a particular activity (Imms et al. 2017). Measures of attendance generally include frequency counts (e.g. how often someone attends a sporting activity), measures of diversity (the number of different activities a person attends) or other measures of time spent doing an activity.

Involvement is defined as 'the experience of participation while attending' (Imms et al. 2017). This definition of the involvement construct was derived from a content analysis of measures used by researchers investigating participation outcomes, and is considered to include 'elements of motivation, persistence, social connection [perhaps], and affect' (Imms et al. 2016). This means that the involvement construct is complex, multidimensional and not necessarily visible to an outside observer.

CONSIDERATIONS WHEN CHOOSING MEASURES OF PARTICIPATION

Chapter 11 provided an overview of the general issues to consider when selecting measures to ensure they are valid and reliable. The multidimensional and complex nature of the participation construct means additional considerations may need to be addressed when choosing an appropriate participation measure, as described below.

The Importance of Life Situations

'Everyday life situations are episodes that occur regularly in the natural environments where children [people] usually spend time' (Adolfsson 2011). All aspects of participation occur within a specific setting or life situation (Imms et al. 2017) and it is the transactional relationship between the individual and the situation or activity setting that characterises participation. The environment and/or life situation will influence the availability of activities and therefore have an effect on how an individual participates (Imms et al. 2017). Individuals are also influential within their situations; for example, a child's interaction during certain activities will impact other's actions, and potentially change the availability of objects or actions within a setting (Davidov et al. 2015). Moreover, a child's participation experiences in one activity setting may further influence their participation in other settings.

The life situation can influence how a child participates or what aspects of participation involvement are visible to others. For example, when watching a movie in a theatre there is an expectation to be quiet and to listen. In contrast, watching a movie at home with friends might involve more discussion about the movie and interaction with peers.

Given all participation occurs within varying life situations, practitioners and researchers need to choose which life situations they wish to focus on during the measurement process. Measurement of the environment is not synonymous with quantifying a child's participation (Imms et al. 2016); however, documenting the relevant setting or life situations in which children attend provides necessary contextual information.

Most measures of participation consider a child's attendance or involvement in particular settings. For example, the Participation and Environment Measure for Children and Youth (PEM-CY) (Coster et al. 2011) considers a child's frequency of attendance and involvement in the home, school and community, as well as assessing the helpfulness of the environment and the available resources. Other measurement tools focus on specific activity types and also assess the various settings in which the activities may be undertaken. For example, the Children's Assessment of Participation and Enjoyment (CAPE) (King et al. 2004) lists 55 activities that occur 'outside of school' with no other limitations (or expectations) applied regarding the environment. The CAPE then asks where the activities were undertaken and with whom, thereby quantifying aspects of the setting further. Choice of the most appropriate measure of attendance or involvement, with consideration to the life situation, therefore depends on whether you wish to assess a child in a consistent or specific life situation or whether you wish to assess participation as the child undertakes a specific activity across a variety of settings.

CULTURAL INFLUENCES

Cultural context includes one's beliefs, language, values and traditions that are held in common with a community or group of people (often of the same ethnicity or religion). Cultural context can influence perceptions of health as well as opportunities for social interaction and participation. More specifically, cultural values can influence life roles and the expectations for level of engagement in different life situations and activities such as sports, social activities and higher education.

Cultural Considerations for Measures

For an assessment to be valid, it must be culturally relevant. This means that the words used and the items themselves must be meaningful to the individual being assessed. Some cultural differences appear obvious, for example, a participation measure developed in Canada or Australia may not be relevant for use in China or Tanzania because of differences in activity patterns, climate or cultural preferences.

Measures must undergo a validation process (and often, translation) when there are questions about the cultural fit of the measure. Some items may need to be added, rephrased and/or eliminated. Following this, the reliability and validity of the newly translated and adapted measure will also need verification (Ullenhag et al. 2012). Generic tools that are not bound by specific items, such as the Canadian Occupational Performance Measure (Law et al. 2014), allow for greater flexibility in their application across cultural contexts.

Cultural Influences on Participation

Participation expectations can vary widely across different communities. For example, one study found that, overall, Druze children in Israel attended fewer leisure activities and had less enjoyment of these activities when compared to Jewish children (Engel-Yeger et al. 2007). Of note, there were gender differences in these two cultural groups when comparing preferences for leisure activities; Druze males showed greater preference for most activity domains when compared to Jewish males, and similarly female Druze children showed higher preferences for skill-based, self-improvement and recreational leisure activities when compared to female Jewish children (Engel-Yeger and Jarus 2008). In another study, Australian adolescents with Asian-speaking backgrounds or youth in urban environments were more sedentary than peers from rural areas or other cultural backgrounds (Hardy et al. 2006).

Participation level, both attendance and involvement, is largely culturally bound.

These examples highlight the influence between and within countries based on religious, ethnic and cultural mores. For young people growing up in countries that differ from their parental cultural norms, this can introduce tension and family conflict when opportunities are available that traditionally would not be, and vice versa. For example, a young Muslim woman making choices for independent living and work in a Western culture may experience difficulties if there are family expectations that she will live at home and provide household labour. In this example, the identified influence is on the 'attendance' aspect of participation. Cultural expectations of role may also influence the involvement aspect of participation. Thus, an important consideration for those wishing to measure participation is whether certain activities are both actually available, and also perceived to be available, depending on cultural background; both can influence participation in various life situations.

THE INFLUENCE OF TIME

Time is an important topic both from the perspective of measurement, and from the perspective of participation. In this section we consider: (1) how the quality of an individual's participation may change over time (e.g. to what extent do people do the same things in different ways as they age, versus changing their participation patterns completely); (2) decisions about frequency of measurement; and (3) the measurement time frame (e.g. reporting on past days, months, years; or moment by moment observation).

Age-Based Participatory Roles

Age is likely to influence the choice of activities, including who chooses the activity (i.e. a parent or the individual themselves), and the way in which an individual participates in a chosen activity (see Chapter 3). There is evidence that participation diversity decreases over time for recreational, active physical and self-improvement activities but increases over time in social activities when measured over a 9-year period (Imms and Adair 2017). Therefore, when choosing measures of participation attendance, consideration should be given to the type of activity as well as the age of the individual in question: a culturally appropriate measure would consider potential activities that an individual of that age might usually attend. For example, very young children are unlikely to visit the theatre or movies while this activity is much more common for teenagers; therefore, a measure that focuses on this activity may not be the best choice to quantify participation attendance over time if beginning in infancy. Likewise, participation in work is highly relevant for adults, but not for young children.

The quantification of participation attendance and involvement for infants and young children is complex. For infants, participation attendance is often decided by their parents, meaning young children may not be in control of the activities in which they participate; this may also be the case for older children who are more severely impaired and less able to make decisions for themselves. Measurement of participation attendance in these cases may instead quantify the activities that the parents or carers prefer to attend and could have strong links to cultural expectations. It may be more useful and valid to assess infants' *involvement* in varying settings. For example, an infant might attend a coffee shop with her parents because this is a preferred parental activity. While it may be important to note the child's attendance, quantification of her engagement and interactions with café staff and other people may provide richer information about this child's participation via the involvement construct.

The involvement construct is complex, and it is not yet clear how *involvement* per se changes with age – do children develop the capacity to be more deeply involved with age, or is that a somewhat stable construct with change shown through the range or complexity of life situations that increase over time? It is possible that participation involvement may have the same hallmarks regardless of age; however, the way in which involvement can be measured differs depending on the age of the individual in question. It is also unreasonable to expect the level of involvement to be the same in every situation – fluctuations are natural – and needed – so how involvement varies over time within an activity and over time across the lifespan is of interest.

Involvement is the experiential component of participation (Imms et al. 2017) and therefore measurement of this construct may consider how and the depth or extent to which a person engages with his or her environment or context while participating in an activity. Very young children interact within their contexts by actions such as facial gestures and reaching for toys, while older children and adolescents might show their involvement by talking to others, physically moving about the setting and interacting with objects or tasks. Measuring involvement for young children may therefore focus on observable actions. While this may also be the case for older children and adults, it is also sometimes possible to ask an older child how involved they were during an activity. Therefore, when choosing measures of participation involvement, it is crucial to consider the individual's age and his/her ability to communicate. The importance of proxy measurement and considerations for selecting the respondent are discussed later in this chapter.

Time and Measurement

The influence of time on participation measurement can be considered in relation to the length of time over which a measure quantifies an individual's participation (e.g. minutes, days, months) and, when using a measure repeatedly, the time-period between occasions of measurement.

Many self-report measures ask about participation over the preceding week, several months or year. For example, the CAPE (King et al. 2004) asks the respondent (the person completing the form) to consider activity participation over the preceding 4 months. This measure relies on a person remembering their average frequency of attendance and enjoyment, thereby introducing possible recall bias to the results. The relatively long length of time might also mean that seasonal variations occur during the 4-month period, thereby complicating the reporting of results.

Time sampling is another method that has been used in the past to quantify participation attendance and involvement. This method is generally conducted over a short period (e.g. 1 hour or 1 week) with observations of 'in-the-moment' participation being made at regular and short intervals (e.g. every 5 minutes for 30 seconds). Seasonal variation will not impact on this form of measurement, but when using time sampling it may be useful to consider whether a child is involved in a 'usual' activity/setting so that a representative sample of participation is obtained.

One of the challenges of repeated, longitudinal measurement is that the longer the period in which participation is to be measured, the more any observed change is likely to be explained by multiple factors which themselves may also be changing. For example, if measuring annual patterns of activity, it is likely that seasonal variation will influence what and how a child participates in various activities (Atkin et al. 2016; Schüttoff and Pawlowski 2018). One clear example is of physical activity participation in temperate countries: participation in outdoor physical activities is generally dependent on weather; that is, children cannot ski in summer and are much less likely to swim at the beach during winter. Previous studies have also shown that children are less active during winter and autumn (Atkin et al. 2016), suggesting that they use their time to participate in more sedentary activities. Given the potential influence of season, it is possible that patterns of participation for the same child would differ if measured at the end of summer compared to the end of winter. This is particularly important if the purpose is to assess participation changes longitudinally; if you were to assess a child at 18-month intervals (i.e. different seasons) it is possible that seasonal variations, as well as any other factors under investigation, might influence the results.

When repeated measurement is of interest, either in practice or research, chosen measures need to be responsive, valid for participants with increasing age, and be able to account for other issues of variability including seasonal or other lifespan transition periods. The timing of measurement longitudinally should be based on theoretical premises (or hypotheses) about when change is expected to occur, rather than simply on a repeated equal interval set period (e.g. 6-monthly). The number of assessments, and therefore the overall length of follow up, also needs to be considered. In research, if we wish to understand the shape of participation change, longitudinal studies require a minimum of three measurement points (Singer and Willett 2003).

MEASURES OF INDIVIDUAL CONSTRUCTS AND MULTIFACTORIAL MEASURES

Participation is a multifactorial concept. Although the fPRC describes the separate constructs of attendance and involvement, as well as the participation-related constructs, it can still be difficult to disentangle the measurement of these aspects. When choosing participation measures consideration should be given to: (1) the constructs of interest for example, attendance, involvement or both; (2) whether it is important to document changes in each construct separately or whether a combined score is sufficient to describe the expected change; and (3) how a measure calculates the resultant 'participation' score and thus how it can be interpreted.

Although some measures provide separate sub-scores for attendance and involvement (e.g. the PEM-CY), there are a number that create a combined score for the two participation constructs. The Child and Adolescent Scale of Participation (CASP) (Bedell 2004) includes items that relate to being there and performing activities in different social contexts, compared to age expected norms, and results in a composite score that essentially includes aspects of attendance and involvement. If participation attendance and/or involvement were the outcome of interest during an intervention trial and the CASP was the chosen the outcome measure, the researchers may find it difficult to interpret whether the intervention influenced either attendance, *or* involvement, *or* both.

THE RESPONDENT AND THE RESPONSE FORMAT

Respondent: Who is Describing the Individual's Participation?

Self-report and proxy-report measures are cost-effective ways to assess populations. For *self-report* measures, respondents are typically asked to read questions or statements on a questionnaire or respond to interview questions that are about their experiences or behaviours, attitudes or beliefs and are asked to select the response that best characterises them. In this case, it would be the children themselves who would be responding to the questions. When using self-report measures, there is some concern that respondents may either under-report or exaggerate their responses. Social desirability bias (i.e. reflecting themselves in ways that are socially acceptable) is a possibility using this approach. Sometimes, questions may not be clear to the respondent and if completing the measure independently (e.g. a mail or online survey), they cannot ask for clarification. However, self-report measures do allow the respondent to provide their own perspective and to describe their experiences or feelings directly. Furthermore, self-report measures enable the evaluators to learn more about specific constructs, such as participation involvement, that are challenging to measure by direct observation.

A *proxy* may be used to respond on behalf of an individual with a disability. This is often the case for children when they are too young or do not have the intellectual and/or language competencies to reliably report for themselves (Varni et al. 2007). Parents are often used as proxy respondents since they know their children best. This is common in high- as well as low- and middle-income countries (Lygnegård et al. 2013). Proxies other than parents can include another relative, a caregiver or a teacher (e.g. participation at school activities).

The extent to which children and, for example, their parents (the proxy) agree on the ratings on a measure will depend on a wide range of factors. Parents spend more time with their children when they are younger and therefore age is one consideration – it may be easier for them to be proxy respondents when their children are younger rather than older. Some constructs are more directly observable (e.g. number of activities completed, frequency of attending) whereas other constructs may be intrinsic (e.g. perceived level of engagement, satisfaction with involvement in the activity) and may be more difficult for a parent or other proxy-respondent to appreciate. The context in which the behaviours of interest occur (e.g. home, school, community) will also influence the opportunities for direct observation by the parent/proxy and therefore may influence the extent of agreement in ratings between an individual and the proxy (Marques et al. 2013; Majnemer et al. 2008). As such, proxy-reports are useful, and are sometimes the only report available, even though they have limitations. They should, however, be considered as secondary data as the report is not coming from the primary source; the individual (Jokovic et al. 2004).

> *Proxy respondent information may not accurately reflect the individual's actual experience.*

Response Format: How is Participation Information Being Collected?

Questionnaires or surveys include a series of written questions that are typically presented in a very structured format. Questions may be open-ended, allowing the respondent to provide information using their own words, or they may be closed, providing specific options from which to select an answer. Examples of closed questions are yes/no responses, responses on a Likert scale (e.g. five levels from strongly disagree to strongly agree), a range within one category (e.g. frequency response options might include: never, once in 4 months, daily), or specific answer options (to yield proportions). In research, the closed question format is more amenable to quantitative descriptive analysis whereas the open-ended question format requires qualitative analysis of content or themes. Qualitative analysis takes longer to complete than quantitative but can provide a more in-depth understanding of the phenomenon of interest. In practice, either format can be used to elicit information for programme planning.

The advantage of questionnaires is their relatively low cost and ease of use with large groups. They can be easily scored if close-ended questions are used and, in research, anonymity is possible. Another advantage is that the respondents can complete the measure when convenient for them without pressure, rather than at a designated time. An important disadvantage is that if the questions are not clear to, or are interpreted differently by different respondents without an administrator available to explain the questions, then the reliability and validity of the measure is jeopardised. It is also important to ensure that the content is culturally appropriate and at a literacy level that is broadly applicable.

Conducting an *interview* allows the evaluator to present a questionnaire (structured or semi-structured) out loud, and therefore provides opportunities to further clarify any questions that the respondent finds unclear. In research, these interviews are typically audio recorded and transcribed for later analysis. Interviews may be conducted either face-to-face or by telephone. Structured interviews follow a specific script or interview guide and may limit opportunities for the respondent to express themselves freely and ask their own questions. Unstructured interviews can take a long time to complete and may not capture all the information of interest. A semi-structured approach is often used as a compromise, to ensure that specific questions are answered, and that the respondent can expand in some areas or respond to more open questions as well. The interview approach may be more amenable to application in different cultural contexts as phrasing can be readily adapted and translators can be utilised if needed. However, this is a more time-consuming and costly approach, when compared to questionnaires.

One example of an interview-based instrument is Picture my Participation (PmP) (Arvidsson et al. 2019; Imms et al. 2014). Administration of this measure involves the use of 'talking mats' or a 'yarning' process in which the child is engaged in a conversation about their daily routines to elicit the frequency of their participation in a range of typical daily activities and the level of their involvement in those activities. The conversation is supported using a mat on which pictures (depicting various activities) are placed while they are talked about. Images that represent varying frequencies and varying amounts of involvement are also used to support the child's thinking. The child describes and selects responses that best fit their experiences and the administrator records the responses.

Direct observations involve having the observer write down what they see during a child's participation, including what the child is doing, with whom, where and how. Alternatively, structured observational checklists can be used where observer time sampling is conducted (e.g. Child Observation in Preschool) (Farran 2014). Direct observations are generally a more exploratory approach, to generate hypotheses and to better understand the factors that may influence, in this case, participation attendance and involvement. It is important to observe the child in situations that represent their real-life context and capture what they usually experience. With respect to participation, this may, or may not, be a practical approach for measurement, but can be extremely rich in better understanding the phenomena captured on self- or proxy-report measures.

MEASURES OF PARTICIPATION

Table 12.1 displays a selection of measures that quantify aspects of participation attendance and/or involvement for children of varying ages. This is not an exhaustive list, instead it is meant to be used as a guide, based on the considerations discussed in this chapter, to help practitioners and researchers to choose an appropriate measure. New measures are being developed regularly but until there is evidence of reliability and validity it is difficult to recommend them for use. The measures shown here have demonstrated evidence for reliability and validity; however, caution is needed when selecting a measure to ensure that it has been found to be psychometrically sound for the specific population and life situation of interest to you (see Chapter 11). The same considerations are needed when selecting measures to use with adults with impairments. The checklist in Box 12.1 provides a quick reminder of issues to consider when choosing a measure of participation attendance or involvement.

CURRENT AND FUTURE CHALLENGES WHEN MEASURING PARTICIPATION ATTENDANCE AND INVOLVEMENT

Participation is a complex and multidimensional concept. The choice of measurement tool influences the ability of a researcher or practitioner to quantify aspects of attendance and involvement and then interpret these results in a meaningful way. Measures of attendance are relatively common and generally well described; measures of involvement are much less common and often operationalise involvement in terms of a child's enjoyment of an activity: this is a somewhat limited expression of involvement (Adair et al. 2018).

Researchers and practitioners are still trying to clarify what it means to be involved and determine whether a subjective concept such as this can be observed and if so, what involvement 'looks' like. It may be that individuals interpret the idea of involvement differently (and report their experiences in different ways), thus further complicating the measurement construct. Currently, the pool of potential measures of involvement is somewhat limited in number and care is needed when choosing measures to ensure that what is chosen addresses involvement, as intended. There is a need for further development of measures of involvement that are suitable for individuals across a range of ages and abilities. Because of the complexity of the construct, development of the content of measures of involvement must consider the perspectives of relevant stakeholders to ensure relevance, comprehensiveness and comprehensibility of any resultant measure (Terwee et al. 2018).

Another challenge of measuring participation is that little information exists about what can be considered as 'ideal' or good participation. In some respects, this challenge arises because participation is heavily influenced by individual and cultural preferences, therefore ideal participation for one child might not be what another child considers to be right for them. For example, one child and family might be interested in attending many activities (increased diversity of attendance) while another might feel that doing one activity more frequently is better. One child may feel they are very involved with their friends when they are part of the group, another will only feel involved if they are the centre of attention. The exact nature of the relationship between attendance and involvement is also not yet well understood. These uncertainties impact on how participation goals are determined, documented, supported and measured in practice and in research – do we know when clients, patients or participants have achieved an 'ideal' or optimal level of participation?

What does 'ideal' participation look like?

There is evidence to suggest that participation during childhood can influence participation in adulthood; for example, adults are less likely to get involved in sports unless they have experienced these

Table 12.1   Potential measures of participation attendance and involvement

Instrument	Definition of purpose according to the developers	fPRC construct			Life situation/activity setting	Measurement timeframe	Population	Respondent/response format
		Attendance	Involvement	Related				
Activity Card Sort (Baum and Edwards 2001): Preschool (Berg and LaVesser 2006) and Paediatric (Mandich et al. 2004) versions	Levels of occupational engagement in daily activities	Current activity score and occupational profile of activities done		'Want to do' score	Activities related to personal care, school/productivity, hobbies/social activities and sports	In the past 4 months	Preschool: 3–6 years; Paediatric: 5–14 years; All diagnostic groups	Pictures used in interview format; self or proxy report
Assessment of Preschool Children's Participation (Petrenchik et al. 2006)	Questionnaire designed to identify activities that a child participates in	Diversity sub-score; intensity sub-score; total score			In the context of play, skill development, active physical recreation and social activities. No specified environment	In the past 4 months	2–5 years 11 months	Questionnaire completed by parents/caregivers
Child and Adolescent Scale of Participation (CASP) (Bedell 2004)	Extent of participation in home, school and community activities	Sub-section and total summary scores (**composite score**)			Home, school and community participation; Home and community living activities	Current	5 years and older; all diagnostic groups (developed for traumatic brain injury)	Questionnaire; self-report, or by parent/caregiver interview
Child Engagement in Daily Life Measure (Chiarello et al. 2014)	To measure the degree in which a child participates in daily activities	Part one frequency sub-score	Part one enjoyment sub-score	Part two score related to consistency of performance	Family and recreational activities and participation in self-care	Current	Originally designed for children with cerebral palsy	Questionnaire completed by parents/caregivers
Children Participation Questionnaire (Rosenberg et al. 2010)	Measure of participation in everyday activities in six areas of occupation according to the Occupational Therapy Practice Framework	Diversity and intensity scores	Enjoyment score	Independence score and parent satisfaction score	Areas of education, social participation, play, leisure, activities of daily living and instrumental activities of daily living	In the past 3 months	4–6 years; all diagnostic groups	Questionnaire completed by parents/caregivers

Table 12.1 (continued....)

Measure							
Children's Assessment of Participation and Enjoyment (CAPE) (King et al. 2004)	Participation in leisure activities outside of mandated school activities	Diversity and intensity scores	Enjoyment score	Preferences, where and with whom scores	Activities outside those mandated at school	In the past 4 months	6–21 years; all diagnostic groups	Questionnaire; Self-report using drawings, or interview format (child or proxy)
Participation and Environment Measures for Young Children (YC-PEM)(Khetani et al. 2013) and Children and Youth (PEM-CY) (Coster et al. 2011)	Participation of children in the home, school and community with consideration of environmental factors that support or hinder participation	Frequency score	Involvement score	Environmental helpfulness and environmental resources scores	Home, school and community	In the past 4 months	5–17 years; all diagnostic groups	Online survey or paper/pencil questionnaire completed by parent/caregiver
Pediatric Rehabilitation Intervention Measure of Engagement (PRIME) (King et al. 2019)	Capture affective, cognitive and behavioural involvement for clients and service providers in the client–provider interaction		Engagement		Paediatric rehabilitation	Observation of a session or a video record of a session	Children, youth and parents involved in rehabilitation	PRIME-O is an observational rating of the client, service provider and interaction; PRIME-SP is a service provider rating of the client
School Function Assessment (SFA) (Coster et al. 1998)	Performance on tasks that support participation in activities at school	Part I: participation in same context as his/her peers (composite score)		Part III: functional performance of activities	School	Current	Kindergarten to Grade 6; all diagnostic groups	Questionnaire completed by school personnel familiar with child's participation
Canadian Occupational Performance Measure (COPM) (Law et al. 2014)	Self-perception of occupational performance	Can be applied to quantifying attendance, involvement or related constructs depending on the application of the tool			Not defined	Flexible	All ages and diagnostic groups	Interview child or caregiver

Note: This table focuses on potential measures of attendance and/or involvement. Some measures also include scales/sub-scales that tap one or more of the related constructs of activity competence, sense of self and preferences. Where that occurs, the information is provided in the 'related' constructs column of the table.

> **Box 12.1**   Checklist of factors to consider when selecting measures
>
> **For measures of participation:**
> - Are you interested in:
>   ☐ Attendance or
>   ☐ Involvement in life situations?
> - Which life situations? _____
>
> **For each measure you consider:**
> - What is the purpose of using the measure?
>   ☐ Does the measure's construct and psychometric properties align with your purpose?
> - Does it include scales measuring other attributes (e.g. environment or preferences) and is that helpful or not needed?
> - Is it suitable for your population of interest?
>   ☐ Is it valid for the diagnostic group?
>   ☐ Is it age appropriate?
>   ☐ Is it culturally appropriate?
> - Is it capturing the timeframe of interest in the child's development?
> - Does the format meet your needs?
>   ☐ Is the respondent appropriate – whose perspective is captured?
>   ☐ Is it feasible to use in terms of cost, time and acceptability?
> - Is it reliable?
>   ☐ Is test–retest reliability established if it is a self-report instrument?
>   ☐ Is rater-reliability established if it is an administered instrument?
>   ☐ If you want to measure change over time, is it a responsive tool?

activities when they were younger (Hirvensalo and Lintunen 2011). In a similar way, the experiences of a child or family are likely to influence their ideals and expectations for future participation (King et al. 2006). However, current evidence about longitudinal change in participation suggests relative stability (Imms and Adair 2017; Lygnegård et al. 2013). As even brief reflection indicates that children and adolescents do in fact change both what they do and their involvement in activities over time, these findings suggest we have a somewhat limited approach to measurement, or that we need to reconceptualise how we approach longitudinal evaluation of participation and participation-related constructs. Measurement may need to focus on shorter duration experiences of involvement as well as longer duration attendances. When thinking longitudinally, we need to ensure we are asking the right questions. Do we want to know 'how much' participation is enough, and if so, is the 'how much' related to the duration of attending specific life situations or activity settings, or is it related to 'how much' involvement is enough?

SUMMARY

This chapter has provided an overview of issues that need to be considered when selecting a measure of participation attendance or involvement. Knowledge about measurement properties in general is required, but important issues related to the life situation of interest, the age of the child, and perspectives related to culture, time, respondent and format will all influence the choices made. The following chapter considers measurement from the perspective of participation as a process, rather than an outcome.

SUMMARY OF KEY IDEAS

- Measures are available that quantify participation attendance – these can support measurement of whether individuals with disability attend the same activities as others.
- There are few measures of involvement available at present.
- Measures of involvement will provide information about the extent to which participation actually occurs when an individual attends particular activity settings or life situations.

REFERENCES

Adair B, Ullenhag A, Rosenbaum P, Granlund M, Keen D, Imms C (2018) Measures used to quantify participation in childhood disability and their alignment with the family of participation-related constructs: a systematic review. *Dev Med Child Neurol* **60**: 1101–1116.

Adolfsson M (2011) Applying the ICF-CY to identify children's everyday life situations: A step towards participation-focused code sets. *Int J Soc Welf* **22**: 195–206.

Arvidsson P, Dada S, Granlund M et al. (2019) Content validity and usefulness of Picture My Participation for measuring participation in children with and without intellectual disability in South Africa and Sweden. *Scand J Occup Ther* **10**: 1–13.

Atkin AJ, Sharp SJ, Harrison F, Brage S, Van Sluijs EMF (2016) Seasonal variation in children's physical activity and sedentary time. *Med Sci Sports Exerc* **48**: 449–456.

Baum CM, Edwards D (2001) *Activity Card Sort*. St Louis, MO: Washington University School of Medicine.

Bedell GM (2004) Developing a follow-up survey focused on participation of children and youth with acquired brain injuries after discharge from inpatient rehabilitation. *Neuro Rehabilitation* **19**: 191–205.

Berg C, LaVesser P (2006) The Preschool Activity Card Sort. *Occu Particip Health* **26**: 143–151.

Chiarello LA, Palisano RJ, McCoy SW et al. (2014) Child Engagement in Daily Life: a measure of participation for young children with cerebral palsy. *Disabil Rehabil* **36**: 1804–1816.

Coster W, Deeney T, Haltiwanger J, Haley S (1998) *School Function Assessment*. Texas: The Psychological Corporation, Harcourt Brace (Therapy Skill Builders).

Coster W, Bedell G, Law M et al. (2011) Psychometric evaluation of the Participation and Environment Measure for Children and Youth. *Dev Med Child Neurol* **53**: 1030–1037.

Davidov M, Knafo-Noam A, Serbin LA, Moss E (2015) The influential child: how children affect their environment and influence their own risk and resilience. *Dev Psychopathol* **27**: 947–951.

Engel-Yeger B, Jarus T (2008) Cultural and gender effects on Israeli children's preferences for activities. *Can J Occup Ther* **75**: 139–148.

Engel-Yeger B, Jarus T, Law M (2007) Impact of culture on children's community participation in Israel. *Am J Occup Ther* **61**: 421–428.

Farran D (2014) *Child Observation in Preschool (COP)*. Nashville, TN: Peabody College/Vanderbilt Universit. https://my.vanderbilt.edu/toolsofthemindevaluation/files/2012/01/New-COP-Manual-051414.pdf [Accessed 13 September].

Hardy LL, Dobbins T, Booth ML, Denney-Wilson E, Okely AD (2006) Sedentary behaviours among Australian adolescents. *Aust N Z J Public Health* **30**: 534–540.

Hirvensalo M, Lintunen T (2011) Life-course perspective for physical activity and sports participation. *Eur Rev Aging Phys Act* **8**: 13–22.

Imms C, Adair B (2017) Participation trajectories: impact of school transitions on children and adolescents with cerebral palsy. *Dev Med Child Neurol* **59**: 174–182.

Imms C, Granlund M, Bornman J, Elliott C (2014) Picture my Participation: Research Version 1.0. Unpublished manual, available from the authors.

Imms C, Adair B, Keen D, Ullenhag A, Rosenbaum P, Granlund M (2016) "Participation": a systematic review of language, definitions, and constructs used in intervention research with children with disabilities. *Dev Med Child Neurol* **58**: 29–38.

Imms C, Granlund M, Wilson PH, Steenbergen B, Rosenbaum PL, Gordon AM (2017) Participation, both a means and an end: a conceptual analysis of processes and outcomes in childhood disability. *Dev Med Child Neurol* **59**: 16–25.

Jokovic A, Locker D, Guyatt G (2004) How well do parents know their children? Implications for proxy reporting of child health-related quality of life. *Qual Life Res* **13**: 1297–1307.

Khetani MA, Coster W, Law M, Bedell GM (2013) *Young Children's Participation and Environment Measure (YC-PEM)*. Fort Collins: Colorado State University.

King G, Law M, King S et al. (2004) *Children's Assessment of Participation and Enjoyment (CAPE) and Preferences for Activities of Children (PAC)*. San Antonio, TX: Harcourt Assessment, Inc.

King G, Law M, Hanna S et al. (2006) Predictors of the leisure and recreation participation of children with physical disabilities: A structural equation modeling analysis. *Child Health Care* **35**: 209–234.

King G, Chiarello LA, Thompson L et al. (2019) Development of an observational measure of therapy engagement for pediatric rehabilitation. *Disabil Rehabil* **41**(1): 86–97.

Law M, Baptiste S, Carswell A, Mccoll MA, Polatajko H, Pollock N (2014) *Canadian Occupational Performance Measure Manual*. Ontario: CAOT Publications ACE.

Lygnegård F, Donohue D, Bornman J, Granlund M, Huus K (2013) A systematic review of generic and special needs of children with disabilities living in poverty settings in low- and middle-income countries. *J Policy Pract* **12**: 296–315.

Majnemer A, Shevell M, Law M, Poulin C, Rosenbaum P (2008) Reliability in the ratings of quality of life between parents and their children of school age with cerebral palsy. *Qual Life Res* **17**: 1163–1171.

Mandich A, Polatajko HJ, Miller L, Baum C (2004) *The Paediatric Activity Card Sort (PACS)*. Ottawa: Canadian Association of Occupational Therapists.

Marques JCB, Oliveira JA, Goulardins JB, Nascimento RO, Lima AMV, Casella EB (2013) Comparison of child self-reports and parent proxy-reports on quality of life of children with attention deficit hyperactivity disorder. *Health Qual Life Outcomes* **11**: 186.

Petrenchik T, Law M, King G, Hurley P, Forhan M, Kertoy M (2006) *Assessment of Preschool Children's Participation (APCP)*. Hamilton, ON: CanChild Centre for Childhood Disability Research, McMaster University.

Rosenberg L, Jarus T, Bart O (2010) Development and initial validation of the Children Participation Questionnaire (CPQ). *Disabil Rehabil* **32**: 1633–1644.

Schüttoff U, Pawlowski T (2018) Seasonal variation in sports participation. *J Sports Sci* **36**: 469–475.

Singer JD, Willett JB 2003 *Applied Longitudinal Data Analysis*. New York: Oxford University Press.

Terwee CB, Prinsen CAC, Chiarotto A et al. (2018) COSMIN methodology for evaluating the content validity of patient-reported outcome measures: a Delphi study. *Qua Life Res* **27**: 1159–1170.

Ullenhag A, Almqvist L, Granlund M, Krumlinde-Sundholm L (2012) Cultural validity of the Children's Assessment of Participation and Enjoyment/Preferences for Activities of Children (CAPE/PAC). *Scand J Occup Ther* **19**: 428–438.

UN General Assembly (2007) Convention on the Rights of Persons with Disabilities: Article 3 – resolution adopted by the General Assembly, 24 January 2007 (A/RES/61/106). Paris: UN General Assembly. https://www.refworld.org/docid/45f973632.html [Accessed 11 September 2019].

UN General Assembly (2007) Convention on the Rights of Persons with Disabilities: Article 30 – resolution adopted by the General Assembly, 24 January 2007 (A/RES/61/106). Paris: UN General Assembly. https://www.refworld.org/docid/45f973632.html [Accessed 11 September 2019].

UN General Assembly (2007) Convention on the Rights of Persons with Disabilities: Article 31 – resolution adopted by the General Assembly, 24 January 2007 (A/RES/61/106). Paris: UN General Assembly. https://www.refworld.org/docid/45f973632.html [Accessed 11 September 2019].

Varni JW, Limbers CA, Burwinkle TM 2007 Parent proxy-report of their children's health-related quality of life: An analysis of 13,878 parents' reliability and validity across age subgroups using the PedsQL™ 4.0 Generic Core Scales. Health Qual Life Outcomes **5**: 2.

WHO (2001) *International Classification of Functioning, Disability and Health: Short Version*. Geneva: World Health Organization.

Measuring Participation as a Means: Participation as a Transactional System and a Process

Gillian King, Mats Granlund and Christine Imms

SETTING THE STAGE

What do we mean by participation as a means and as a transactional system? In this chapter we consider how to measure participation as a system of variables changing in relation to one another over time. Think about driving a car on a journey. Your experience will be affected by your driving and navigational skills, the time of day and year (is it late night in winter, or early on a spring morning?), whether you have passengers and who they are (e.g. your grandmother, your boss), your feelings about the anticipated destination (are you tired or excited?; are you going to the dentist?), the road conditions (are you on a busy snow-covered highway or a quiet country road?), and the condition of the car. Thus, your journey is affected by many variables related to both you and the situation (including the passengers, road, and car), which may change in importance throughout your journey and affect one another, reflecting the idea of a system of variables in transaction over time. For example, your driving speed will be affected by the road conditions, and your passengers might affect your navigational skills.

Additionally, this system of variables can be considered and measured from different time perspectives. Your journey can be thought of in relation to the present, future or past: in-the-moment, in anticipation or in remembrance. Your in-the-moment experiences likely encompass various feelings and anticipations. If you were looking back on a fairly long journey, you might think about the events and experiences that made your journey noteworthy, such as all the things that went wrong.

In this chapter, we consider participation in this way – as the experienced, remembered and anticipated journey – and the things affecting the journey.

AIMS OF THE CHAPTER AND LINK TO PRACTICE

Chapter 12 described a range of tools that can measure participation attendance and involvement as an outcome of therapy, education or experience. The goal of the present chapter is to provide the reader with ways of thinking about assessment and measurement from a transactional and systems perspective: that is, focused on participation as a process. The intent is to assist service providers to design quality participation interventions from a process-oriented perspective, and to help them to assess whether interventions are in fact 'quality programmes'. This requires measuring not only participation outcomes, but also aspects of the intervention itself, including its active ingredients and processes. To be able to do this, we need a shared understanding of what is meant by transactions between the person and their environment.

Person–Environment Transactions

By transaction we mean the bi-directional influence of person and environment. The literature includes many terms to describe elements of the environment, including situation, activity setting, niche and context. For clarity, we have defined our use of these general and more specific environment terms, predominantly informed by Bronfenbrenner (1979), Rauthmann (2015) and Rauthmann et al. (2015) as described in Table 13.1. Our conceptualisations of environmental entities are pertinent to both the actual and virtual world. The concepts are ordered from broader and more stable phenomena at the top of the table to more person-centred and less stable phenomena at the bottom.

According to our process-oriented perspective, transactions loop in cycles over time at all levels: environment, context, situation, activity setting and niche. Therefore, the starting place for considering a transaction can be the person or any of the environmental entities. Because both are always implicated in a transaction, it is important to measure aspects of the situation/environment as well as the person's participation experience or related intrapersonal variables. Participation-related outcomes (sense of self,

Table 13.1	Defining constructs related to the environment
Term	**Definition**
Environment	Physical, socio-cultural, institutional, political features and structures in which people live and conduct their lives (Bronfenbrenner 1979; WHO 2001) that are typically stable over time (Rauthmann et al. 2015). Environments contain multiple activity settings, and can be seen as habitual or enduring places, for example, home, work-place, school (Rauthmann et al. 2015), or structures; for example, legal or political systems (Bronfenbrenner 1979)
Context	Context is an abstract construct (Rauthmann et al. 2015) containing situated meaning whereby both the objective and subjective elements of the environment and participatory experience come together. Along with observable dimensions, the 'environmental context' brings in the perceived elements of the social or physical environment; 'situational context' brings in the meaning or value ascribed to the activity setting
Situation	A fluctuating and dynamic circumstance in people's life streams (Rauthmann 2015). 'Situational entities include *occurrence, situation, episode, life event* or *typical situation*' (Rauthmann et al. 2015, p. 18). A typical situation is similar to the idea of 'life situation' proposed by the International Classification of Functioning, Disability and Health and defined by Adolfsson as 'episodes that occur regularly in the natural environments where children usually spend time' (Adolfsson et al. 2010, p. 34)
Activity setting	Activity settings are places where people 'do things' (King et al. 2013, p. 1578) or things happen, and can be measured at one point in time and over time in an aggregated or sequential manner. In Rauthmann's terms, activity settings can be occurrences or situations, depending on duration
Niche	A place where someone thrives (Seligman and Csikszentmihalyi 2000), implying a goodness-of-fit between the person and the activity setting. People select niches that they believe will provide them with certain experiences or outcomes (Wachs 1996). Developmental niches refer to the physical and social settings in which a child lives, the culturally regulated customs of child care and rearing, and the psychology of the caretakers (Super and Harkness 1986)

activity competence or preferences) are dependent on experiences, the opportunities for experiences that are provided, and the supports and resources available – that is, the environmental entity, whether it be a one-off occurrence or series of episodes.

A PROGRAMMATIC PERSPECTIVE TO PARTICIPATION

In health and education literature, measurement of participation is typically focused on an individual, but we can adopt a programme or environmental design lens to understand participation as a designed or optimised process: a means to an end. Inclusive spaces and immersive environments provide useful examples for thinking about what we mean. Inclusive spaces, such as the early childhood education settings described by Björck-Åkesson et al. (2017), meet universal design principles to be free of physical barriers; they are characterised by their welcoming atmosphere; child-centred and friendly approaches; and have furniture, equipment and/or materials that are suitable for all children. Thus any child has the opportunity to exercise choice and to experience engagement in the activity setting. Immersive programmes, such as residential immersive life skills programmes (King et al. 2016a), focus on explicitly designing (and measuring) programme opportunities and intervention strategies that aim to promote participation within the programme, contributing to future participatory and person-centred participation-related outcomes.

To assess transactions, we need to understand what is provided, as well as what is experienced by both the individual and others in the situation. Programmes (educational, psychological, therapeutic, recreational) can be considered as a series of situations. Situational characteristics influence what different children – with and without disabilities – are feeling, thinking and doing in-the-moment (during an occasion) and over time (i.e. sequential episodes or in repeated activity settings) in the programme. In addition, children's subjective experiences and observed behaviours are influenced by how children are interacting with one another and the structures of the situation.

> *What can be measured transactionally in an inclusive space, immersive programme, or other participation-focused intervention?*

If participation is considered from a 'process-oriented, transactional, and systems perspective' then we may be able to identify and measure crucial person- and situation-related variables, and their mechanisms of transaction, to optimise children's participation. These participation outcomes will in turn influence changes in the child's self-determination, self-efficacy and other capacities. This perspective encompasses how situations influence the individual, how the individual's reactions influence others and their situations or environments, and how participation experiences are linked to the changing and adapting self, and life roles (King et al. 2018b).

PERSPECTIVES INFLUENCING MEASUREMENT

Throughout life, people are involved in different life situations that change with their age, expectancies and life roles. In addition, the characteristics of the person (such as activity competence, sense of self and preferences) change with time and age. These dynamic environmental factors and person characteristics affect the construction of the activities in which a person takes part and is engaged in, through life. In a transactional process there are ongoing mutual influences between the child and the environment. Transactional processes can be captured using measures of participation and factors related to participation, which involve both the child and other people in the environment, when the measures are used repeatedly over time.

In this section, we use the terms 'involvement' (reflecting the fPRC) and 'engagement' synonymously. 'Being engaged is both a driver of transactions and an outcome of transactions'. Children who are frequently engaged tend to interact more intensively with the environment, often in a positive way (Sjoman et al. 2016). They interact with other people and navigate the environment to find and construct activity settings that make it possible for them to use their skills. Additionally, they try to avoid activity settings that do not fit with their skills and preferences. In this way, different children may construct different activity settings within the same situation, reflecting individualised patterns of transaction.

When highly engaged in interactions that fit the child, the child learns new skills and may subsequently perceive wellbeing (Aydogan 2012). Children's engagement not only leads to outcomes in terms of learned skills and wellbeing, but also elicits and influences the engagement of other people, which in turn 'drives' new transactions (Sameroff 2009). Other people become engaged by interacting with children who show an interest and active participation in activities. They then tend to invite these children to already established activity settings and to co-create new activity settings that fit the child. Positive transactional processes can be observed in various situational entities, from single occurrences in a specific activity to enduring environments such as school, home and even society.

Assessing the Characteristics of the Situation

In assessing transactional processes, it is very important to assess characteristics of the environment and how these characteristics affect the child and are affected by the child. Rauthmann et al.'s (2015) 'taxonomy of situations' can be used to identify what to assess – abstraction level, duration and dynamicity versus stability – in relation to the types of situational entities (see Table 13.2).

The 'abstraction criterion', or level (i.e. situational entities vary from the highly concrete to the highly abstract), is related to what Bronfenbrenner (1979) describes as ecological levels; from the interactions here and now between the child and the environment, to societal structures such as culture, laws and regulations and attitudes. 'Duration' is the criterion that describes the time spent in different situations, which affects the impact of the situation on the functioning of the person. Measurable aspects of 'duration' include the frequency of attendance, duration of attendance, diversity of situations attended and intensity of the situation attended. Duration is a central aspect when participation attendance is assessed. The criterion 'dynamicity versus stability' concerns how a situation varies over time, from a brief dynamic occurrence in a specific activity to a highly stable typical situation.

In relation to interventions aimed at enhancing engagement in children with disabilities the situational entities 'occurrence', 'situation', 'episode' and 'typical situation' are especially interesting. In Table 13.2, some examples of the four situational entities and the enduring environment are provided.

Each of the situational entities puts different demands on how and what to assess and how to intervene in order to enhance the child's participation. Assessing 'occurrences' can be important for collecting information about how frequently something happens, which can start or sustain transactional processes. For example, we know that children who seldom initiate contact with peers tend to exhibit lower engagement overall and are infrequently exposed to opportunities to participate in peer interactions (Odom et al. 1990). Occurrences may be best assessed through observations or self-report.

Situations provide the opportunity to take an in-depth look at a particular aspect of participation, such as the experience of a birthday party (informal) or of a school outing.

Episodes can be very important to assess as they provide information about how to initiate and start a transactional process between the child and other people. For example, in preschool, peer groups are usually formed within a week after the semester starts. If a child spends almost all the time with a personal assistant rather than with peers, peer groups may have formed before the child is encouraged to interact with other children. Episodes, such as the first week of school, can be observed but also discussed or asked about in a questionnaire or interview.

Table 13.2 Situational and environmental entities: Criteria, examples and measurement approaches

| Entity | Rauthmann criteria[a] | | | Example | Measurement approaches |
	Abstraction	Duration	Dynamicity/stability		
Occurrence[a]	Extremely concrete in specific activity setting	Brief, a few seconds	Highly unstable, occurrence may vary over activities, hours or days	Child initiates interaction with peers; Child initiates play with found objects in the garden	*Assessment of multiple facets of experience in-the-moment* Examples: Self-report measures of experiences Structured observations
Situation[a]	Concrete in environment (home); may include a few activity settings	Short, an hour or two	Unstable and dynamic, may include both predictable and unpredictable activities	Child attends informal birthday party in friend's home	*Assessment of the experience of a defined situation* Examples: Self-report measures of belonging Structured observations of a variety of behaviours indicative of social inclusion
Episode[a]	Concrete in environment (school) but several activity settings occur	Relatively short period, such as one week	Dynamic in activity settings attended but with some stability in terms of environment	Child spends first week at new school with teacher and peers	*Assessment of the occurrence or experience of a discrete type of episode* Examples: Self-report of the experience of the first week of school Structured observations of, for example, peer interactions at recess
Typical situation[a]	Abstract in the sense that the pattern is unknown	Repeated; for example, happens before lunch every day in preschool	Stable in that it reoccurs in a predictable manner in a specific environment	Child spends time with peers in child-constructed play	*Assessment of the experience of a defined situation* Examples: Qualitative assessment of participation experiences Structured observations of others, including staff actions
Enduring environments	Very abstract	Long duration	Stable	Child's sense of participation at school	*Assessment over a longer time frame* Examples: Proxy measures of participation experiences (e.g. at school) Assessments of community integration or social inclusion

[a] Situational and environment entities and criteria as defined by Rauthmann et al. (2015).

Typical situations may be important as the comprise activities in which a planned participation intervention can be implemented that is aimed at eliciting and sustaining transactional processes. Typical situations, such as child-constructed play, can be observed, discussed and assessed through questionnaires. Norm- or criterion-referenced tests are seldom applicable.

Along with identifying the situational entity in focus, we also need to consider their measurable characteristics. Objective assessable elements include place, objects, activity, people, and time (Batorowicz et al. 2016). Individual experiences of a situation, however, may vary based on the meaning carried in the style and content (Rauthmann 2015) of the situation.

For example, the 'situational style' may be:

- formal (or informal);
- active (or passive);
- constrained (or free); or
- involving (or uninvolving).

The 'situational content' may be experienced by an individual as:

- duty (i.e. work oriented);
- adversarial (i.e. competitive);
- friendly, positive (relaxed, pleasant); or
- negative (frightening, unpleasant).

All these aspects can have both social and physical qualities. Information about how situational style can be designed (or influenced), and situational content experienced as growth enhancing, is important to our understanding of how to use participation as a means to promote positive future participation outcomes and development.

MEASURING ASPECTS OF PARTICIPATION RELATED TO CLINICAL PRACTICE

The two dimensions of participation – attendance and involvement – can be applied to two parallel processes in intervention. One process is about how to ensure that the child and the family are attending and involved throughout the intervention process: from identifying their challenges to evaluating their goal attainment. The other process is about the participation issue that brings the child and family to the practitioner. In the two processes, participation in the intervention and formulation of a participation goal, different aspects of how we assess participation and participation-related constructs are important. Through the remainder of the chapter, measures that might be used to support understanding participation as a process are identified, and further described in Table 13.3.

Involvement in Assessment

How assessment tools and measures are used can enhance the active participation of the child and parent(s) in the process. In this respect, child and parent participation starts as soon as interviews and assessment instruments are used to identify the aspects of participation that will be addressed. A key issue is whether or not the child and family are explicitly aware that assessment is occurring (Björck-Åkesson et al. 2000). This is usually self-evident when tests and criterion-referenced instruments are used. However, it is not as self-evident when the assessment involves observing or otherwise gauging the child's participation patterns in activities, child-parent interaction or environmental barriers and facilitators. Such assessment is frequently informal with professionals collecting information from

Table 13.3 Example measures of situations, environments and outcomes that support understanding of 'participation as means'

	Instrument	Purpose	What is measured	Example use
1	Children's Assessment of Participation and Enjoyment and Preferences for Activities of Children (King et al. 2004)	Assess the multidimensional nature of participation in activities outside school, including objective and subjective elements	Diversity; Intensity; With whom; Where; Enjoyment; Preference	Discuss activities that are rated high on preference/enjoyment but low on attendance (diversity/intensity) to identify potential participation restrictions
2	Structured participation interview (Arvidsson et al. 2014)	Assess performance (frequency) and importance of participation in across-life situations	Frequency and importance of participation in activities from nine ICF activity/participation domains	Discuss activities that are rated high on importance but low on frequency of attendance to identify potential participation restrictions
3	Goal Attainment Scaling (Kiresuk et al. 1994)	Set and assess an individualised outcome (goal) using a standardised 5-level scale	Goal content determined by client/caregiver; levels assessed from 'current' (no change expected) to 'much more than expected' (best outcome)	GAS can be used as a means to support the person and the caregivers to clarify their participation attendance and involvement expectations
4	Child Engagement Questionnaire (McWilliam 1991)	Evaluate amount of time spent interacting in the environment in a developmentally and contextually appropriate manner	Engagement (or 'competency' in the fPRC)	To guide staff to actively observe the child's engagement in preschool settings
5	Participation and Environment Measure for Children and Youth (Coster et al. 2012)	Measure participation in the home, school and community with consideration of environmental factors	Attendance, Involvement, Environmental helpfulness and resources	To capture changes/differences in participation in different environments
6	Pediatric Rehabilitation Observational Measure of Fidelity (Di Rezze et al. 2013)	Examine the fidelity of intervention in a generic manner	Fit of programme content to intended intervention	To capture indicators of fidelity in paediatric rehabilitation intervention programmes
7	Service Provider Strategies Checklist (King et al. 2016a)	Evaluate service provider use of strategies – an aspect of process fidelity	Use of teaching/learning techniques, physical/handling interventions, and cognitive, socially-mediated, and non-intrusive strategies	To capture active ingredients within intervention programmes
8	Inclusive Early Childhood Education Environment Self-reflection Tool (Björck-Åkesson et al. 2017)	Identify and measure characteristics reflecting the quality of inclusive early childhood education settings	Structure of programme environment	Staff use tool to reflect on the inclusiveness of their programme's social, learning and physical environment

(Continued)

Table 13.3 (Continued)

	Instrument	Purpose	What is measured	Example use
9	The Measure of Environmental Qualities of Activity Settings (MEQAS) (King et al. 2016b)	Assess the nature of the opportunities provided by activity settings – an aspect of structural fidelity	Extent to which activity settings afford opportunities for: choice, privacy/relaxation, personal growth, physical activity, co-operative group activity, interactions with adults and with peers	Use to determine important qualities of developmentally favourable activity and programme environments
10	State Hope Scale (Snyder et al. 1996)	Assesses sense of goal directed determination and planning to meet goals, that is, a snapshot of current goal directed thinking	Measures current goal directed thinking (agency) and actions (pathways to goals)	Measure of the adapting self to demonstrate outcomes from participation programmes on motivation for future action
11	Dimensions of Mastery Questionnaire (Morgan et al. 2018)	Assesses the persistence and/or reactions/feelings that drive someone to attempt to master a challenging task or skill	Cognitive/object persistence Gross motor persistence Social persistence with adults and children/peers Mastery pleasure Negative reaction to challenge	Measure of the adapting self
12	Self-perception scales (Harter 1982)	Evaluate self-esteem, or self-perceived competence and global self-worth	Scholastic competence Social acceptance Athletic competence Physical appearance Behavioural conduct Global self-worth	Measure the adapting self/sense of self (fPRC) to demonstrate participation-related outcomes from participation programmes

observations and 'small talk' without explicitly informing parents and children that assessment is occurring, and often no instruments are used.

If information is gathered in this informal way there is no pedagogical effect of assessment. This leads to a second key issue. Do the questions asked, or the observations made, require or encourage a response from the child or parent? What can children and parents learn from responding to questions in an interview or questionnaire? Can children and parents understand how the questions asked are related to participation? Does the child have the opportunity to provide his/her perspective? Assessment serves multiple purposes and collecting information is just one. Assessment is also a learning opportunity for the child and family – positive or negative – and, when positive, is a way to build a common frame of reference for children, parents and professionals (see Chapter 14).

> *It is difficult for children and parents to engage in, and learn from, the assessment process if they do not realise it is happening.*

Involvement in Intervention

In addition to being a goal for intervention, participation can be means to an end in any intervention focusing on the child. By increasing involvement in intervention, outcomes related to an individual's activity competence or sense of self can be enhanced. One of the most common reasons for clinical interventions demonstrating small effects is low adherence to the planned intervention methods. Low adherence might be an indicator of low involvement by children and parents. By enhancing involvement in the intervention process, outcomes may be stronger. A simple problem solving model will be used to illustrate the process of involvement in co-designing individualised intervention and evaluation (adapted from Björck-Åkesson et al. 1996). The model contains seven steps:

A. Identifying participation challenges;
B. Developing hypothetical explanations;
C. Prioritising the participation challenge to intervene with;
D. Goal setting;
E. Designing the intervention methods;
F. Implementing the method; and
G. Evaluating goal attainment.

A. Identifying Participation Challenges

A problem or challenge has been defined as the experienced gap between a current state and a desired state (Dunst et al. 1988). A participation challenge can be expressed in several ways such as:

• attending one or several situations too seldom
• never attending one or several situations; or
• attending one or a few situations too frequently.

Challenges can also concern the level of involvement in the same way, from seldom being engaged in one or more situations to being highly engaged but only in a very restricted type of situation.

Applying this definition of problem/challenge raises several ethical concerns. 'Who decides what constitutes a participation problem?' Is the decision based on interviewing the person, observing the person, proxy ratings, interviews with parents, or self-ratings or self-reports? Because participation contains the subjective involvement dimension it is important that, if possible, the person him/herself decides what constitutes a participation challenge. However, the individual's lack of experience and current participation restrictions can lead to a lack of information about what participation opportunities are available or what is possible. Therefore, it is likely that information from the person as well as others in the person's environment will be needed.

'Challenges or experiences tend to come in clusters' (Sameroff 2009). For example, participating very infrequently in a specific social situation tends to increase the probability that other social situations are attended with low frequency. This clustering tendency makes it important to survey patterns of partici-

> **LINK TO MEASURE**
> *See item 1, Table 13.3.*

> **LINK TO MEASURE**
> *See item 2, Table 13.3.*

pation rather than only single situations. It is also important to support the person in identifying challenges to understand what their perceived participation challenges have in common. One means for doing this is to talk with the person about their challenges by comparing ratings of the attendance and involvement dimensions of participation When reviewing the ratings from measures like CAPE/PAC (King et al. 2004) and the Structured Participation Interview (Arvidsson et al. 2014), activities that are rated high on enjoyment/importance but low on attendance are especially important to discuss. It is possible that the combined attendance-involvement index can be described as a measure of perceived participation restriction (Arvidsson et al. 2014).

B. Developing Hypothetical Explanations

When several participation challenges have been identified it is time to come up with several hypothetical explanations for them. Typically, this is undertaken when practitioners assess children using a range of measures thought to tap factors related to the issue at hand. According to Rusk et al. (2018), most problems with everyday functioning are related to several influences that, when orchestrated, impact functioning. In the fPRC framework, the attendance and involvement dimensions of participation are hypothesised to be influenced by factors intrinsic to the person (activity competence, sense of self and preferences), by factors in the situation, and by factors in the environment that exist independent of the person.

It is important to assess the influencing factors separately and to discuss how they interact with each other. From a transactional perspective, person-based and situational explanations of issues are interrelated. Therefore each explanation focused on the person has to be supplemented by situational/environmental explanations. For example, if a child's cognitive functioning is assessed, then, to find a hypothetical explanation, the results have to be related to how other people adapt to the child in terms of verbal complexity, the type of activities offered, and so on.

'If people are actively involved in explaining their participation challenges, their autonomy in solving the problems increases' (Pittman et al. 2003). By knowing the explanations, parents and children are more able to personally design and test different interventions (i.e. solutions). It is especially important to identify hypothetical explanations that can affect several participation challenges. Lack of transportation is, for example, one frequently occurring explanation for low attendance, while low responsiveness of adults is a relatively frequent explanation for low engagement/involvement. The more hypothetical explanations that are identified, the easier it is to propose a multimodal/multidimensional intervention. This is important, because interventions commonly only address one explanation at a time (e.g. training skills only) and therefore are unlikely to lead to sustainable changes in participation (Rusk et al. 2018).

C. Prioritising The Participation Challenge To Intervene With

Addressing the explicit priorities of the person and the family is very important. It is also important to facilitate understanding of patterns of participation and hypothetical explanations to participation patterns. For example, if transportation is an explanation to many participation restrictions in the community for an adolescent with mild intellectual disability, it might be better to focus intervention on supporting the person in using public transport rather than solely on providing someone to accompany the person to a few community activities every second week.

D. Goal Setting

Sometimes it is difficult for the person or the family to prioritise among challenges. In such instances it might be helpful to mix prioritising with goal setting. For example, the person can be asked to concretely describe how the situation and participation would be improved if a certain challenge was addressed. Developing descriptions of goal attainment can be facilitated by using a Goal Attainment Scale (GAS, Kiresuk et al. 1994). In this instance, the GAS is not primarily seen as a measurement instrument but rather as a means to support the person and the parents/caregivers to clarify their expectations.

> LINK TO MEASURE
> See item 3, Table 13.3.

Participation goals can be formulated on several situational/environmental levels, from occasions (e.g. increasing the frequency of use of participation enhancing actions such as initiating interactions with other children) to targeting participation in a new environment (e.g. facilitating supported employment). If possible, goals should be formulated so that it is possible to experience and/or observe positive changes within just a few weeks.

E. Designing the Intervention Methods

In designing methods or solutions, the child and/or parents (depending on the child's age) are guided through a reasoning process where they try to see how the different explanations can be used to design solutions. This is possible when explanations are illustrated by the results of assessments. If the explanations only exist in the professional's mind, it is very difficult for the person and parents to understand the mechanisms of the intervention method. If they don't understand the mechanisms, they become dependent on the professionals and it is difficult for them to adapt or change the methods if they are not working well. It is more likely that the solutions will lead to goal attainment if several explanations and solutions are combined (Rusk et al. 2018).

F. Implementing the Method

Implementation of solutions requires that the person, as well as parents and others who are taking part in implementation, are motivated, have the knowledge necessary to be autonomous in implementing, and receive feedback on how it is going. Instruments used to assess participation challenges can also be used to support implementation, for example the Child Engagement Questionnaire (McWilliam 1991) can be used to support staff in actively observing the child's engagement. To be used effectively, professionals have to ask for information, provide feedback and discuss how the implementation is working. Usually the

> LINK TO MEASURE
> See item 4, Table 13.3.

child, parents and other actors in the child's natural setting will experience some difficulties with implementation, especially within the first 2 weeks. It is therefore especially important to provide feedback in this time period to enhance motivation or engagement with implementing the solution.

G. Evaluating Goal Attainment

How goal attainment is evaluated is partly dependent on the situational level of the participation challenge. As shown in Table 13.2, goals related to occurrences, specific situations and episodes are probably best evaluated by intervention-specific observational measures or self-reports. Typical, recurring situations can be evaluated by situation-specific assessments both of the participation challenge and other aspects of the situation (e.g. staff actions when children are involved in free play in preschool). At the level of the environment, several proxy measures and assessments exist that can be used to assess changes in

LINK TO MEASURE
See item 5, Table 13.3.

participation within each environment such as home, school or leisure [e.g. Participation and Environment Measure for Children and Youth (Coster et al. 2012); see also Chapter 12].

Section Summary

Participation is always contextualised and contains both the more objective dimension of attendance and the more subjective dimension of involvement. Involvement can be operationalised as engagement 'here and now' or as ratings or reports made before or after taking part in a situation – whether that situation is therapy or another life situation. Participation challenges and hypothetical explanations to participation challenges can be identified on several situational levels, from brief occurrences to relatively stable events to recurring typical situations or even enduring environments. Assessment methods and instruments match the different types of situations to different degrees.

MEASURING THE ACTIVE INGREDIENTS AND PROCESSES OF PARTICIPATION-ORIENTED INTERVENTION PROGRAMMES

In paediatric rehabilitation there is growing interest in defining, operationalising and measuring the key ingredients and processes of programmes (i.e. group therapy programmes such as life skills or arts-mediated programmes, rather than one-on-one therapy). In addition to measuring outcomes, measuring process is an important aspect of evidence-based practice (Peterson et al. 1982). In both treatment process literature (Armitage et al. 2017) and literature on theory-based programme evaluation (Harachi et al. 1999) there is an interest in identifying active ingredients and programme processes, as well as the client change mechanisms by which these elements of programme delivery affect desired outcomes. For example, instructional practice (or training) is a programme process, whereas the underlying operative mechanism refers to the response these activities generate in the client, such as increased knowledge or increased feelings of self-efficacy.

In this section, we consider how to measure three aspects related to participation from a transactional systems perspective: the programme environment, the adapting self and context–mechanism–outcome patterns of participation. Box 13.1 illustrates how the programme theory underlying a youth transitions programme serves to identify possible active ingredients and client change mechanisms underlying youth outcomes. The example highlights measurement of programme **opportunities**, service provider **strategy use**, youth **experiences** (client change mechanisms) and youth **outcomes**.

Measuring the Programme 'Environment'

There are relatively few measures of optimal programme environments conducive to enhancing children's participation outcomes. If we take a systems view of participation, the importance of considering the environment becomes evident, pointing to the need to measure environmental affordances and the nature of the strategies used by service providers delivering programmes to children and youth with disabilities.

What aspects of the programme 'environment' are thought to bring about positive participation experiences? What aspects of programme format, content and delivery engage children in ways that enhance positive participation outcomes?

> **Box 13.1 The independence programme**
>
> *Description* This residential immersive youth life skills programme provides opportunities for youth with disabilities to develop and practice the life skills they will need in adult life. Youth attend an away-from-home group programme for 3 weeks. The programme takes place in a college residence and provides instruction in life skills, multiple experiential opportunities to practice these skills, and appreciable opportunities for youth to interact with other youth outside of scheduled programme activities.
>
> *Programme theory* The programme is based on an ecological and experiential approach. Opportunities provided by immersion in real-life, supportive and growth-enhancing activity settings are thought to set the stage for youth experiences involving personal growth, choice and social interaction that lead, over time and when youth return to their home and community, to enhanced awareness of strengths, sense of self-identity, a broadened sense of life opportunities and other positive developmental benefits.
>
> *Measurement of key ingredients, change processes and outcomes* Using mixed methods, studies have pointed to the importance of: creating a supportive programme atmosphere with multiple **opportunities** for social interaction, choice and personal growth; using socially-mediated, teaching/learning and non-intrusive **strategies** to support, encourage and engage youth; and, intentionally fostering youth **experiences** of social belonging, choice and control, psychological engagement and meaningful interactions (King et al. 2016a). Qualitative case studies are being used to link the findings to different trajectories of change, and to youth benefits or **outcomes** involving awareness of new opportunities, sense of hope for the future, self-determination, milieu selection and the creation of new goals.

Important qualities, attributes or active ingredients of the programme environment have been examined using measures of fidelity. Fidelity measures indicate whether a programme is in fact delivered as intended and are typically observational. Process aspects of fidelity capture service provider behaviours and intervention strategies, whereas structural aspects include the nature of the programme's opportunities. In a programme purporting to be client-directed, do service providers interact with children using strategies that reflect this philosophy, and are there adequate opportunities for children to make choices?

Table 13.3 provides examples of programme measures that can be used to measure important active ingredients in real-life or video-recorded intervention sessions, including multiple sessions of intervention. Some measures capture elements of the programme processes such as the Pediatric Rehabilitation Observational Measure of Fidelity (Di Rezze et al. 2013) or the Service Provider Strategies Checklist (King et al. 2016a).

LINK TO MEASURE
See items 6 & 7, Table 13.3.

Other measures, such as the Inclusive Early Childhood Education Environment Self-Reflectiontool (Björck-Åkesson et al. 2017) and the Measure of Environmental Qualities of Activity Settings (MEQAS) (King et al. 2016b), address programme structures or the opportunities of activity settings.

LINK TO MEASURE
See items 8 & 9, Table 13.3.

Measuring 'The Adapting Self'

From a transactional systems perspective and the fPRC, it is important to be able to capture changes to the self in response to changing situations and environments, including programme environments. Here we consider changes in the self that arise from participation-oriented intervention. We use the term 'the adapting self' to indicate changes to self-perceptions of capacities, self-concept, self-identity and expectations for the future, all of which can be considered integral to change due to intervention.

Changes in self-perceptions are often examined in research, as they are considered necessary for sustainable and transferable participatory changes. We view 'the adapting self' as fundamental to personal change through intervention, and as part of a system of variables implicated in changes to participation in real-life. Similarly, Kang and colleagues' (2014) model of optimal participation emphasises the importance of self-perceptions and participation experiences. The model highlights the dynamic interaction of physical, social and self-engagement and attributes of the child, family and environment. Thus, both this model and the fPRC provide a strong rationale for examining changes in the self (e.g. changes in self-concept, self-identity and self-awareness) as 'indicators' of mechanisms underlying clinical change. Furthermore, 'the adapting self' can be seen as a marker of self-regulatory processes leading to adaptive benefits (King et al. 2018b).

Self-variables with state-like qualities amenable to change and with implications for future action are important to consider and measure, such as self-efficacy, mastery motivation, self-determination, self-concept and sense of hope. Such future-directed self-variables are key to

> **LINK TO MEASURE**
> *See items 10, 11 & 12, in Table 13.3.*

demonstrating positive outcomes from participation programmes because they have a motivational or self-regulatory aspect. Changes in these self-perceptions can be measured. Measures used in paediatric rehabilitation include the State Hope Scale (Snyder et al. 1996), the Dimensions of Mastery Questionnaire (Morgan et al. 2018) and Harter's (1982) measure of self-concept.

From a systems perspective, by quantitatively measuring important aspects of the self at different points in time, and also measuring aspects of the environment, we can determine whether the self is indeed changing, and in response to which set of experiential opportunities. Qualitative methods can also be used to understand 'the adapting self', as illustrated by a recent study exploring mechanisms of change for children participating in therapeutic horse riding (Martin et al. 2018). This study used interviews and participant-observation to develop a grounded theory illustrating mechanisms of change.

To investigate the nature of the adapting self, we require measures appropriate for children to complete, methods or measures to obtain family perspectives on changes to their child or youth's sense of self, and we need to measure these changes at various time points, given that time may be critical in allowing the repeated effects and reflections needed to generate a change in one's sense of self.

Measuring Context–Mechanism–Outcome Patterns of Participation

In the previous sections, we considered how to measure aspects of the programme environment and 'the adapting self', both of which are important in a transactional systems view of participation. In this final section, we consider the need to look at patterns, unfolding over time, comprising a number of participation-related person and situational/environmental variables, mechanisms of client change and participation outcomes. Specifically, we consider the clinical utility of understanding and measuring context–mechanism–outcome (CMO) linkages (Hewitt et al. 2014) and thus pathways to participation outcomes.

The notion of CMO linkages reflects a realist perspective on how things work. Context refers to the situation or programme environment – the contextual variables that trigger client change mechanisms. Mechanisms refer to a wide range of processes. Outcomes are the end result. Consider how a mastery experience, a positive interaction with a peer, or 'being believed in' by someone can influence how a child sees her/his self, has a sense of new possibilities, or has new confidence, and how those 'processes' lead to seeking or taking new participation opportunities, with cascading/cumulative effects over time. In our programme theory example in Box 13.1, the CMO linkages of interest involve programme opportunities and service provider strategies (context), self-change due to experiential learning (mechanisms) and a variety of developmental benefits for youth (outcome).

At present, there are few studies of CMO linkages in paediatric rehabilitation; however, the findings of existing studies show the potential of this approach for measuring the complex phenomenon of participation. We informally reviewed paediatric rehabilitation studies of child or youth participation that explicitly investigated at least two of the components of context, mechanism and outcome. We found a mix of qualitative and quantitative studies examining a range of participation-related phenomena, including the factors and processes affecting children's perceptions of their physical activity participation (Arnell et al. 2017), the context, mechanisms and outcomes of a participation-focused physical activity intervention (Willis et al. 2018), and the processes and outcomes of a therapeutic horse riding programme (Martin et al. 2018). Other studies examined links between learning engagement and learning outcomes in a lab simulation of preschool learning situations (Halliday et al. 2018), the processes and outcomes of youth engagement in a solution-focused coaching intervention targeting participation goals (King et al. 2018a), and the programme opportunities and service provider strategies linked to youth experiences (King et al. 2016a).

The context variables in these studies (operationalised and measured, rather than assumed) included opportunities for experiences, service provider strategies and service variables such as service intensity and family-centred care. Thus, context variables ranged from micro structural aspects (strategies) to more macro service variables (intensity, duration, type of service), reflecting some of the active ingredients discussed previously. Client change mechanisms (inferred qualitatively or directly measured) included motivation, engagement, self-efficacy and self-confidence, and experiences related to self-determination theory (mastery or success, learning or personal growth; autonomy, agency or choice; belonging or social interaction). Outcomes included self-efficacy and self-variables, participation (including attainment of participation goals), friendships and learning. Thus, the processes of interest in these studies were motivation-related, and there was overlap between process and outcome (i.e. an outcome in one study was considered a process in another).

These findings suggest the necessity of paying attention to the measurement of context in studies of participation. The findings also indicate the growing interest in directly examining client change mechanisms reflecting person–environment transactions over time, and the varied nature of participation outcomes.

CMO linkages imply the operation of a group of variables affecting change in complex interventions, as described in the Synergistic Change Model (Rusk et al. 2018). Thus, one way of examining CMO linkages is to measure a constellation of variables using a battery of tools assessing person, situation–environment, mechanism–process and outcomes; all related to a particular participation context. Examining CMO linkages will allow us to deconstruct the nature of 'optimal' participation in various contexts, its determinants, and its sequelae (and how these in turn influence future person-situation transactions). This work may indicate constellations of variables that reveal important patterns of participation variables, and inform the ways and means in which we intervene to bring these about.

FUTURE DIRECTIONS

Considering participation as a process involves acknowledging and working with complexity. This challenge for practice and research is real, and involves being able to consider multiple dimensions in the design and evaluation of participation-promoting interventions and activity settings. Current evidence for interventions to promote participation outcomes indicates that carefully selected multiple strategies that target the individual and elements of the setting are effective (see Part IV, Chapter 17). For example, interventions that (1) focus on intrinsically motivating activities (meaningful participation goals); (2) enable access and attendance at relevant activities (through modification of the setting); (3) provide peer or other mentoring (engaging alongside, believing in one another) and support (aimed at negotiating for positive accommodations required by the individual to take part); and (4) facilitate practice of needed skills, can result in increased self-efficacy that can support future sustained participation in desired leisure activities.

Rusk et al.'s (2018) Synergistic Change Model provides theoretical support for the notion of 'targeting mutually reinforcing elements' (p. 8) to achieve lasting change. Other mechanisms of change that might be considered in complex and dynamic systems include targeting 'pivotal elements'; for example, engagement experiences that might lead to new strengths or 'leveraging existing strengths and values' (p. 7). The field needs research that provides clarity about the nature of the key mechanisms that have demonstrated empirical relationships with child/youth outcomes. As another future direction, measuring CMO linkages is important as it provides us with knowledge about how participation interventions work. This knowledge reinforces the importance of enabling participation in context and over the lifespan.

Some of the questions to address in future research and practice include: What experiences are provided by participation in context? How will we address the unique nature of participation satisfaction, along with the shifts and trade-offs that we know can occur with changing circumstances? How do we understand the participation of an individual in isolation (as is common in research and practice) when the reality is individuals are influential within their settings and contexts and their actions and choices influence the situation for others (Davidov et al. 2015)? Does what we learn about participation as a process influence how we conceptualise the construct?

CONCLUSION

Although there appears to be general acceptance of the notion that participation is both a process and an outcome, clarity about what constitutes the 'process' is needed. Taking a transactional, systems approach to participation and participation intervention highlights elements of both the person and the situation that need to be in focus when designing effective interventions. This chapter provided ways to consider participation as a process with a focus on both what to measure and how to measure it. Part IV of the book explores participation as either a dependent (the outcome) or independent (the process) variable in interventions.

SUMMARY OF KEY IDEAS

- Participation can be measured as a system of variables in the person and the environment changing in relation to one another over time, that is, transactions.
- Transactions occur between the person and various situational entities, in both real-world and therapy environments.
- How we measure participation will differ for different situational entities, such as occurrences, situations, episodes, and also for enduring environments.
- Examining context–mechanism–outcome linkages may be a useful approach to capture the complexities of the participation process.

REFERENCES

Adolfsson M, Malmqvist J, Pless M, Granuld M (2011) Identifying child functioning from an ICF-CY perspective: everyday life situations explored in measures of participation. *Disabil Rehabil* **33**: 1230–1244.

Armitage S, Swallow V, Kolehmainen N (2017) Ingredients and change processes in occupational therapy for children: a grounded theory study. *Scand J Occup Ther* **24**: 208–213.

Arnell S, Jerlinder K, Lundqvist L (2017) Perceptions of physical activity participation among adolescents with autism spectrum disorders: A conceptual model of conditional participation. *J Autism Dev Disord* **48**(5): 1792–1802.

Arvidsson P, Granlund M, Thyberg I, Thyberg M (2014) Important aspects of participation and participation restrictions in people with a mild intellectual disability. *Disabil Rehabil* **36**: 1264–1272.

Aydogan C (2012) *Influences of Instructional and Emotinal Classroom Environments and Learning Engagement on Low-Income Children's Achievement in the Prekindergarten Year.* Nashville, TN: Vanderbilt University.

Batorowicz B, King G, Mishra L, Missiuna C (2016) An integrated model of social environment and social context for pediatric rehabilitation. *Disabil Rehabil* **38**: 1204–1215.

Björck-Åkesson E, Granlund M, Olsson C (1996) Collaborative problem solving in communication interventions. In: Von Tetchner S, Hygum-Jensen M (Eds) *Augmentative and Alternative Communication – European Perspectives.* London: Whurr.

Björck-Åkesson E, Granlund M, Simeonsson R (2000) Assessment philosophies and practices in Sweden. In: Guralnick M (Ed) *Interdisciplinary Clinical Assessment of Young Children with Developmental Disabilities.* Baltimore: Paul H. Brookes.

Björck-Åkesson E, Kyriazopoulou M, Giné C, Bartolo P (2017) *Inclusive Early Childhood Education Environment Self-Reflection Tool.* Odense: European Agency for Special Needs and Inclusive Education.

Bronfenbrenner U (1979) *The Ecology of Human Development: Experiments by Nature and Design.* Cambridge, MA; Harvard University Press.

Coster W, Law M, Bedell G, Khetani M, Cousins M, Teplicky R (2012) Development of the participation and environment measure for children and youth: conceptual basis. *Disabil Rehabil* **34**: 238–246.

Davidov M, Knafo-Noam A, Serbin LA, Moss E (2015) The influential child: how children affect their environment and influence their own risk and resilience. *Dev Psychopathol* **27**: 947–951.

Di Rezze B, Law M, Eva K, Pollock N, Gorter JW (2013) Development of a generic fidelity measure for rehabilitation intervention research for children with physical disabilities. *Dev Med Child Neurol* **55**: 737–744.

Dunst CJ, Trivette CM, Deal AG (1988) *Enabling and Empowering Families.* Cambridge, MA: Brookline Books.

Halliday SE, Calkins SD, Leerkes EM (2018) Measuring preschool learning engagement in the laboratory. *J Exp Child Psychol* **167**: 93–116.

Harachi TW, Abbott RD, Catalano RF, Haggerty KP, Fleming CB (1999) Opening the black box: using process evaluation measures to assess implementation and theory building. *Am J Community Psychol* **27**: 711–731.

Harter S (1982) The Perceived Competence Scale for children. *Child Dev* **53**: 87–97.

Hewitt G, Sims S, Harris R (2014) Using realist synthesis to understand the mechanisms of interprofessional teamwork in health and social care. *J Interprof Care* **28**: 501–506.

Kang LJ, Palisano RJ, King GA, Chiarello LA (2014) A multidimensional model of optimal participation of children with physical disabilities. *Disabil Rehabil* **36**: 1735–1741.

King GA, Law M, King S et al. (2004) *Children's Assessment of Participation and Enjoyment and Preferences for Activities of Kids.* San Antonio, TX: PsychCorp.

King G, Rigby P, Batorowicz B (2013) Conceptualizing participation in context for children and youth with disabilities: an activity setting perspective. *Disabil Rehabil* **35**: 1578–1585.

King G, Kingsnorth S, McPherson A et al. (2016a). Residential immersive life skills programs for youth with physical disabilities: A pilot study of program opportunities, intervention strategies, and youth experiences. *Res Dev Disabil* **55**: 242–255.

King G, Rigby P, Avery L (2016b). Revised Measure of Environmental Qualities of Activity Settings (MEQAS) for youth leisure and life skills activity settings. *Disabil Rehabil* **38**: 1509–1520.

King G, Schwellnus H, Keenan S, Chiarello LA (2018a) Youth engagement in pediatric rehabilitation: service providers' perceptions in a real-time study of solution-focused coaching for participation goals. *Phys Occup Ther Pediatr* **38**: 527–547.

King G, Seko Y, Chiarello L, Thompson L, Hartman L (2018b) Building blocks of resiliency in pediatric rehabilitation: A framework of health-related adversities, self-capacities, self-regulatory processes, and adaptive benefits. *Disabil Rehabil* **14**: 1–10.

Kiresuk TJ, Smith A, Cardillo JE (1994) *Goal Attainment Scaling: Applications, Theory and Measurement.* Hillsdale, NJ: L. Erlbaum Associates.

Martin R, Graham F, Taylor W, Levack W (2018) Mechanisms of change for children participating in therapeutic horse riding: A grounded theory. *Phys Occup Ther Pediatr* **38**(5): 510–526.

McWilliam RA (1991) *Child Engagement Questionnaire: Instrument*. Chapel Hill, NC: Frank Porter Graham Child Development Center, University of North Carolina.

Morgan GA, Wang J, Barrett KC, Liao H, Wang P, Huang S, Jozsa K (2018) *The Revised Dimensions of Mastery Questionnaire (DMQ 18)*. Fort Collins, CO: Colorado State University.

Odom S, Peterson C, McConnell S, Ostrosky M (1990) Ecobehavioural analysis of early intervention/specialized classroom settings and peer social interaction. *Educ Treat Child* **13**: 316–330.

Peterson L, Homer AL, Wonderlich SA (1982) The integrity of independent variables in behavior analysis. *J Appl Behav Anal* **15**: 477–492.

Pittman K, Irby M, Tolman J, Tohalem N, Ferber T (2003) *Preventing Problems, Promoting Development, Encouraging Engagement: Compelling Priorities or Inseparable Goals?* Based on Pittman K, Irby M (1996) *Preventing Problems or Promoting Development?* Washington DC: The Forum for Youth Investment, Impact Strategies, Inc. http://citeseerx.ist.psu.edu/viewdoc/download?doi=10.1.1.471.1224&rep=rep1&type=pdf [Accessed 7 October 2019].

Rauthmann JF (2015) Structuring situational information – a roadmap of the multiple pathways to different situational taxonomies. *Eur Psychol* **20**: 176–189.

Rauthmann JF, Sherman RA, Fuller D (2015) New horizons in research on psychological situations and environments. *Eur J Pers* **29**: 382–432.

Rusk RD, Vella-Brodrick DA, Waters L (2018) A complex dynamic systems approach to lasting positive change: the synergistic change model. *J Posit Psychol* **13**: 406–418.

Sameroff AJ (2009) *The Transactional Model of Development: How Children and Contexts Shape Each Other*. Washington, DC: American Psychological Association.

Seligman MEP, Csikszentmihalyi M (2000) Positive psychology. An introduction. *Am Psychol* **55**: 5–14.

Sjoman M, Granlund M, Almqvist L (2016) Interaction processes as a mediating factor between children's externalized behaviour difficulties and engagement in preschool. *Early Child Dev Care* **186**: 1649–1663.

Snyder CR, Sympson SC, Ybasco FC, Borders TF, Babyak MA, Higgins RL (1996) Development and validation of the State Hope Scale. *J Pers Soc Psychol* **70**: 321–335.

Super CM, Harkness S (1986) The developmental niche: A conceptualization at the interface of child and culture. *Int J Behav Dev* **9**: 545–569.

Wachs TD (1996) Known and potential processes underlying developmental trajectories in childhood and adolescence. *Dev Psychol* **32**: 796–801.

WHO (2001) *International Classification of Functioning, Disability and Health: Short Version*. Geneva: World Health Organization.

Willis CE, Reid S, Elliott C, Rosenberg M, Nyquist A, Jahnsen R, Girdler S (2018) A realist evaluation of a physical activity participation intervention for children and youth with disabilities: what works, for whom, in what circumstances, and how? *BMC Pediatr* **18**: 113.

Measurement Challenges

Christine Imms, Jessica M Jarvis, Mary A Khetani and Bridget O'Connor

This chapter summarises important challenges to measuring participation that must be addressed to advance participation-focused work in clinical practice. At present, there are challenges to knowing what, when and where to assess participation, and to selecting the most appropriate instrument or process. Most importantly, we propose that clinicians need to be repeatedly challenged to reflect on and address *how* they implement assessment processes with children and their families.

KNOWING WHAT TO ASSESS, AND WHERE AND WHEN TO ASSESS IT: THE COMPLEXITY OF CONTEXT

Our attempt to unpack contextual factors that shape children's participation has revealed that most studies to date focus on modelling children's participation as an outcome and employ gross estimates of extrinsic factors, excluding data on intrinsic factors altogether in their analyses. While these studies offer great value in establishing the role of a child's environment on their participation, this approach does not yield comprehensive and granular knowledge about the relative impact of specific contextual factors on participation.

Practitioners can benefit from knowing which contextual factors are more salient in shaping a child's participation across time. Most studies examine context through general environmental measures. Some studies emphasise select features of the child's environment (Clarke et al. 2011), others adopt a multidimensional assessment of environment (Albrecht and Khetani 2017). In either case, researchers use one or more sum scores to capture environmental impact on participation (e.g. caregiver perceptions of home environmental support) (Albrecht and Khetani 2017; Anaby et al. 2014; Khetani et al. 2018a). It might be more clinically meaningful to examine contextual factors as individual items, or by deriving multiple summary scores (e.g. summary scores representing micro-, meso- and macro-levels of environmental impacts), to build knowledge that can shape participation-focused interventions.

In addition to what we assess, when we assess is important to consider. Most studies to date examine contextual factors using cross-sectional study designs, providing limited guidance for practice. Future research would benefit from a longitudinal approach to understand how these factors influence each other over time as this knowledge is needed to guide practice. Few studies examine participation change (Anaby et al. 2012; Khetani et al. 2018a; Imms and Adair 2017), and their follow-up period may have been too short to detect change (Khetani et al. 2018a). Technology-based approaches to data collection (Khetani et al. 2018b), particularly when integrated within electronic data capture systems, may be useful in harmonising data collection for these needed studies (Khetani 2017).

> *Longitudinal research is needed to understand the complex interplay of participation and context over time.*

Longitudinal study designs also offer new analytic opportunities. Developmental scientists often frame studies using a person–process–context–time model and transactional perspective (Bronfenbrenner and Morris 2006; Sameroff and Mackenzie 2003): novel methods for examining these relationships longitudinally. It is possible we can glean from approaches developed in this field (e.g. cross-lagged panel models, sequential cohort designs) the bidirectional linkages between intrinsic and extrinsic factors over time. These approaches capture intrinsic factors specific to the caregiver and child over time. One growing body of developmental studies examines reciprocal pathways between positive parent–child transactions and children's developing social-emotional adjustment (Lunkenheimer et al. 2013). While these studies acknowledge parenting occurs in the context of the home environment (Bradley 2015), their home environment measure – of cognitive stimulation and emotional support – may not capture the most salient aspects for children with neurodisability. The methodological approach, however, remains useful for examining how intrinsic and extrinsic factors shape children's participation over time.

Accelerating knowledge about children's participation requires careful consideration regarding how to measure both extrinsic and intrinsic factors and report contextual factors (e.g. individual items or summary scores). These decisions, along with selection of appropriate study methodology (e.g. cross-sectional versus longitudinal) and consideration of analytic models for contextual variables (e.g. mediating variable, outcome variable), will advance the field.

SELECTING THE MOST APPROPRIATE TOOL, INSTRUMENT OR PROCESS

We are often guilty of measuring what we can measure rather than what we need to measure. This can be a problem because 'what we measure shapes what we collectively strive to pursue' (Stiglitz et al. 2009, p. 9). For example, if our primary measure is at the level of body function or skilled performance, that is what we tend to pursue. If we wish to pursue participation outcomes, then that should shape what we measure. A systematic review of measures of participation suggests we are trying to do this in childhood disability research and practice (Adair et al. 2018). Although the review identified 309 measures, few measures included the involvement construct. This is an immediate challenge. If what you measure is what you learn, and we do not have adequate measures of participation involvement, then we likely have inadequate understanding of the experience of involvement.

This assumption is supported by the fact that of the 11 'involvement' measures reviewed, over half measured enjoyment (Adair et al. 2018). While important, enjoyment does not sufficiently capture involvement. The Participation and Environment Measures capture 'involvement', which at its peak is defined as 'your child is actively engaged most of the time. He/she interacts and/or is helpful for most of the activity' (Coster et al. 2011; Khetani 2015). In these measures, the word 'engaged' is used to define involvement, suggesting that 'involvement' and 'engagement' might be synonyms.

Review of 13 measures of 'engagement' that use observation of behaviour as the assessment method, designed for young children, supports the notion that the construct of engagement has cognitive (thinking about what you are doing), affective (how you feel about what you are doing) and behavioural (what you are doing) components. Although this provides a more detailed understanding of engagement, it is not yet clear whether the constructs of involvement and engagement are synonymous. Currently we view involvement as a multidimensional construct describing the experience of participation that has elements of engagement, which itself is multidimensional (e.g. orientation to, or action with, objects and/or people), persistence (e.g. time spent, sustained effort), perhaps social connection (interactions with others and/or a sense of belonging; but you can also participate in activities all by yourself) and affect (which includes more than the idea of enjoyment).

The key questions going forward are:

- Is involvement as a construct observable:
  - at the level of the brain?
  - in individual behaviour?
  - between people?
  - between ecological systems?
- Who should rate it and how? Or, how else should it be measured?
- What are the multiple dimensions, and how can they be rated in a way that gives credence to the complexity and importance of the construct?

Solving this measurement problem is crucial, as involvement is the fundamental participatory outcome. Of course, those with childhood onset neurodisability should be able to attend the same situations as others, but being involved while attending is the element that makes the effort worthwhile and can shift the lived experience to being positive and growth enhancing.

Involvement is the fundamental participatory outcome, so we need to know how to measure it.

In Chapter 9, therapy was described as one life situation that those with childhood onset disability might experience. The experience of assessment in practice is the third key challenge for us to address.

LINK TO VIGNETTE 14.1
'Jack in the Box', p. 170.

APPROACHING ASSESSMENT FROM A STRENGTHS-BASED PERSPECTIVE: THE CHALLENGE OF *'HOW'*

The principles of family-centred care (King et al. 2006) are endorsed as 'how we should operate' as practitioners. Whether practitioners adopt a relational practice approach (Epsi-Sherwindt 2008) or a participatory practice approach (Dunst et al. 2002), their use of a family-centred frame supports more positive outcomes for children and families (Moore et al. 2009; Trivette et al. 2010). This occurs by involving our clients – including the individual and family members – in ways that support their commitment and investment in care (Bright et al. 2015), and in ways that value and respect their goals and preferences.

One of the earliest opportunities for practitioners to enact family-centred care is during assessment. Information is gathered and interpreted to guide professional reasoning about priorities and recommendations for intervention (or prognosis). Assessment occurs routinely in practice, either using formal processes (and we may do this explicitly or not), or implicitly as we make observations and form judgements. In Chapter 13, the importance of making assessment explicit from a pedagogical perspective was highlighted. Along with this key factor lies the imperative that we undertake all assessment with great care.

'Involvement' in assessment is a transactional exchange among clinicians, children, parents, and the structures (activity, objects, time) of the assessment that impacts all those involved. We know that practitioner engagement in formal assessment is impacted by their level of comfort and confidence in engaging with parents around assessment (O'Connor et al. 2019b). To understand this further, we conducted a qualitative study involving in-depth interviews with 14 parents who reflected on and described their experiences with allied health assessment (O'Connor et al. 2019a), resulting in the Steering Wheel for Collaborative Assessment (see Fig. 14.1). The Steering Wheel has a central hub with four radiating spokes to an inner rim and outer rim. The hub contains two central themes: protection, and framing assessment positively. Most central is 'protection' where parents act to protect their child's being, identity and representation through assessment, along with their own psychological wellbeing during diagnostic and assessment processes.

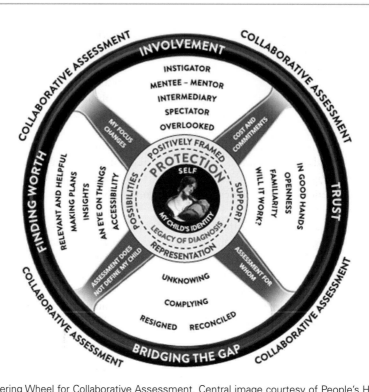

Figure 14.1 Steering Wheel for Collaborative Assessment. Central image courtesy of People's History Museum. Reprinted from O'Connor et al. 2019a, by permission of Taylor & Francis Ltd, http://www.tandfonline.com.

No matter what we choose to assess, how we assess the child is critical.

In the Steering Wheel, framing assessment positively wraps around protection and is connected by a 'porous' line to indicate the potential influence of assessment on parents' need to protect. We propose the way assessment and diagnosis is framed, strongly influences parents need to protect with enduring impacts on collaboration and building capacity with parents.

The themes illustrated that a parent's need to protect is magnified by negative assessment interactions that threaten their child's identity, revive feelings of grief and erode optimism, making collaboration with the therapist to enable involvement in the assessment process difficult. In these situations, parents may avoid assessment interactions or feel they can only participate as a resigned spectator of their child's assessment. Assessment may hold little worth and decrease parent motivation to implement recommendations.

In contrast, positively framed assessment interactions, that focus on a child's strengths, reduces the parent's need to protect; thereby opening opportunities for parents to be involved in the assessment process and develop a positive partnership. When framed positively, parents may reconcile the limitations of the assessment process and feel able to choose how they want to be involved according to their circumstances, and priorities. Assessment in this instance is collaborative, and builds capacity, as represented by the outermost rim of the figure.

The Steering Wheel metaphor implies that the assessment process is driven, with choices made about where to go and the route to be taken. Assessment determines the directions for therapy interventions – a process driven traditionally by the therapist or rehabilitation team. Within a capacity-building paradigm, one can ask who is holding the wheel and how tightly – the therapist, the parent and child or both?

Assessment is a learning process for parents and their child that perhaps requires therapists to not only let the child and family choose their desired destination, but to also loosen their grip on the wheel when navigating to a valued destination. If the Steering Wheel is shared, by making the assessment process transparent, parents may be empowered with relevant information that enables their job of parenting.

When thinking carefully about participation attendance and involvement in therapy as a life situation, it becomes apparent that therapy might not be 'mostly harmless'. Recent work focused on engagement in therapy provides an important set of principles and practices about how to engage with clients in therapeutic interactions (D'Arrigo et al. 2017, 2018). Applying self-determination theory suggests we need to support autonomy, relatedness and competence in the individual and their family.

The notion of engaging in therapy as an affective (emotional connection, positive affect, enthusiasm), behavioural (asking questions to appraise recommendations prior to uptake) and cognitive (effort, readiness for change) commitment, describes a range of positive energising traits and efforts. These ideas are consistent with the stories of some parents in O'Connor et al.'s (2019a) study who felt they were in good hands and could work together with their therapist and be involved in assessment to support the things they valued for their child. Those parents' experiences though, sat in contrast to others who felt an eroding sense of optimism and felt like spectators in a disconnected process of assessment that was done by and for the therapist and his or her professional team.

Despite advancements in implementing family-centred care, insufficient focus may have been given to 'how to' involve parents and children in formal assessment. The Pediatric Rehabilitation Intervention Measure of Engagement (PRIME) suite of measures were developed to support our understanding of engagement in therapy, including assessment (King et al. 2019). These measures have the potential to assist us in understanding our own contributions to optimal engagement. Focusing on how to engage with children and families in assessment is complex. The checklist in Box 14.1 provides a list of questions that practitioners can reflect on when preparing for assessment with families that might support their positive involvement.

Box 14.1 Reflecting on involving parents and children in the assessment process: A checklist for practitioners

Steering Wheel checklist for collaborative assessment

FIRST CONSIDER

Do I know:

- Why I'm gathering this assessment information, e.g. early detection, diagnosis, surveillance, guide therapy, evaluate therapy?
- Who the assessment information is for-parent, therapist, service, funders, researcher?
- How the assessment information will be useful to parents and their child?

Am I aware of:

- The family's therapy 'ethos', current focus and aspirations for their child?
- Previous disempowering experiences (including diagnosis) in the health system?
- The possible emotional and pragmatic costs of attending?
- What this parent thinks and knows about formalised assessment in therapy?
- The potential harms from this assessment and how to mitigate these e.g. language, task administration, scoring and implications?
- How to positively frame the assessment process and findings from a strengths perspective, i.e. positively represent the child, protect individual identity and the parent, identify possibilities, suggest ways forward and next steps?

(Continued on next page)

Box 14.1   (Continued)

THEN COLLABORATE

DECIDING TOGETHER   **BRIDGING THE GAP**

Have I

- Made time to specifically discuss assessment with the parent?
- Provided general information about what formal assessment is and why it is used?
- Asked the parent how they feel about their child being formally assessed?
- How their child manages and responds to being 'tested'?
- Acknowledged that formal assessment can be emotionally difficult for some parents?

Have I

- Provided specific and easy to understand information about the assessment, i.e. its name and what it assesses?
- Discussed the outcomes anticipated from the assessment?
- Given examples of the types of tasks their child will be asked to do, or types of questions if a parent questionnaire?
- Shown the parents (and child) the score sheets and how it is scored?
- Discussed how the assessment information can be interpreted (using common terms)?
- Discussed how the information is related to their child's therapy?
- Confirmed this assessment aligns with the parent's current focus, aspirations or goals?
- Identified aspects of this assessment that may be emotionally difficult, e.g. deficit-based terms, images, pass-fail scoring, less than anticipated results?
- Reassured the parent that the assessment findings do not define who their child is?
- Provided written information about the assessment for parents to consider?
- Confirmed the decision: the parent is comfortable and mentally ready; would prefer it to be done later; or, not at all?

PLANNING TOGETHER   **INVOLVEMENT**

Have I

- Asked about any issues the parent might anticipate for their child during the assessment?
- Discussed strategies to make the assessment more manageable and enjoyable for the child and parent, e.g. where, when, who is present, things they don't like, positions to avoid, use of visuals, fun things to include and ways to encourage?
- Asked about their child's behavioural cues that indicate pain, anxiety, stress, fatigue?
- Discussed what to bring, e.g. clothing, hoists, transfer board, favourite toys or items, food and drink?
- Suggested practical ways the parent and child can be involved (if desired) that don't jeopardise reliability and scoring, e.g. recording results; holding the infant during test?
- Gained consent for electronic material and who receives copies of the written report?
- Asked who the parent would like present when discussing the assessment and written report?

DOING TOGETHER   **DEVELOPING TRUST**

Have I

- Checked in to see if this is a 'good' day (for parent and/or child) to do the assessment?
- Given parent 'permission' to indicate if any concerns during the assessment?
- Clarified the child behavioural cues with the parent if unsure?
- Kept the score sheet visible to the parent while assessing?
- Been available to discuss or clarify questions with parent questionnaires?
- Found ways for the parent to stay close and involved during handling of their infant?
- Given older children or parents the option to be involved in the assessment when possible, e.g. setting up items, recording scores, taking photos?

(*Continued on next page*)

Box 14.1   (Continued)

- Framed the assessment dialogue and items positively, i.e.
  - □ used strengths-based language, i.e. highlighting what the child CAN do and interests.
  - □ made items playful, fun, engaging and efficient.
  - □ ensured a sense of achievement with each item.
- Checked mid-way to see how the assessment is going for the parent and their child?
- Articulated what I'm doing and thinking while assessing whenever possible and appropriate?
- Drawn attention to the child's strengths?

DISCUSSING TOGETHER   **FINDING WORTH**

Have I

- Asked the parent (and child) about the assessment experience-what they noticed and thought?
- Discussed findings face-to face using everyday language that is positive and inclusive (not stigmatising)?
- Contextualised the findings from a strength (not deficit) perspective, i.e. how the findings relate to their child's development, participation and the six F's (Function, Friends, Fitness, Fun, Family, Future)?
- Discussed findings in relation to:
  - □ parent goals and aspirations for their child.
  - □ child interests, home, school and community.
  - □ a therapy plan that accommodates family routines, resources and activities.
- Provided parents with a written summary or report that;
  - □ uses understandable language and explains profession-specific terms and acronyms.
  - □ includes a summary of the assessment purpose and findings.
  - □ interprets findings in terms of promoting child development.
  - □ explains how the findings contribute towards the parents' and child's priorities.

Summary

Measurement of participation has come a long way since publication of the International Classification of Functioning Disability and Health (ICF) in 2001. Our focus now needs to be on measuring transactions among people in context over time, participation involvement as an outcome, and how we effectively and compassionately involve children and parents in the assessment process.

SUMMARY OF KEY IDEAS

- Generating evidence for participation-focused practice requires a thoughtful approach to capturing involvement and contextual factors across time.
- Researchers and practitioners must find ways that involve children and their parents, and that support their commitment and investment in therapy.
- Positively framed assessments provide opportunities for parents to inform their child's therapy. In turn, this collaborative approach reinforces transparency and empowers parents with knowledge that enables their parenting self-efficacy.

ACKNOWLEDGEMENTS

We thank Erin Albrecht and Evgenia Popova for their contributions regarding current methodologies in research and practice, and Claire Kerr, Nora Shields and Brooke Adair for their contributions toward development of the Steering Wheel for Collaborative Assessment.

REFERENCES

Adair B, Ullenhag A, Rosenbaum P, Granlund M, Keen D, Imms C (2018) Measures used to quantify participation in childhood disability and their alignment with the family of participation-related constructs: a systematic review. *Dev Med Child Neurol* **60**: 1101–1116.

Albrecht EC, Khetani MA (2017) Environmental impact on young children's participation in home-based activities. *Dev Med Child Neurol* **59**: 388–394.

Anaby D, Law M, Hanna S, Dematteo C (2012) Predictors of change in participation rates following acquired brain injury: results of a longitudinal study. *Dev Med Child Neurol* **54**: 339–346.

Anaby D, Law M, Coster W et al. (2014) The mediating role of the environment in explaining participation of children and youth with and without disabilities across home, school and community. *Arch Phys Med Rehabil* **95**: 908–917.

Bradley RH (2015) Constructing and adapting causal and formative measures of family settings: The HOME inventory as illustration. *J Fam Theory Rev* **7**: 381–414.

Bright FA, Kayes NM, Worrall L, McPherson KM (2015) A conceptual review of engagement in healthcare and rehabilitation. *Disabil Rehabil* **37**: 643–654.

Bronfenbrenner U, Morris P (2006) The bioecological model of human development. In: Damon W, Lerner R (Ed) *Theoretical Models of Human Development. Handbook of Child Psychology, vol. 1.* New York, NY: Wiley.

Clarke MT, Newton C, Griffiths T, Price K, Lysley A, Petrides KV (2011) Factors associated with the participation of children with complex communication needs. *Res Dev Disabil* **32**: 774–780.

Coster W, Bedell G, Law M et al. (2011) Psychometric evaluation of the Participation and Environment Measure for Children and Youth. *Dev Med Child Neurol* **53**: 1030–1037.

D'Arrigo R, Ziviani J, Poulsen AA, Copley J, King G (2017) Child and parent engagement in therapy: what is the key? *Aust Occup Ther J* **64**: 340–343.

D'Arrigo R, Ziviani J, Poulsen AA, Copley J, King G (2018) Measures of parent engagement for children receiving developmental or rehabilitation interventions: A systematic review. *Phys Occup Ther Pediatr* **38**: 18–38.

Dunst CJ, Boyd K, Trivette CM, Hamby D (2002) Family-oriented program models and professional helpgiving practices. *Fam Relat* **51**: 221–229.

Epsi-Sherwindt M (2008) Family-centred practice: collaboration, competence and evidence. *Support Learn* **23**: 136–143.

Imms C, Adair B (2017) Participation trajectories: impact of school transitions on children and adolescents with cerebral palsy. *Dev Med Child Neurol* **59**: 174–182.

Khetani MA (2015) Validation of environmental content in the Young Children's Participation and Environment Measure. *Arch Phys Med Rehabil* **96**: 317–322.

Khetani MA (2017) Capturing change: participation trajectories in cerebral palsy during life transitions. *Dev Med Child Neurol* **59**: 118–119.

Khetani MA, Albrecht EC, Jarvis JM, Pogorzelski D, Cheng E, Choong K (2018a). Determinants of change in home participation among critically ill children. *Dev Med Child Neurol* **60**: 793–800.

Khetani MA, McManus BM, Arestad K et al. (2018b). Technology-based functional assessment in early childhood intervention: a pilot study. *Pilot Feasibility Stud* **4**: 65.

King G, Meyer K, King G, Meyer K (2006) Service integration and co-ordination: a framework of approaches for the delivery of co-ordinated care to children with disabilities and their families. *Child Care Health Dev* **32**: 477–492.

King G, Chiarello LA, Thompson L et al. (2019) Development of an observational measure of therapy engagement for pediatric rehabilitation. *Disabil Rehabil* **41**(1): 86–97.

Lunkenheimer ES, Kemp CJ, Albrecht EC (2013) Contingencies in mother–child teaching interactions and behavior regulation and dysregulation in early childhood. *Soc Dev* **22**: 319–339.

Moore MH, Mah JK, Trute B (2009) Family-centred care and health-related quality of life of patients in paediatric neurosciences. *Child Care Health Dev* **35**: 454–461.

O'Connor B, Kerr C, Shields N, Adair B, Imms C (2019a) Steering towards collaborative assessment: a qualitative study of parents' experiences of evidence-based assessment practices for their child with cerebral palsy. *Disabil Rehabil* **23**: 1–10.

O'Connor B, Kerr C, Shields N, Imms C (2019b) Understanding allied health practitioners' use of evidence-based assessments for children with cerebral palsy: a mixed methods study. *Disabil Rehabil* **41**: 53–65.

Sameroff AJ, Mackenzie MJ (2003) Research strategies for capturing transactional models of development: the limits of the possible. *Dev Psychopathol* **15**: 613–640.

Stiglitz JE, Sen A, Fitoussi JP (2009) *Report by the Commission on the Measurement of Economic Performance and Social Progress*. Brussels: European Commission.

Trivette CM, Dunst CJ, Hamby D (2010) Influences of family-systems intervention practices on parent-child interactions and child development. *Top Early Child Spec Educ* **30**: 3–19.

This powerful story places our role as practitioners in the assessment experience in the spotlight. No matter *what* we choose to assess, *how* we do it is critical. Every therapeutic exchange is a participatory transaction among those in the situation along with the contextual elements of objects, activities and time. No therapeutic exchange is more important than assessment where judgement is always implied or indeed highly evident. As you read, consider how the context (including practitioners) influences ongoing child and family involvement in assessment along with participation-related constructs such as sense of self.

Jack in the Box (Australia)

Bridget O'Connor

Fear and dread. This is what comes to mind when I think about assessment. I'm Jack's mother and Jack's my 5-year-old boy. Assessment unfortunately, brings back memories of the worst night of my life – the night Jack stopped breathing. We threw ourselves into the car and rushed to the hospital with no seat belts and no baby seat. The police pulled us over on the way, but we sped off towards the hospital, so when we arrived it was chaos – police and doctors everywhere, everyone huddled around my child except me, I couldn't see him, and nobody told us what was going on … and then our child was gone. Then the questions started. I slowly realised they thought we had done something terrible to our baby and that we could lose our baby. They wouldn't let us out of their sight. It wasn't until after the MRI results came through that they realised his seizures were coming from a malformation in his brain, and we were no longer suspects. They showed us his damaged brain on the MRI, the tubes came out eventually and we left the hospital along with every ounce of trust we once had, and a sense of shame. All I knew was I would never lose control again.

Different therapists contacted us after we got home. They were all very nice, but I always felt on guard in our appointments, not knowing what was being judged and what this might mean for Jack and us. Each time, I felt the tension rising in me in the days before Jack's appointments – that fear of again being out of control. At these appointments the therapists were always looking, and I was always wondering – what were they looking for and what were they seeing and thinking? I hated handing him over, particularly when they took his clothes off and he was laying there half naked on the floor. I often felt like scooping him up and running out of those appointments, but I made myself stay, just in case there was something they said that might be helpful for Jack. I just sat on the edge of my chair looking on.

I remember an early assessment of Jack. It seemed like the therapist was trying to figure out what was inside a parcel that had arrived unexpectedly. They tapped Jack's knees, tugged and turned his little arms, tipped him this way and that way, trying to see what was inside my little Jack in the box. The therapist kept her sheet of paper and pen tucked in next to her on the other side, away from me. I couldn't quite see what was on it, but it looked like there were little stick figures of frogs with heads and legs bent in all different directions – sideways, forwards and backwards. She circled the little 'frogs' that didn't bare any resemblance to my baby. Maybe she had a secret code that I wasn't meant to know about or wouldn't understand. Eventually Jack had had enough, and I had too. I leant forward and thankfully she passed my Jack in the box back to me. She gathered her frog pictures together and arranged our next appointment time. The only time available was when my partner had his next job interview, so again he couldn't come. I never knew what to tell him or my Mum about these assessments as I had no idea, really, what they had ascertained from it all. It was all so foreign to me. I guess I looked for different things – the smile of recognition, the relaxation of his body when I soothed him, the change in his cry that let me know he was hungry, the hand that recently caressed my hand while he drank – this was the Jack in the box I knew and loved, I didn't see the boy with a malformed brain.

A few months later we had an appointment to see our paediatrician – again the looming dread, but this time it was only to check his weight just like they do for all kids. My partner and I waited patiently in the consulting room with Jack on my lap while the paediatrician read a letter from our therapist. She mentioned a letter, but I hadn't received it yet. Now he's roaming the internet looking for things on the computer. As he scrolls down the screen he slowly nods at the screen and says 'Yes, I guess he does fit the description of cerebral palsy – he definitely has a disorder of posture and movement'. He went on 'It's a bit early to say how severe it will be but from the therapist's assessment and score (the frog one, I guess) he's likely to be a 4 or a 5'. 'What do you mean a 4 or a 5?' I asked. He swung the computer screen around for us to see. There were pictures of children in wheelchairs and frames, and others running upstairs. He pointed at the children in the wheelchair pictures next to the 4 and the 5. My Jack had been reduced to a number, I thought – that was very odd. My ears buzzed as I sat Jack on my partner's lap and stood up. I didn't know where I was going but I had to get out of there. I felt so left out in the dark, like I was the last person to know and the lid had been closed on my Jack in the box. I wasn't sure I could go on with this stuff and therapy anymore – it just didn't seem worth it.

PART IV

Participation Interventions

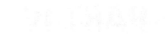

Enabling Participation: Innovations and Advancements

Dido Green

In previous sections we outlined underlying concepts and contexts for participation and considered the challenges of measurement. This part of the book will focus on how to promote participation, presenting innovations and advancements in interventions. This chapter will begin by addressing concepts of enablement, intervention and therapy, and consider these in relation to participation across different contexts. A broader perspective, that considers direct and indirect actions which influence 'enablement' will also be presented to extend the notion of rehabilitation to consider empowerment rather than specific therapeutic actions only.

ENABLEMENT

The transactional nature of participation involving environmental and socialisation processes as well as personal factors, including resiliency (King et al. 2018), provides multiple entry points for interventions that aim to enable participation. Classically, we think of interventions in rehabilitation as psychological, physical and or environmental, which may be led or guided by health or social care professionals. Constructs of client-centred practice introduced the dimension of empowerment in which the client (as child, adult and/or carer) is provided with information along with choices and empowered to make decisions regarding the treatments they receive (Malin and Teasdale 1991). Client-centred practice and methods supporting empowerment may be influenced by information provided by society at the macro level, professionals at the meso level (service/institutional) or led by individuals (parent and child) at the micro level; the latter increasingly influenced by the internet and self-help organisations. Thus, the messages delivered via societal 'nudges', evidenced in policies and publicity and more recently, social media trends, extend the boundaries of rehabilitation to consider direct and indirect enabling actions.

Empowerment supports individuals to be in control of their lives, thus allowing for independent actions of the child and family for self-management and self-directed interventions.

'Enablement' includes multiple dynamically interacting components, moving us away from Cartesian Dualism in which there is a distinct separation of mind and body. Thus, any intervention framework must integrate the physical and emotional experiences of the individual with the attitudes and expectations of society. Enabling greater participation for children and young people with disabilities requires promotion of both attendance and involvement; the latter including elements of engagement, motivation, persistence, social connection and affect (Imms et al. 2017).

ENGAGEMENT

Engagement is a complex multidimensional concept that has multiple meanings depending on the differing perspectives of individuals. In previous chapters we have seen both distinctions made between involvement and engagement and the terms used interchangeably. Engagement may be evidenced through the focus of attention, persistence and effort within a task or activity. Involvement, while embracing engagement, may incorporate a greater social dimension via interactions with others and sense of belonging, as well as the emotional content of the moment. When we consider engagement in intervention, the experiences of the individual form the foundation for considering participation as 'involvement in meaningful life situations'. Engagement may be observed with respect to the initiation and persistence in actions or absorption with or within particular activities. However, the motivations for engagement will be dependent on past experiences and future expectations. Engagement may be considered at a micro (individual) level as well as group (meso) and societal (macro) levels.

At the micro level, Bright and colleagues (2017), show engagement in healthcare and rehabilitation to be a co-constructed process between clinician and patient in which practitioner engagement influences patient engagement and vice versa. At the meso level, in which interventions may take place within specialised groups (e.g. after school clubs) or be embedded within regular daily contexts (e.g. within the school setting), the dynamics of the group need to be taken into consideration. At the macro level, interventions to promote participation are predominately addressing access and attendance rather than engagement per se. However,

LINK TO VIGNETTE 5.1
'The Mothers' Wishes and Dreams', p. 55.

interventions extending from the organisation and management of health services and institutions to government legislation and policies may directly or indirectly impact on societal attitudes to influence interactions in the community. Organisational and institutional structures contribute to opportunities that are accessible within the community and also indirectly influence expectations that individuals and their families may have, for example, to play in a park or attend university, despite significant physical or intellectual difficulties. An exemplar in shifting expectations is the Inclusive University, an empowerment project between The International Trump Institute for Continuing Education in Developmental Disabilities of Beit Issie Shapiro and Bar Ilan University in Israel. The Inclusive University offers academic programmes for individuals with learning and adjustment disabilities; integrating these students within usual undergraduate courses for which they earn academic credits. This programme supports social integration of students with intellectual difficulties; strengthening their self-image and confidence as well as changing attitudes and expectations for learning of these adults (Hozmi 2009).

How information is delivered to promote access to healthcare services or community activities may vary from the subliminal messages of advertising to more overt public health campaigns. More recently, consumer movements have seen the demand for patients' rights to information to be met and for them to influence the way in which health professionals research, design and deliver services, leading to co-production across research and implementation activities (Chapter 10). This has an effect of shifting responsibility for health promotion and participation (in culturally determined 'healthy activities') towards the individual, along with an onus on society to enable those with disabilities (or their parents) to have a voice and opportunities for active involvement in societies' decisions.

Enabling participation thus involves multiple layers that need to be considered across macro-, meso- and micro-levels. Figure 15.1 illustrates the dynamic interactions across these multiple layers, for the individual and the contexts for participation, on a time-scape in which temporal elements also influence expectations. The connections illustrated in this figure reflect the co-dependency as well as transactions between enabling – engaging aspects of cultures and attitudes and intervening – empowering aspects that occur across institutional and political contexts, whether these be within the family, at school, within therapy, in the community or at a societal level (see Part II). For example, an intervention designed to

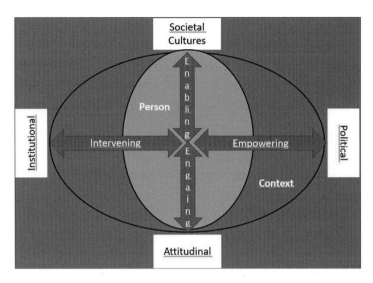

Figure 15.1   Interactions between macro-, meso- and micro-levels for interventions to enable participation.

improve independence through increased mobility using a wheelchair, will only be effective if society provides wheelchair access along with the attitude to allow wheelchair users to be involved in community activities. Being taken to a supermarket in a wheelchair does not enable participation in 'shopping' on its own. Attitudinal interventions, along with access interventions, might be needed at both the meso and macro levels. The Disability Matters e-learning programme is designed to shift attitudes towards disabled individuals (Royal College Paediatrics Child Health 2015). Designed by disabled young people, parent carers and other experts, the Disability Matters multiple short e-learning sessions aim to enhance understanding and provide practical advice about supporting disabled young people and their families to achieve meaningful outcomes. Topics range from understanding pain, communication and mobility needs to decision making and advocacy. Other multi-faceted pro-

Positive societal attitudes are fundamental for enabling participation and engaging disabled individuals in their communities.

gramme examples include Partnering for Change (Missiuna et al. 2012), that offers interdisciplinary interventions at the macro-, meso- and micro-levels and the MATCH framework that promotes the following approach: Modify the task, Alter your expectations, Teach Strategies, Change the environment and Help by understanding (Pollock and Missiuna 2016).

PARTICIPATION AS A DESIRED OUTCOME OR AS A PROCESS

Participation may be viewed as 'the means' or 'the ends' of interventions (Imms et al. 2016). Therapeutic interventions have tended to focus on a desired end-point, defined on or by a specific dimension rather than active engagement in meaningful life situations. We have seen from the previous section on measurement, how difficult this concept can be to pin down into measurable units. Distinguishing between capacity and participation can be equally challenging. In a review of interventions designed to improve physical activity participation many, if not most, studies measured physical activity levels (e.g. steps taken)

These young people chose to use the term 'disabled young people' to set the disability within the environment rather than within the individual.

rather than participation outcomes (Reedman et al. 2017). Empowerment and enablement can only occur when the individuals (children and or their carers) retain some autonomy for decision making during the period of treatment, along with acceptance of responsibility for decisions (Malin and Teasdale 1991). These are critical components of interventions enabling participation.

Extending from Part III, in which measurement was in focus, Part IV of the book includes the most current participatory intervention research. The following chapters explore participation as either the process (or means) to other outcomes (i.e. the independent variable) or as the outcome (i.e. the dependent variable). The transactional nature of participation, across spatial and temporal contexts, and multi-disciplinary approaches are critical functions of the interventions in this section.

SUMMARY OF KEY IDEAS

- Enabling participation involves numerous transactional processes across macro-, meso- and micro-levels, providing multiple platforms on which an intervention may occur.
- Interventions enabling participation may focus on participation as a desired outcome and/or as the process.
- Enabling participation requires involvement and engagement as well as empowerment supported by providing autonomy for choice and decision making.

REFERENCES

Bright FA, Kayes NM, Cummins C, Worrall LM, McPherson KM (2017) Co-constructing engagement in stroke rehabilitation: a qualitative study exploring how practitioner engagement can influence patient engagement. *Clin Rehabil* **31**: 1396–1405.

Hozmi B (2009) Accessible academic studies for adults with learning and adjustment disabilities. *Issues Edu Rehabil* **24**: 5–13.

Imms C, Granlund M, Wilson PH, Steenbergen B, Rosenbaum PL, Gordon AM (2017) Participation, both a means and an end: a conceptual analysis of processes and outcomes in childhood disability. *Dev Med Child Neurol* **59**: 16–25.

Imms C, Adair B, Keen D, Ullenhag A, Rosenbaum P, Granlund M (2016) "Participation": a systematic review of language, definitions, and constructs used in intervention research with children with disabilities. *Dev Med Child Neurol* **58**: 29–38.

King G, Imms C, Stewart D, Freeman M, Nguyen T (2018) A transactional framework for pediatric rehabilitation: shifting the focus to situated contexts, transactional processes, and adaptive developmental outcomes. *Disabil Rehabil* **40**: 1829–1841.

Malin N, Teasdale K (1991) Caring versus empowerment: considerations for nursing practice. *J Adv Nurs* **16**: 657–662.

Missiuna CA, Pollock NA, Levac DE et al. (2012) Partnering for change: an innovative school-based occupational therapy service delivery model for children with developmental coordination disorder. *Can J Occup Ther* **79**: 41–50.

Pollock N, Missiuna C (2016) *MATCH Flyers: A Resource for Educators*. Hamilton: CanChild Centre for Childhood Disability Research, McMaster University. http://elearning.canchild.ca/dcd_workshop/match.html [Accessed 13 September 2019].

Reedman S, Boyd RN, Sakzewski L (2017) The efficacy of interventions to increase physical activity participation of children with cerebral palsy: a systematic review and meta-analysis. *Dev Med Child Neurol* **59**: 1011–1018.

Royal College of Paediatrics and Child Health (2015). *Disability Matters e-Learning, e-Learning for Healthcare*. London: Royal College of Paediatrics and Child Health. https://www.disabilitymatters.org.uk/ [Accessed 7 April 2018].

Providing Opportunities for Participation: A Focus on the Environment

Dana Anaby

THE IMPACT OF THE ENVIRONMENT ON CHILDREN'S PARTICIPATION

Current perspectives on disabilities, as illustrated by the International Classification of Functioning, Disability and Health (ICF) (WHO 2007), place importance on the environment and conceptualise participation restriction as a form of disability, resulting from of the dynamic interaction between a person's health condition and their environment. With accumulating evidence, it has become clear that the environment plays a key role in shaping children's participation (Hammal et al. 2004; Law et al. 2007; Colver et al. 2011). To illustrate, a scoping review (Anaby et al. 2013) indicated that each domain of the environment within the ICF influenced participation as a facilitator and/or barrier. Most common facilitators were social support from family and friends and geographic location (i.e. one's district), whereas the most common barriers were attitudes, followed by physical accessibility, services and policies, and lack of support by staff and service providers. Unique barriers also emerged in the literature indicating parents' lack of time and lack of access to information. Structural models testing the impact of the environment on participation in the presence of other important factors reveal the mediating role of the environment in explaining levels of participation frequency and involvement among both children and youth with disabilities aged 5–17 years (Anaby et al. 2014), as well as among younger children (<6 years) with developmental disabilities (Albrecht and Khetani 2017). In other words, the environment as a mediating factor consistently alleviates or intensifies the impact of a child's condition (in terms of complexity or severity) on their levels of participation across different settings: at home, school and in the community. The effect of the environment was most pronounced in the community setting where the most common barriers involved the demands of the activity (cognitive, physical and social) and most common supports included the availability of resources in terms of programmes, services and information (Bedell et al. 2013). Such evidence further suggests that the environment is a promising target of intervention and strengthens the idea of context-based therapies (Darrah et al. 2011). This is of great importance as in many cases the environment is more amenable to change as compared to the child's functional ability or their body functions.

HOW ARE WE DOING IN PRACTICE?

A Canada-wide survey (Anaby et al. 2017a) revealed that occupational therapists and physical therapists spend less intervention time, that is, 2–15%, directed to the participation (e.g. leisure, community-based activities, bike riding, playing hockey) of school-age children with cerebral palsy; compared to task-oriented activities such as daily living and mobility, which were well-addressed (up to 56% of therapy time), and body functions/structures (e.g. muscle strength, joint mobility, attention) which received up to 42% of therapy time. While these clinicians addressed aspects of the environment in their treatment plan (19–37%), they mostly focused on the physical environment (e.g. home accessibility, equipment related to mobility). Other important facets of the environment such as social support, attitudes of others and institutional factors such as availability of programmes, although known to impact participation (Anaby et al. 2013), received little attention. A knowledge-to-practice gap highlights the need to bring about a change in practice towards a greater emphasis on all aspects of participation and on the broad facets of the environment. Recent research evidence about effective interventions to improve children's participation by changing aspects of their environment exists, as illustrated below, and can facilitate a shift in the way rehabilitation practice is delivered and packaged.

THE ENVIRONMENT AS A PROMISING TARGET AREA OF INTERVENTION FOR PROMOTING PARTICIPATION: THE PREP APPROACH

Law and Darrah (2014) in their writings on emerging therapy approaches, including context-therapy which has demonstrated effectiveness among young children with cerebral palsy (Law et al. 2011), call for goal-directed interventions that are ecological in nature and occur within the child's immediate environment (i.e. where they live, learn and play). These scholars shifted away from traditional impairment-focused interventions, as it was found that remediating impairment deficits/body functions does not necessarily translate into improved functional independence and 'real-life' participation (Novak et al. 2013). Within this paradigm, therapists are encouraged to 'step-out' of the rehabilitation centre/therapy room towards the child's natural environment (home, school, community), enabling children to participate in desired activities with the capacities they have, just 'as they are'. This can be achieved by modifying aspects of the environment and/or the requirements of the activity as well as by coaching the family, among other stakeholders, on solution-based strategies for removing barriers and building on existing supports.

Therapists need to step into children's naturally occurring contexts to enable participation.

The Pathways and Resources for Engagement and Participation (PREP) (Law et al. 2016) is an innovative strength-based, client-centred practice model that draws on these principles. It is designed to enhance participation in different settings and life situations (or contexts of participation) among clients with various conditions throughout their lifespan/at all ages, by changing aspects of their environment only. This chapter focuses on the application of the PREP approach in improving leisure community-based activities among youth who are living with a physical disability.

WHAT STEPS ARE INVOLVED IN PREP?

The PREP intervention follows a five-step approach, including: Make Goals, Map Out a Plan, Make it Happen, Measure Processes and Outcomes and Move Forward. Further information about this approach can be found in the PREP manual (Law et al. 2016). Within this process, the therapist meets with the child and their family at their home/community in order to identify three specific activities in which the youth wants to participate, yet finds difficult. The PREP addresses a range of activity types, based on the youth's preferences, from structured recreational activities done with others (youth film group, cooking club, programming, computer animation, music club) or skill-based one-on-one activities (guitar, piano, swimming) as well as sports/physical related activities (boccia, wheelchair basketball, sludge hockey, yoga, dancing) to informal unstructured social activities (walking, going to the mall with friends, attending sporting events or concerts). In many cases, youth prefer to join a mainstream programme that is open to all rather than join an adapted programme which is also enabled through the PREP.

The PREP intervention addresses any activity of choice through a five-step approach, and by incorporating collaboration, engagement, coaching and building of a participation team.

The therapist then *collaborates* with the client and *engages* them in identifying and implementing solution-based strategies for removing environmental barriers and leveraging existing supports. Effective strategies to minimise barriers vary, extending beyond physical accessibility or the built environment and include other modifiable aspects such as attitudinal, social and institutional factors. Examples include improving physical accessibility; adapting activity equipment; finding available programmes; providing information about transportation services to and from other local resources (libraries, community centres); informing community agencies about how they could adapt their programmes and provide accessible services; improving attitudes of others through education and training; reaching out to nongovernmental organisations (NGOs) (volunteers to accompany youth to activities, equipment, funding) for support; advocating for the client (letters, job postings, champion for inclusion by modifying existing programmes to allow access to all); as well as addressing financial constraints.

This collaborative process incorporates elements of *coaching* such as engaged discussion and ongoing exchange of information with the purpose of increasing the family's knowledge base and skills and enhancing their ability to solve problems. The primary outcome of the PREP focuses on the client's level of performance in each selected activity as measured using the performance scale of the Canadian Occupational Performance Measure (COPM).

One of the key ingredients of the PREP is *building a participation team* by reaching out and working collaboratively with all relevant stakeholders. This includes family members, friends, neighbours, teachers, volunteers, college students, community instructors, programme coordinators, vendors, other healthcare professionals, among others – those who bring knowledge and provide support. The following case study illustrates how the therapist brought together a strong participation team and built a new community resource to assist Ella in participating in her chosen activity – playing music with others.

CASE STUDY

Ella's Aspiration to Play Music in a Social Context

Ella is a 13-year-old girl, an only child, who lives with both parents in a small neighbourhood and attends a specialised school for children with disabilities. Ella's diagnosis involves a global developmental delay secondary to a metabolic disorder and cortical visual impairment. She is non-verbal, has difficulty learning and sustaining her attention and has delayed responses to environmental stimuli. For mobility, she relies on a caregiver to push her in a wheelchair, but she is able to participate during transfers. Ella is fully dependent on her parents for all hygiene, dressing and toileting needs. She is also dependent for all household chores and medical needs. Ella has difficulty using her hands to carry out fine motor tasks. She inconsistently nods her head to answer simple yes/no questions.

Overall participation patterns and interests: Ella participates mostly in home-based activities such as listening to music (parents report she is happiest and most focused with music), watching videos and movies and listening to stories on her iPad. Her parents take her to the local mall or a coffee shop a few times each week but she does not participate in any other community-based activities. On weekends, the family retreats to a country house away from the city. They do not have other family living nearby and Ella does not have other friends.

Environmental barriers: Identified barriers include the physical layout, demands of the activity (physical, cognitive, social) and attitudes of community members. Resources are also lacking in terms of access to transportation, inclusive programmes and services, and time available to support Ella's participation.

Supports: At home, an extremely dedicated family; at school, a multi-disciplinary rehabilitation team is involved in her care.

PREP Intervention

Ella's goal was *to listen to and play music with others in a social setting.*

Identified barriers: No programmes in the community for her age/needs and no friends with common interests. The therapist contacted local music centres and met with directors to discuss suitability of programmes and accommodations that can be made for Ella yet was *met with reluctance to make accommodations for her.*

INTERVENTION STRATEGIES:

- Therapist contacted local high school and met with the principal to present Ella's strengths and needs and to discuss potential collaborations.
- Principal connected the therapist with the **Glee Club** and six students volunteered to spend time with Ella doing music-related activities on a weekly basis.
- Coaching volunteers: a presentation led by the parents about the project and Ella's needs, strengths, likes and dislikes in music was conducted and included training on strategies for interacting with Ella.
- Site visit was made to determine accessibility: school facility was used for a singing/music group with Ella (basement was selected as it was quiet, allowed focused attention and access via ramp).
- Moving forward: therapist met with parents, high school vice principal and student service providers to discuss the *continuation* of an after-school music programme for Ella post-intervention. Through this discussion, roles of all involved were clarified and a strategy for upcoming seasons was put in place.

Results

Ella, with the help of her parents, rated her **performance** before the intervention as 6 on the COPM 10-point scale, as 8 following the intervention and as 9 and during follow-up (week 36). Figure 16.1 illustrates changes in performance over time across three chosen activities, including playing music with peers.

Ella's **involvement** in community activities, measured on a 5-point scale of the PEM-CY (Participation and Environment Measure for Children and Youth), increased from 1 pre-intervention to 4.6 post-intervention. **Number of community-based activities** in which Ella participated also increased from only one activity (out of 10) before the intervention to five activities post-intervention. **Number of**

environmental barriers to participation in the community setting decreased from 6 to 4 (out of 9). **Number of resources** available to support participation increased from 2 (out of 7) during baseline to 5 post-intervention.

Creating a new resource: The local high school is now looking into creating a volunteer programme focused on enabling participation, similar to what was accomplished by for Ella.

Mother's testimonial: 'I just want to say 10 000 times thank you to everybody, everybody. That was absolutely fabulous, you couldn't help me more than you've done, that's for sure. Ella is, she's thrilled every time I mention just the programme, or we go there, she knows the people, they became really like friends to her. And, inclusion, what can be more satisfying for a child like her to feel that she's accepted the way she is. Nothing.'

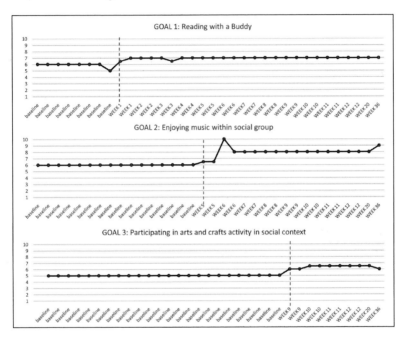

Figure 16.1 Change in levels of performance in three activities chosen by Ella.
Note: Dotted vertical line indicates the timepoint in which each intervention started.

EVIDENCE OF THE EFFECTIVENESS OF THE PREP

To date, there is growing evidence to support the effectiveness of the PREP in enhancing youth participation in chosen activities (e.g. riding a bike, shopping with friends, joining a music club); particularly among those living with a physical disability (Law et al. 2015; Anaby et al. 2016, 2018). To illustrate, through an interrupted time series study (n = 28) (Anaby et al. 2018), a clinically and statistically significant improvement (p < 0.001) of more than 2 points on the COPM scale was observed across 79 activities identified by the youth. Levels of performance were maintained during follow-up. Overall, the intervention was most effective for boys and those with a higher number of functional issues. Aspects of cost-effectiveness were also observed, with an average of 6.5 hours needed to accomplish each goal/activity over a period of 4 weeks.

The PREP was also positively perceived by both parents whose child received this intervention (Anaby et al. 2017b) and by clinicians who implemented it, both among youth with mobility restriction in Canada (Anaby et al. 2015) as well as among children in the United Kingdom enrolled in neuro-rehabilitation following a brain injury (Burrough 2017). In a qualitative study (Anaby et al. 2017b), parents discussed the multiple benefits of the intervention extending beyond the accomplishment of the chosen activities targeted in the intervention. Through individual interviews (Anaby et al. 2015), clinicians acknowledged the various aspects of the environment that serve as barriers and that can be modified with a special focus on the attitudinal barriers (i.e. lack of knowledge and/or willingness of programme instructors and directors to accommodate for the youth needs). This required a lot of advocacy on the side of the therapists as well as education and training of community-based stakeholders about how they can provide accessible services. Indeed, clinicians' experience using the PREP led to a new refreshing take on their therapeutic role as a facilitator, advocate, educator and team collaborator (Anaby et al. 2015); one that creates social opportunities for engagement (e.g. friends, peer groups, family, wider community) (Burrough 2017).

Benefits of the PREP intervention included an improvement at the physical, social and emotional level as well as in autonomy.

Recent studies provide preliminary evidence of the additional benefits resulting from this participation-based intervention. Using the Aday app (Kroksmark and Nordell 2018), a time-geography 24-hour activity diary, we have found significant differences in overall participation patterns before and after the PREP intervention. Specifically, following the PREP, youth were engaged in less digital media, in more study-related activities, and spent more time in activities with friends (Anaby et al. 2019b). In addition, a pilot study of young adults with physical disabilities demonstrated an improvement in body functions (e.g. motor, affective and cognitive) underlining the specific chosen activity (e.g. swimming, badminton, playing the piano) following the PREP intervention. Improvement was observed in the cognitive and affective aspects of body functions such as anxiety and attention followed by an improvement in motor function such as muscle strength and reaching (Anaby et al. 2019a).

These findings support a shift in practice towards 'top down' community-based ecological interventions that involve 'real world' meaningful activities.

CONCLUSION AND DISCUSSION

With accumulating evidence, the environment has gained recognition as being key to children's participation. This suggests a paradigm shift in practice towards therapy approaches that move away from solely focusing change on aspects of the child, or trying to fix the child's deficits or impairments, towards activity-based, child-engaging approaches that occur in real-life situations – those that are chosen by and are meaningful for the child, youth and their family. Such patient-oriented approaches, endorsed by the Institute of Medicine, are enjoyable, socially engaging, guided by the child's/youth's preferences, occur within their natural environment and include the people or peers with whom the child wants to participate. These interventions hold promise, as they are perceived as motivating to the youth, and can thus promote adherence to healthcare treatment and sustainability following their completion. Furthermore, since these interventions incorporate elements of coaching and an exchange of information on solution-based strategies for removing environmental barriers, they can build the capacity of children and parents to become problem-solvers and self-advocators. Thereby, children and their families can be empowered to apply these strategies to future activities or participation goals. Indeed, including a component of education in the form of coaching appears to enhance aspects of participation (Adair et al. 2015) as is evident in the OPC Model (Occupational Performance Coaching) which was found effective in improving participation of young children (Graham et al. 2010).

Aligned with the family of environmental-based interventions described in this chapter, that is, context-therapy and PREP, a recent approach has emerged called TEAM (Teens making Environmental and Activity Modifications; see Chapter 17) aimed at improving the knowledge of youth with intellectual disabilities about strategies for modifying their environment. Having a range of therapeutic options is important as it can contribute to customised care that is more responsive to the needs, resources and preferences of the youth and families. Focusing change on the environment appears to be practical, effective and efficient in improving participation in an array of activities, and thereby contributes to the improvement of the provision of paediatric rehabilitation services.

SUMMARY OF KEY IDEAS

- The environment is key to children's participation and can serve as an effective target of intervention.
- Solution-based intervention strategies for removing environmental barriers, guided by the PREP approach, are effective in improving and maintaining adolescents' participation.
- Participation-based interventions can result in multiple benefits (e.g. changes in the youth overall daily patterns, social and emotional growth, physical improvement and greater autonomy) and may also impact body function level outcomes.
- A shift in clinical practice is required towards a greater focus on participation and the environment.

REFERENCES

Adair B, Ullenhag A, Keen D, Granlund M, Imms C (2015) The effect of interventions aimed at improving participation outcomes for children with disabilities: a systematic review. *Dev Med Child Neurol* **57**: 1093–1104.

Albrecht EC, Khetani MA (2017) Environmental impact on young children's participation in home-based activities. *Dev Med Child Neurol* **59**: 388–394.

Anaby D, Hand C, Bradley L et al. (2013) The effect of the environment on participation of children and youth with disabilities: a scoping review. *Disabil Rehabil* **35**: 1589–1598.

Anaby D, Law M, Coster W et al. (2014) The mediating role of the environment in explaining participation of children and youth with and without disabilities across home, school, and community. *Arch Phys Med Rehabil* **95**: 908–917.

Anaby D, Law M, Teplicky R, Turner L (2015) Focusing on the environment to improve youth participation: experiences and perspectives of occupational therapists. *Int J Environ Res Public Health* **12**: 13388–13398.

Anaby DR, Law MC, Majnemer A, Feldman D (2016) Opening doors to participation of youth with physical disabilities: an intervention study. *Can J Occup Ther* **83**: 83–90.

Anaby D, Korner-Bitensky N, Steven E et al. (2017a). Current rehabilitation practices for children with cerebral palsy: focus and gaps. *Phys Occup Ther Pediatr* **37**: 1–15.

Anaby D, Mercerat C, Tremblay S (2017b). Enhancing youth participation using the PREP intervention: parents' perspectives. *Int J Environ Res Public Health* **14**: 14.

Anaby DR, Law M, Feldman D, Majnemer A, Avery L (2018) The effectiveness of the Pathways and Resources for Engagement and Participation (PREP) intervention: improving participation of adolescents with physical disabilities. *Dev Med Child Neurol* **60**: 513–519.

Anaby D, Avery L, Gorter JW et al. (2019a) Improving body functions through participation in community activities among young people with physical disabilities. *Dev Med Child Neurol* doi:10.1111/dmcn.14382.

Anaby D, Vrotsou K, Kroksmark U, Ellegård K (2019b) Changes in participation patterns of youth with physical disabilities following the Pathways and Resources for Engagement and Participation intervention: A time-geography approach. *Scand J Occup Ther* **20**: 1–9.

Bedell G, Coster W, Law M et al. (2013) Community participation, supports, and barriers of school-age children with and without disabilities. *Arch Phys Med Rehabil* **94**: 315–323.

Burrough M (2017) Implementing a participation-focussed intervention: "Pathways and Resources for Engagement and Participation" (PREP) protocol in children's neurorehabilitation. Oral presentation. *Royal College of Occupational Therapists Children, Young People and Families Annual National Conference.* 9 November 2017. Leeds, UK.

Colver AF, Dickinson HO, Parkinson K et al. (2011) Access of children with cerebral palsy to the physical, social and attitudinal environment they need: a cross-sectional European study. *Disabil Rehabil* **33**: 28–35.

Darrah J, Law MC, Pollock N et al. (2011) Context therapy: a new intervention approach for children with cerebral palsy. *Dev Med Child Neurol* **53**: 615–620.

Graham F, Rodger S, Ziviani J (2010) Enabling occupational performance of children through coaching parents: three case reports. *Phys Occup Ther Pediatr* **30**: 4–15.

Hammal D, Jarvis SN, Colver AF (2004) Participation of children with cerebral palsy is influenced by where they live. *Dev Med Child Neurol* **46**: 292–298.

Kroksmark U, Nordell K (2018) *Aday Life Contexts Evaluation* [Online]. Gothenburg: Aday. https://aday.se/ [Accessed 27 September 2019].

Law M, Darrah J (2014) Emerging therapy approaches: an emphasis on function. *J Child Neurol* **29**: 1101–1107.

Law M, Petrenchik T, King G, Hurley P (2007) Perceived environmental barriers to recreational, community, and school participation for children and youth with physical disabilities. *Arch Phys Med Rehabil* **88**: 1636–1642.

Law MC, Darrah J, Pollock N et al. (2011) Focus on function: a cluster, randomized controlled trial comparing child- versus context-focused intervention for young children with cerebral palsy. *Dev Med Child Neurol* **53**: 621–629.

Law M, Anaby D, Imms C, Teplicky R, Turner L (2015) Improving the participation of youth with physical disabilities in community activities: an interrupted time series design. *Aust Occup Ther J* **62**: 105–115.

Law M, Anaby D, Teplicky R, Turner L (2016) *Pathways and Resources for Engagement and Participation (PREP): A Practice Model for Occupational Therapists* [Online]. Hamilton: CanChild. https://www.canchild.ca/en/shop/25-prep [Accessed 13 September 2019].

Novak I, McIntyre S, Morgan C et al. (2013) A systematic review of interventions for children with cerebral palsy: state of the evidence. *Dev Med Child Neurol* **55**: 885–910.

WHO (2007) *International Classification of Functioning, Disability and Health: Children and Youth Version.* Geneva: World Health Organization.

Enhancing Participation Outcomes in Community Contexts

Nora Shields, Ai-Wen Hwang and Jessica Kramer

Previous chapters have discussed participation, including definitions and outcome measures using the International Classification of Functioning Disability and Health – Children and Youth (ICF) (WHO 2007) and the family of participation-related constructs (Imms et al. 2016) frameworks. In this chapter, we focus on the translation of these theories and knowledge into practice with three programmes delivered in natural, community-based settings that target participation as an outcome.

Interventions striving to facilitate participation require learning and behavioural change both in individuals with disability and those in their social environment. This reflects an understanding that learning and development is a result of dynamic transactions among the individual with disability and those charged with facilitating their development and growth (Sameroff and MacKenzie 2003) including people in their communities. Over time, people with disability experience multiple transactions among themselves, their environment, and significant others (Imms et al. 2016). Successful facilitation of participation depends on the environment including those individuals who support the individual with the disability.

The three programmes, which have been developed in different parts of the world, exemplify essential components of participation: being present to participate in the community with peers, and the individual's experience of participation in that context. These exemplars also illustrate the diversity of participation interventions across childhood stages and cultural contexts. We first describe the characteristics of each programme and second describe four characteristics common across programmes that facilitate participation:

- building skills;
- social learning;
- empowerment; and
- challenging attitudes about disability.

EXAMPLE 1. ROUTINES-BASED ENGAGEMENT CLASSROOM MODEL (RECM): SUPPORTING FAMILIES, EDUCATORS AND YOUNG CHILDREN IN PRESCHOOL AND DAY-CARE SETTINGS

What is the Routines-Based Engagement Classroom Model?

This model is designed within the conceptual frameworks of 'Participation-based therapy' and the 'Routines-based model' (McWilliam 2010). RECM is a unified, community-based, culturally appropriate and practical programme used in preschools and day-care centres in Taiwan to support children and families, educators and professionals. The goal is to enhance children's engagement in classrooms by building capacity in teaching, caring for and parenting children.

Programme development was based on a previous study of the Routines-based model with home visiting (Hwang et al. 2013) and a series of pilot studies (Su et al. 2017; Hwang et al. 2018). The community-based applications of RECM have been adopted in research with young children with autism spectrum disorder. The preliminary protocol of RECM was further operationalised to include outcomes monitoring by international collaboration with worldwide scholars to select and apply the measures in preschools. The implementation steps are shown in Table 17.1.

Who Can Participate?

RECM is designed for preschool and day-care settings. The participants include children aged 2–6 years, and their families, educators and staff in these settings, and other professionals. Each preschool is assigned a primary service provider for the children whose educators and parents need support for child care, teaching or parenting. The primary service provider is the health or education professional who has comprehensive information about the families. The primary service provider also provides support in the classroom context, rather than taking the children out of the classroom to provide therapy de-contextually. Children and families are followed from the child's first transition from home to preschool until the child's second transition from preschool to elementary (primary) school.

Table 17.1   The protocols and corresponding strategies for the routines-based classroom engagement model (RECM) programme

Steps	Strategies	Description
Step 1	Gathering information	The primary service providers (PSPs) and other non-PSPs conduct the routines-based interviews for needs assessment. The caregivers (parents/classroom teachers) **share information** about routines, needs and concerns (1.5–2 hours)
Step 2	Collaborative goal setting	The family members are supported/coached by the PSPs to identify **functional goals**
Step 3	Joint-planning of the intervention	The PSPs **collaborate with/coach caregivers** through **joint-planning**
Step 4	Embedded intervention	The PSPs **collaboratively consult with caregivers** with the strategies **embedded** in **classrooms/family routines** based on **systematic observation** to address the functional goals
Step 5	Caregiver–professional partnership for outcome and process evaluation	At the end of the semester, the PSPs and the caregivers (classroom educators/parents) **work together** to **examine the achievement of the functional goals** with the goal attainment scale (GAS), the Canadian Occupational Performance Measure (COPM) and Goal Functionality III to assess the individualised goals as the outcomes for children
Step 6	Successful transition	The PSPs interview the **children** about their **views of transition** (from preschool/centre to elementary school) before and 4–6 months after transition

Who are the Primary Service Providers?

The primary service providers conducting the RECM programme are professionals, including therapists, medical practitioners, special education teachers and social workers. Each participating centre has a primary service provider who is supported by other professionals called non-primary service providers.

EXAMPLE 2. PROJECT TEAM (TEENS MAKING ENVIRONMENT AND ACTIVITY MODIFICATIONS): TEACHING TRANSITION AGE YOUTH WITH DEVELOPMENTAL DISABILITIES TO IDENTIFY AND RESOLVE ENVIRONMENTAL BARRIERS TO PARTICIPATION

What is Project TEAM?

Project TEAM is a multi-component intervention from the United States that teaches transition age youth with developmental disabilities to identify environmental barriers and supports, generate solutions to resolve barriers, and request modifications that facilitate participation at school, work, and the community. Project TEAM is uniquely designed to support youth who may have co-occurring cognitive impairments and/or intellectual disabilities. It is co-facilitated by a licensed health professional (e.g. occupational therapist, social worker, teacher, nurse) and a person with a disability (advocate) with prior advocacy experience. In combination, the professional and advocate foster an environment conducive to learning and that takes a positive orientation towards disability. The 12-week intervention includes three components: individualised goal setting, a group curriculum and peer mentoring.

Before the first group session, youth identify an individualised participation goal. Youth choose a valued everyday life situation in which they desire to increase the frequency, quality or independence of engagement. Youth set goals related to leisure and social activities, vocational or employment roles, independent living, education and advanced training, or community participation and mobility. They also attend one community-based outing (Levin and Kramer 2015) related to the goal to identify environmental barriers and implement modifications with the support of a facilitator.

The group curriculum includes eight modules that teach concepts necessary to identify and resolve environmental barriers using the problem solving process called the 'Game Plan'. The modules include multi-modal learning activities ranging from didactic discussions, interactive visual slide presentations, games and role playing. An intervention manual provides detailed directions for each learning activity, and the key elements necessary to facilitate youths' learning. At the conclusion of each module, youth apply these concepts to their individualised participation goal and complete one additional step of the problem solving process.

Each youth in Project TEAM is matched with a peer mentor, or a youth who previously completed Project TEAM. Ideally, peer mentors have expertise or skills that can support the youth's attainment of the participation goal (Kramer et al. 2018). Peer mentors provide weekly e-mentoring using the phone, video chat or internet messaging platform. Each week's mentoring session is guided by a participation topic, such as eating at a favourite restaurant, being a part of school activities or having a job (Levin and Kramer 2015). With the support of the peer mentor, youth practice applying the Game Plan to these additional participation scenarios.

Project TEAM is a theory-driven and evidence-based intervention. All components follow a specific protocol that therapists, peer mentors and youth follow sequentially. Project TEAM was designed in partnership with teens and young adults with developmental disabilities to ensure the format and content is salient to youths' everyday experiences and needs (Kramer et al. 2013). Four theoretical approaches underlay the design of Project TEAM: universal design for learning, experiential learning, cognitive-behavioural techniques, and peer and social learning (Kramer 2015). The components are designed to operationalise these theories and are hypothesised to activate the mechanisms that lead to changes in youth's capacity to problem solve and address environmental barriers to participation.

Who Can Participate?

Project TEAM takes a comprehensive approach to conceptualising the environment and recognises the unique impact of environment demands on each individual. Project TEAM is appropriate for youth with a range of cognitive, motor and sensory abilities and needs. All materials and activities incorporate visuals to support learning and comprehension and provide a variety of avenues for expressing ideas (e.g. written, spoken, drawings). Youth with and without intellectual disabilities, including those with moderate level intellectual disability can engage in the intervention and learn the Game Plan problem solving process (Kramer et al. 2018).

Project TEAM research has included youth and young adults preparing for transition to adulthood, who are aged 14–21 (Kramer et al. 2018). These youth experience increased opportunities to demonstrate independence and engage in a range of leisure, social, educational and vocational activities across contexts. Youth with some previous exposure to these activities may be better able to identify a meaningful personal participation goal and have previous experiences with environmental barriers and supports that they can use as a self-reference during the training.

What is the Game Plan?

The Game Plan is a four-step problem solving approach: Goal, Plan, Do and Check. Each step includes a self-talk question, along with a visual image and kinaesthetic motion to promote internalisation and recall. The Game Plan worksheet further breaks down the steps needed to successfully identify barriers, supports and potential solutions (Table 17.2). For example, in Plan Step 1, youth decide if any of 11 categories of the environment help or make it harder for them to participate in their desired activity. In Plan Step 2, youth select from six potential strategies to address identified barriers. The environmental categories and strategies were derived from a meta-synthesis exploring youths' perceptions of participation, and with input from youth who co-developed Project TEAM (Kramer et al. 2012, 2013).

EXAMPLE 3. FITSKILLS: A STUDENT-MENTORED PHYSICAL ACTIVITY PROGRAMME FOR YOUTH WITH DISABILITY

What is FitSkills?

FitSkills is an evidence-based, community-based, physical activity programme for young people with disability aged 13–30 years (Shields et al. 2018). In FitSkills a young person with disability is matched with a student mentor and the pair exercise together at their local gym (a one-to-one programme). The programme runs over 12 weeks with two sessions per week (24 sessions total). The exercise content is individually tailored to the young person with disability and prescribed according to international best practice guidelines from the American College of Sports Medicine.

FitSkills was developed from qualitative studies, randomised controlled trials and knowledge translation studies (Mahy et al. 2010; Shields and Taylor 2010; Shields et al. 2013b). Key to its success is the mutual benefit experienced by the young person with disability and the student mentor; the young

Table 17.2 Project TEAM's Game Plan problem solving approach

Step	Self-talk question	Worksheet steps	UDL features	
			Visual image	Kinesthetic motion
Goal	What activity would I like to do?	Youth identify an individualised participation goal based. They may write or draw their goal		Shoulder shrug, asking question
Step 1	What parts of the environment help me or make it hard for me?	Youth evaluate 11 environmental demands and determine if they are barriers or supports to participation in their goal: things, inside places, outside places, people, services and organisations, rules, technology, ground, entrances and exits, signs and information, light, sound and smell		Thumbs up and down
Step 2	What strategy can I use to change the environment?	Identify the strategy that can reduce and/or remove the specific barrier(s): change the rules, change spaces, teach others about abilities and needs, ask for help, use technology or things, plan ahead		Pointing to head in thinking motion
Step 3	Would using this strategy change this activity for other people?	Determine how family, friends, co-workers, supervisor or boss, teachers or staff, or other community members may be impacted by the strategy		Gesturing/pointing to others
Do	Who do I talk to about making this change?	Identify the disability rights law that provides legal protections for the selected strategy. Write an advocacy script to request the desired change		Hand making talking motion
Check	Can I do this activity now?	Youth self-evaluate goal attainment and decide if additional barriers exist		Make a check with finger

person with disability gets the support they need to participate in exercise and the student develops a deeper understanding of disability (Shields et al. 2013a). FitSkills operates as a fee-for-service programme. A coordinator manages the programme day-to-day including participant and mentor recruitment and matching, mentor training and supervision, and access to community gymnasia.

Who Can Participate?

Young people with any type of disability can participate if they are well enough to do moderate intensity exercise and can follow simple verbal instructions. After an expression of interest has been received, there is a screening process (including obtaining medical clearance if necessary) to identify if there is any safety or medical reason a young person should not participate. For example, having an unstable medical condition or behavioural concerns that would put the student mentor or other gym users at unnecessary risk.

Who are the Student Mentors?

Initially, the student mentors were entry-level physiotherapy and exercise physiology students. We have extended the role to entry-level students from all year levels across a range of health disciplines including occupational therapy, speech and language therapy, podiatry and dietetics. Student mentors need to have a current working with children check and a police check to ensure there are no legal reasons they cannot work with vulnerable populations. They are not required to have experience working in disability. Student mentors are matched with young people with disability based on their availability and where they live. Some matches are based on gender where a young person with disability or their family have requested this.

Student mentors complete a training session (approximately 3 hours) prior to commencing the programme. Training includes discussion about working with a young person with disability, the exercise programme (including a practical session at a gym), occupational health and safety requirements, advice on managing difficult situations and safe-guarding children legal requirements. Each student mentor receives a printed training manual. Mentors engage in ongoing mentoring during the programme with the programme coordinator who is an experienced paediatric physiotherapist.

HOW THESE INTERVENTIONS FACILITATE PARTICIPATION

RECM, Project TEAM and FitSkills target intrinsic and extrinsic factors that influence participation as per the family of participation-related constructs (fPRC). In this section, we describe how these interventions foster participation across the life course.

RECM, Project TEAM and FitSkills are three evidence-based approaches for enabling participation in community contexts and environments.

By targeting intrinsic factors that influence participation, these three interventions lead to individual developmental changes that foster attendance and involvement in community-based contexts. First, RECM, Project TEAM and FitSkills address activity competence by equipping individuals with disabilities with *skills* that facilitate participation. Second, these interventions address a person's intrapersonal sense of self via *social learning* approaches that strive to enhance their confidence and self-esteem. These simultaneous changes in one's sense of self and activity competence change the experience of participation (Imms et al. 2016). As one's experience of participation changes, with the support provided in the intervention, a person gains a sense of *empowerment,* or increased agency to further influence one's own participation. The three interventions also address extrinsic factors that influence participation. By directly or indirectly addressing *others' attitudes about disability,* the interventions change the participation opportunities provided to individuals with disabilities. Third, we will consider how these interventions fit within and across broader cultural environments and discuss how they may be adopted in other countries and cultures.

Building Skills

RECM, Project TEAM and FitSkills all focus on skill development. However, the types of skills developed and the individual targeted for skill development varies with the life-stage.

LINK TO VIGNETTE 17.1
'School Lunches in Japan', p. 55.

ROUTINES-BASED ENGAGEMENT CLASSROOM MODEL

In RECM, service providers use a coaching approach to improve other professionals' and parents' skills to support children's engagement in everyday classroom routines. RECM builds service provider's capacity to deliver family-centred services (family-centredness) and develops caregivers' and children's skills to support participation in everyday routines (functionality). The primary service providers provide the caregivers, including educators in children's classrooms and parents, with emotional, information and material support in the classroom or at home. A coaching approach is used in addition to routines-based interviews with caregivers, and systematic observation of educators and children in classroom. These approaches help caregivers clarify the problems they are concerned about. In addition, at least one home visit is completed to help the primary service providers understand the natural environment that shapes the child's functional ability. It is only after these processes have been completed (interviews, observation in classroom, home visit) that primary service providers share their suggestions.

RECM also attends to the social-emotional development of all preschool children, including children with disabilities. In Taiwanese preschools, developing cognitive and motor skills is emphasised over social-emotional skills. Diverse programmes and training are available to develop cognitive and motor skills but there are few specific programmes designed to develop social-emotional skills in the classroom. This provided a strong rationale to embed social skills learning in classroom routines through the RECM programme. RECM is based on social development theories (Moore 2007) which proposes children's social relationships with others both in the present and in the future are influenced by the type and quality of relationships among the adults surrounding the child. As adults interact with each other and with children, children learn through observing and modelling adult interactions. Social and emotional development is hard to teach, but, children can develop social-emotional skills when they can practice interactions that have been modelled by adults in their daily routines.

PROJECT TEAM

Project TEAM provides youth with disability with the skills needed to identify and resolve environmental barriers to participation in desired activities. The Game Plan problem solving process incorporates self-talk questions, derived from meta-cognitive and cognitive-behavioural approaches that support internalisation of knowledge and generalisation to other situations (Meichenbaum 1977). The Game Plan provides a structured framework with 11 environment categories to help youth learn the skills to identify barriers and supports. Additionally, the Game Plan teaches youth how to use six strategies to resolve identified barriers.

Project TEAM curriculum also teaches youth advocacy skills needed to request changes in their environment. The curriculum introduces an 'advocating for change' social script that youth individualise to include the specific barriers that impact their participation, and the strategy that will resolve that barrier. Youth who completed Project TEAM had a significant increase in their knowledge of environmental barriers and modification strategies, and a significant increase in their ability to apply the Game Plan to problem solve a barrier to participation (Kramer et al. 2018). More importantly, 6 weeks after Project TEAM, youth had significantly higher goal attainment compared to youth who set participation goals without support over a comparable period (Kramer et al. 2018). These findings suggest youth generalised the knowledge and skills acquired in Project TEAM to their everyday lives.

FITSKILLS

FitSkills teaches youth with disability the physical and social skills needed to participate in exercise so they can develop confidence, establish an exercise routine and make positive changes in their health behaviour.

The name FitSkills was chosen to emphasise the programme's purpose in building skills in addition to providing an opportunity for young people with disability to exercise. The programme is targeted at young people with disability who have never participated in exercise and who might need to develop 'skills' to participate. The physical skills they learn relate to how to exercise and how to use gym equipment. The social skills participants develop include navigating a new environment (community gym), meeting new people, how to co-exist in a shared space and the social norms expected. FitSkills was found to support participation in youth with disability by assisting their access to community facilities and to build their skills and capability for community participation (Shields et al. 2018).

Student mentors also develop skills. Research shows students reported developing communication skills, building rapport, giving instructions, modifying communication style, motivation techniques and professional skills, including leadership skills, managing relationships, organisational skills, 'duty-of-care', working with children and problem solving (Shields et al. 2013a, 2014b).

Social Learning

Bandura's Social Learning Theory posits people learn from one another through observation, imitation and modelling (Bandura 1977). RECM, Project TEAM and FitSkills all involve a social learning component. The context and people targeted in these programmes highlight different ways social learning can be used to increase participation across different age ranges.

ROUTINES-BASED ENGAGEMENT CLASSROOM MODEL

In RECM, social learning happens at multiple levels, including children, educators/parents, and primary service providers. Preschool educators play a dual role because they are both professionals and caregivers. They are supported by the primary service providers to offer rich learning opportunities to children in their classrooms. Preschool educators serving a RECM classroom develop social skills in three dimensions: their openness towards receiving strategies, acceptance of families from diverse backgrounds and willingness to follow the children's lead in the classroom.

RECM provides families with the skills they need to be involved in their child's preschool education. Families are encouraged to be involved and to share their opinions with the children's educators about the programme's design. Families are encouraged to use their strengths and to collaborate with educators to promote children's engagement in the classroom. The primary service providers also help families identify existing social relations using an ecomap or to build new relationships with other parents, educators and professionals.

PROJECT TEAM

The Project TEAM group curriculum facilitates social learning where youth are encouraged to share their experiences, identify things they have in common and use their experiences to help others attain their goals. Weekly formalised social learning via e-mentoring compliments this informal social learning. In Project TEAM, each e-mentoring session is organised around seven objectives. These objectives are operationalised into a mentoring 'script', and foster the mentoring relationship (e.g. discuss favourite activities and interests), mobilise the mentor's expertise (e.g. mentor provides examples from his/her own life), and provide mentees assistance with application and generalisation of Project TEAM concepts (e.g. support to practice the Game Plan problem solving process). The script facilitates a successful peer mentoring experience with mentors who have a range of disabilities; a feasibility evaluation of 42 peer mentoring relationships found youth were actively engaged during 94% of all objectives and mentors achieved 87% of objectives (Kramer et al. 2018).

FITSKILLS

As with RECM and Project TEAM, a social learning approach is also fundamental to FitSkills. Matching a young person with disability with a student mentor to positively influence each other's lives is a critical part of the programme. Student mentors provide the social support young people with disability need to participate in exercise (Mahy et al. 2010), while young people with disability provide mentors with the opportunity to learn about living with a disability (Shields et al. 2013a). A pertinent point is that the student mentor is not a personal trainer; rather they exercise together with the young person with disability. This is important to making the relationship between the young person with disability and the student mentor equitable and akin to a peer relationship. As one participant said: 'It made a big difference having someone … that I got along with and, having someone, I have to go to the gym 'cause someone's waiting for me.'

FitSkills shows how social learning at the community level can help address the problem of non-participation in exercise among youth with disability. Community partnerships are an essential element. Programme design, development and delivery involved consumer input and collaboration with community partners including community recreation facilities, disability advocacy groups and local government. FitSkills aims to promote social inclusion (rather than segregation or integration) by facilitating exercise participation that is no different from what is experienced by youth without disabilities. The programme fosters civic values in young people training to be health professionals by encouraging them to volunteer to support youth with disability in their own community.

Empowerment

Through skills development and social learning, preschool children (RECM), adolescents (Project TEAM) and young adults (FitSkills) are empowered to participate in their respective communities. Empowerment is the process of promoting self-actualisation and enhancing an individual's influence over their lives and the lives of others (Christens et al. 2011). In each programme, empowerment is realised in a different way by different target groups.

ROUTINES-BASED ENGAGEMENT CLASSROOM MODEL

In RECM, the aim is to empower educators, parents and children by building a relationship between the primary service providers and caregivers, between educators and children in the classroom, and between parents and children. Empowerment through relationship building is supported by the six steps of the RECM programme that incorporate the concepts of strengths-based, goal-oriented, collaborative goal setting and self-determination of participation-based therapy (Palisano et al. 2012). The steps gather information through routines-based interviews (in Step 1), collaborative goal setting (Step 2), joint-planning of the intervention (Step 3), embedded intervention (Step 4), caregiver–professional partnership for outcome and process evaluation (Step 5), and successful transition (Step 6). These steps enable caregivers (educators or parents) to feel comfortable expressing themselves, and to make informed decisions about the child and family goals by collaborating with the primary service providers. All six steps of the programme follow a similar pattern of coaching to empower the educators and the parents and thereby increase their confidence in their skills, or problem solving. The research indicates caregivers (including educators and parents) who are confident and engaged benefit children's participation (Leonard et al. 2017) by being able to express their parenting ideas, and by advocating for the full inclusion and integration of their children in society in the future (Palisano et al. 2012).

PROJECT TEAM

Youth equipped with the knowledge and skills to resolve environmental barriers to their desired goals are more likely to feel empowered. In Project TEAM, youth are exposed to disability rights laws that posit inclusion and access as a human right. Project TEAM was designed in the United States, and thus the curriculum focuses on laws ensuring access for people with disabilities in education (IDEA), employment law (ADA, Rehab Act), government funded programmes (Rehab Act), and public accommodations (ADA). One youth completing Project TEAM shared: 'I definitely like learning about disability rights laws because I knew the ADA and the IDEA existed, but I didn't know the purpose'. Understanding the purpose of these laws aims to empower youth with disabilities to request changes that will increase their participation in valued everyday life situations.

FitSkills

FitSkills aims to empower young people with disability to exercise in their local community (Shields et al. 2018). Youth with disability often have low expectations about exercise participation. FitSkills has high expectations of participants and emphasises their ability to participate in high intensity community-based exercise. The programme aims to empower youth with disability to challenge perceptions that young people with disability should not participate in strenuous exercise, by offering them the opportunity to show themselves, their families and their communities just what they can do. In the words of one participant, 'It was good to actually see just what I was capable of.'

FitSkills encourages independence as the programme is completed one to one with a mentor who is not a family member, helping to build resilience and increase social connectedness. These outcomes are particularly important for youth with disability who are at higher risk of health problems and who often have small social networks. It is also important for their families, who frequently shoulder the burden of care. As one parent said: 'I think it's been good for [my daughter] to get into a routine of going somewhere else with someone else to do exercise.' A longer term aim of FitSkills is to empower young people with disability to choose positive health behaviours. The programme duration is 12 weeks: short enough to commit to, but long enough to establish a new routine of engagement in physical activity and to achieve the physiological benefits of exercise participation. FitSkills is deliberately set in a real-world community context, so participants can experience their own locality. The rationale is to empower young people with disability to continue to exercise in their local community or engage in another physical activity on an ongoing basis. Up to 50% of participants in our feasibility study continued to exercise either at the gym or in other community-based physical activities after FitSkills (Shields et al. 2018).

By increasing the opportunities for children, youth and young adults to participate, RECM, Project TEAM and FitSkills facilitate a change in the attitudes of others towards disability.

Challenging Attitudes about Disability

Consistent with the fPRC and social learning, participation is influenced by extrinsic factors. However, participation also influences extrinsic factors.

Routines-Based Engagement Classroom Model

RECM directly changes the attitudes of professionals, educators, families and peers towards children with disability. The coaching approach used by the primary service providers supports educators, including those without disability training or experience, to generate strategies supporting children's attainment of functional goals in the classroom context. Primary service providers also facilitate parents' involvement in the planning and intervention process. Parents, in addition to gaining knowledge, can also help educators better understand each child's unique strengths and needs. When caregivers (educators and parents) understand how to better support the inclusion of children with disabilities in classroom routines, this may lead to changes in attitudes to disability. Further, inclusive classrooms allow children with and without disabilities to learn and play together, potentially changing the children's attitudes about disability and further fostering acceptance and inclusion.

Project TEAM

Project TEAM changes youth with disabilities' attitudes and beliefs about the relationship between their disability and participation in society. Although frameworks such as the ICF have increased practitioners' attention to the impact of the environment on a youth's participation, society's predominant approach to understanding disability is to attribute activity and participation restrictions to impairments in body structures and functions. Youth with disabilities are explicitly and implicitly exposed to these assumptions through media, health services and interactions with others. Therefore, youth with disabilities may also attribute participation restrictions to their disability. The Game Plan self-talk questions are designed to shift attributions of participation restrictions away from impairments to environmental barriers (Meichenbaum 1977). The explicit focus on the environment in the Game Plan reminds youth to attend to the impact of the physical, social, policy and sensory environment on participation. The strategies taught in Project TEAM make a direct change in the environment (change the rules, change spaces), or modify the youth's response to the environmental barrier (teach others about abilities and needs, ask for help, use technology or things, plan ahead). Complimented by modelling from peers and mentors, Project TEAM may help youth acquire a new attitude about the origins of challenges they encounter at school, community and work, and may empower youth to address those challenges through environmental modification and accommodations.

FitSkills

FitSkills is a catalyst for positive societal change around disability. The lack of visibility of youth with disability in community settings perpetuates negative societal attitudes towards disability. FitSkills aims to impact the wider community by increasing the visibility of youth with disability in community settings by their increased exercise participation. It is often assumed health professionals, particularly those working as therapists, have a positive attitude towards disability, but the reality is that health professionals' attitudes mirror those of society. Poor attitudes toward disability among health professionals is problematic as it can have a negative impact on the health services and care received by people with disability and can negatively impact workforce availability. Student mentors benefit by getting to know a young person with disability in an everyday context rather than a health context. This assists mentors to develop a richer understanding of living with a disability. Studies show students mentors who participate in FitSkills have more positive attitudes towards disability, are more confident around people with disability, and express a greater desire to work with people with disability in the future (Shields et al. 2014a, 2014b). Therefore, FitSkills encourages future health professionals to consider working in the disability sector when they graduate; an important outcome given the shortage of specialists in this area.

CULTURAL ADAPTATION

Culture is defined as the unique ideas, customs and social behaviour of a particular people or society, and links closely to the concept of social environment as defined in the fPRC. RECM, Project TEAM and FitSkills focus on empowerment, social learning, and building skills and can facilitate participation across cultures. However, each programme may require adaptation prior to adoption in other cultural contexts.

Routines-Based Engagement Classroom Model

RECM was designed for implementation in a cultural and policy context where inclusive education and 'push-in' services (e.g. where therapists provide therapy in the classroom) are not the norm. The primary service providers in RECM are attempting to transform services in which direct hands-on, pull-out therapies are believed to be the most beneficial. RECM may be most relevant in other cultural and policy contexts that also do not have inclusive education or push-in therapy as the primary service delivery model. One challenge is that consultation or non-direct services, especially for children with childhood-onset disability, are not ordinarily reimbursable in Taiwan and this may also be the case in other countries. However, family-centred practice is increasingly recognised as best practice and promoted by the government in Taiwan and health funding models are changing as a result. This may also be the case internationally.

Project TEAM

The specific laws introduced in Project TEAM would require revision for adoption in other countries. A further consideration is the extent to which other countries have robust, regulated disability rights laws. Countries without such laws may have a cultural context incongruent with the basic premise of Project TEAM; such a difference could impact the appropriateness and ultimate effectiveness of the intervention. However, youth with disabilities may still benefit from exposure to an environment-based perspective to understanding disability and completion of Project TEAM with peers may lead to advocacy for changes in policies and systems in their local context.

FitSkills

In FitSkills, the exercise occurs at a community gym because in Australia, most metropolitan and regional government councils own community gym facilities accessible by members of the public at reasonable cost. This may not be the case in other areas (e.g. rural and remote areas) or in other countries where this type of infrastructure either does not exist or is owned and run for-profit and so can only be accessed at high cost. The other aspect of FitSkills that may require adaptation in other cultural contexts is the participation of a student as mentor. This characteristic limits programme availability to areas where students live. However, involving student mentors tests the idea that a relatively low-skilled assistant could support exercise participation for youth with disability and suggests the potential for others such as community volunteers, friends, family members or paid support workers to take on this role if they can access appropriate support.

CONCLUSION

This chapter illustrates how interventions targeting participation can address the shifting needs of children with disabilities as they develop from early childhood to early adulthood. The life-course perspective taken in this chapter demonstrates how the outcome of 'participation' must adapt to social, cultural and contextual demands of each phase of development. Fostering participation of young children in preschool requires practitioners to equip teachers and parents with the skills for including all children, including those with disabilities, in positive learning environments and routines. As youth prepare for adulthood and increase their ability to engage in more complex activities, practitioners must shift their attention to empower and develop the competence and positive sense of self young adults need to engage in their communities, including secondary education, work and independent living. For adults, interventions that build their social networks and other supports to foster meaningful involvement in the community and leisure activities are needed. The RECM, Project TEAM and FitSkills interventions presented share the attributes of building skills, espousing social learning, fostering empowerment and changing cultural norms that ultimately promote participation across the life course for those with disability.

SUMMARY OF KEY IDEAS

- Interventions to facilitate participation require learning and behavioural change both in individuals with disability and those in their social environment.
- Children, adolescents and young adults with disability are empowered to participate in their respective communities through skills development and social learning.
- Interventions such as RECM, Project TEAM and FitSkills all address empowerment, social learning and skill building that can facilitate participation across cultures; however, individual programmes may require adaptation prior to adoption in other contexts.

ACKNOWLEDGEMENTS

RECM was funded by the by the Ministry of Science and Technology (MOST-105-2314-B-182-012 and MOST-106-2314-B-182-047), Chang Gung University and Chang Gung Memorial Hospital.

Project TEAM was developed with a grant from the Deborah Munroe Noonan Memorial Research Fund, the National Institute on Disability, Independent Living, and Rehabilitation Research (90IF0032-01-00), and the National Center for Medical Rehabilitation Research, National Institute of Child Health and Human Development/National Institute Neurological Disorders and Stroke, National Institutes of Health (K12 HD055931).

FitSkills was funded by H+L Hecht Trust and the Joanne Tubb Foundation, and received in-kind support from Disability Sport and Recreation.

REFERENCES

Bandura A (Ed) (1977) *Social Learning Theory*. Englewood Cliffs, NJ: Prentice-Hall.

Bradley RH, Whiteside-Mansell L, Casey PH, Barrett K (2010) Impact of a two-generation early education program on parenting processes at age 18. *J Fam Psychol* **24**: 478–484.

Christens BD, Peterson NA, Speer PW (2011) Community participation and psychological empowerment: testing reciprocal causality using a cross-lagged panel design and latent constructs. *Health Educ Behav* **38**: 339–347.

Dennis CL (2003) Peer support within a health care context: a concept analysis. *Int J Nurs Stud* **40**: 321–332.

Hwang AW, Chao MY, Liu SW (2013) A randomized controlled trial of routines-based early intervention for children with or at risk for developmental delay. *Res Dev Disabil* **34**: 3112–3123.

Hwang AW, Hsu YW, Su HC, McWilliam R (2018) *Case Studies in Implementing Routines-based Early Intervention and Its Cross-cultural Adaptation*. The 9th Conference of Services for People with Intellectual Disability in the Four Chinese-speaking areas. Parents' Association of Persons with Intellectual Disability. Taipei, Taiwan. 21–23 May 2018.

Imms C, Adair B, Keen D, Ullenhag A, Rosenbaum P, Granlund M (2016) "Participation": a systematic review of language, definitions, and constructs used in intervention research with children with disabilities. *Dev Med Child Neurol* **58**: 29–38.

Kramer JM (2015) Identifying and evaluating the therapeutic strategies used during a manualized self-advocacy intervention for transition-age youth. *OTJR (Thorofare, NJ)* **35**: 23–33.

Kramer JM, Ryan CT, Moore R, Schwartz A (2018) Feasibility of electronic peer mentoring for transition-age youth and young adults with intellectual and developmental disabilities: Project Teens making Environment and Activity Modifications. *J Appl Res Intellect Disabil* **31**: e118–e129.

Kramer J, Barth Y, Curtis K et al. (2013) Involving youth with disabilities in the development and evaluation of a new advocacy training: project TEAM. *Disabil Rehabil* **35**: 614–622.

Kramer JM, Olsen S, Mermelstein M, Balcells A, Liljenquist K (2012) Youth with disabilities' perspectives of the environment and participation: a qualitative meta-synthesis. *Child Care Health Dev* **38**: 763–777.

Kramer JM, Roemer K, Liljenquist K, Shin J, Hart S (2014) Formative evaluation of project TEAM (Teens making Environment and Activity Modifications). *Intellect Dev Disabil* **52**: 258–272.

Kramer JM, Helfrich C, Levin M et al. (2018) Initial evaluation of the effects of an environmental-focused problem-solving intervention for transition-age young people with developmental disabilities: project TEAM. *Dev Med Child Neurol* **60**: 801–809.

Leonard JA, Lee Y, Schulz LE (2017) Infants make more attempts to achieve a goal when they see adults persist. *Science* **357**: 1290–1294.

Levin M, Kramer JM (2015) Key elements supporting goal attainment for transition-age young adults: A case study illustration from Project TEAM. *Inclusion* **3**: 145–161.

McDonald KE, Balcazar FE, Keys CB (2005) Youth with disabilities. In: Dubois DL, Karcher MJ (Eds) *Handbook of Youth Mentoring*. Thousand Oaks, CA: Sage.

McWilliam RA (2010) *Routines-Based Early Intervention-Supporting Young Children and Their Families*. Maryland: Paul H. Brookes Publishing.

Mahy J, Shields N, Taylor N, Dodd KJ (2010) Barrier & facilitators to physical activity in adults with DS. *J Intellect Disabil Res* **54**: 795–805.

Meichenbaum D (1977) *Cognitive-Behavioral Modification: An Integrative Approach*. New York: Plenum Press.

Moore T (2007) *The Nature and Role of Relationships in Early Childhood Intervention Services*. Presented at the Second Conference of the International Society on Early Intervention, Zagreb, Croatia, 14–16 June 2007.

Palisano RJ, Chiarello LA, King GA, Novak I, Stoner T, Fiss A (2012) Participation-based therapy for children with physical disabilities. *Disabil Rehabil* **34**: 1041–1052.

Sameroff AJ, MacKenzie MJ (2003) Research strategies for capturing transactional models of development: the limits of the possible. *Dev Psychopathol* **15**: 613–640.

Shields N, Taylor NF (2010) Effects of a student-led progressive resistance training program on muscle strength and physical function in adolescents with Down syndrome. *J Physiother* **56**: 187–193.

Shields N, Taylor NF (2014a) Contact with young adults with disability led to a positive change in attitudes to disability among physiotherapy students. *Physiother Can* **66**: 298–305.

Shields N, Taylor NF (2014b) Physiotherapy students' self-reported assessment of professional behaviours and skills while working with young people with disability. *Disabil Rehabil* **36**: 1834–1839.

Shields N, Bruder A, Taylor NF, Angelo T (2013a) Getting fit for practice: an innovative paediatric clinical placement provided physiotherapy students opportunities for skill development. *Physiotherapy* **99**: 159–164.

Shields N, Taylor NF, Wee E, Wollersheim D, O'Shea SD, Fernhall B (2013b) A community-based strength training programme increases muscle strength and physical activity in young people with Down syndrome: a randomised controlled trial. *Res Dev Disabil* **34**: 4385–4394.

Shields N, van den Boos R, Buhlert-Smith K, Prendergast L, Taylor NF (2018) A community-based exercise program to increase participation in physical activities among youth with disability: a feasibility study. *Disabil Rehabil* **41**(10): 1152–1159.

Su HC, Chiang HY, Su HC, Chu HY, Hwang AW (2017) *The Practice Model for Nonprofit Preschools on Implementing Routines-Based Model in Inclusive Education*. The 18th International Conference and Workshops of Early Intervention Profession for Children with Developmental Delays. Taiwan Association of Child Development and Early Intervention. Taichung, Taiwan: National Taichung University of Education, 3–5 Nov 2018.

World Health Organization (2007) *International Classification of Functioning, Disability and Health: Children & Youth Version (ICF-CY)*. Geneva: World Health Organization.

The following vignette follows Rinta through his early school years as he learns to manage his developmental conditions within school. As you read, consider how the balance between participation as means (being included in usual settings) and participation as ends (separated to learn skills with a specialist) is managed and how choice and control are negotiated among key people.

School Lunches in Japan (Japan)

Manabu Saito and Motohide Miyahara

Rinta has acetonemic syndrome characterised by multiple vomiting. At daycare, his teacher reported: 'Rinta is delayed in language development, often plays alone, and has difficulties following rules when playing in groups'. A 5-year-old health check-up diagnosed Rinta with autism spectrum disorder, attention-deficit–hyperactivity disorder (ADHD) and developmental coordination disorder. Rinta's intelligence quotient was within the normal range, but he showed difficulties with verbal expression and easily gave up attempts to make himself understood.

When Rinta entered primary school, his parents wished to keep his disorders private, as is common with Japanese parents, and decided not to inform the school of his conditions. Rinta was placed in a regular classroom. After the first day of the school, Rinta said, 'I don't want to go to school'. The school teachers commented during the parent–teacher interview before the summer holiday, 'Rinta takes a long time to complete all sorts of tasks. He vomited twice during school lunches. He doesn't seem to like [compulsory] school lunch'.

The Japanese school lunch is a highly organised group activity in which Japanese pupils are expected to perform (see Fig. V17.1): pupil helpers on duty bring food to the classroom and serve food to each pupil

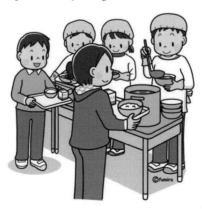

Figure V17.1 Compulsory school lunch; reprinted with permission © fumira. A colour version of this figure can be seen in the plate section.

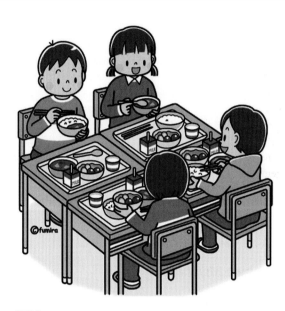

Figure V17.2 The school lunch; reprinted with permission © fumira.
A colour version of this figure can be seen in the plate section.

waiting in a queue, pupils take their plate to their study desk; all pupils in the home classroom say prayers aloud together before and after eating; all pupils are expected to eat all the food on the plate within a set time at the desk in the classroom, and put away their own dishes (see Fig. V17.2). Lunch is supervised by the homeroom teacher.

After the summer holiday, increased tantrums, at times frozen in catatonia, impeded participation in home life. Rinta was reluctant to go to school. His child psychiatrist (MS) prescribed medication for ADHD and proposed play therapy to support Rinta's ability to express himself verbally and emotionally. In the beginning, he expressed violent scenes and violence in play, and thus seemed to release his anger. Coincidentally, Rinta's aggressive behaviours gradually decreased at home.

In the second year of primary school, Rinta obsessively tried to conform to the regime of school lunch because he believed he would be scolded and something horrible would happen if he failed. The frequency of Rinta's food aversions increased and his psychiatrist proposed that Rinta should take his time to eat in the school nurse's room. This proposal was accepted by the school as a special exception.

In this second year, Rinta was placed in a special support class where he studied one hour each school day; developing a bond with a teacher. During a clinic visit Rinta was able to explain to his psychiatrist, that:

> Sensei (the teacher) thinks I pressure myself too hard and I get overwhelmed in my homeroom class. So, I am placed in the special support class to slow down and study at my own pace … I want to spend more time at school than one hour in the special support class.

To make his verbalised wish come true, the psychiatrist requested for Rinta to spend more hours in the special support class, which was granted.

During play therapy a few months later, Rinta was able to describe the events in the play adequately. When it was suggested to terminate play therapy, Rinta insisted 'I want to continue a little bit longer' and his play therapy continued.

In Year 3, Rinta was able to speak about his thoughts and feelings during play therapy. This therapy was terminated in December. Current treatment is limited to his attention problem. His food aversion rarely occurs, and Rinta can eat all his school lunch in the homeroom every day. This vignette highlights the importance of individualising interventions within the school environments. Sensitivity to the balance between inclusion in 'compulsory' (non-discretionary) activities, whilst recognising the need to build skills and performance capacity to enable participation, can be a challenge as in the case for Rinta and other children with different needs. To meet the challenge, a school intervention strategy should be directed to accommodate a wide variety of children, including students with neurodisability to acquire social skills and adapt to a strict school regime gradually at their own pace and to allow for individual decision-making and environmental arrangements.

Participatory Interventions: Interventions Situated in Meaningful Contexts

Citlali López-Ortiz, Reidun Jahnsen and Dido Green

INTRODUCTION

> *I am always chosen last for teams at school and the other team always gloat as they know they are going to win*
>
> – Lisa aged 11, with hemiplegia

Interventions that actively involve individuals performing meaningful activities within relevant contexts and environments not only have ecological validity but are inherently participatory. Enabling access to 'real-world' experiences such as clubs, camps, forums, fairs and specialist events may, on the one hand, be the direct outcome of an intervention and, on the other, enable change processes to be embedded within the participatory occasions. Opportunities to 'take the therapy out of therapy', by repositioning interventions within 'real' or typical activities, offers a different perspective to intervention design with potential for non-intrusive therapeutic strategies. This section focuses on interventions involving different types of participation such as drama, sport or other activities, rather than therapies focusing on increasing skills or environmental changes to enable participation.

PARTICIPATORY INTERVENTIONS

What do we mean when we use the term 'participatory interventions'? With interventions that focus on participation as an *outcome*, the goals of intervention are directed toward increased attendance in meaningful life activities along with opportunities for being involved while attending. Thus, these interventions may focus on increasing individual capacity and or environmental modifications to enable participation. In contrast, we can consider interventions in which participation is the *means* (as well as the ends). As such, intrinsic factors are of paramount importance in the design of these interventions in which individual experiences, including memories and anticipated 'journeys', are integral features with the person situated within contexts of relevance. Participatory interventions work to facilitate involvement of the individual in transaction within momentary situations and more enduring interactions

Although skills are built, and environments may be adapted, these occur within and through the participatory process rather than in preparation for an anticipated participation outcome.

and within the same or differing environments. Emphasis is placed on the context of participation which is accepted by the individual as representative of regular or typical places where people 'do things' (King et al. 2013, p. 1578). The selected contexts, activity settings and niches (see Chapter 4) are those which the person believes will provide them with desired experiences or outcomes or are the physical and social settings in which a child lives. The focus is on the experiences and opportunities for engaging in different life situations.

The next section illustrates different examples that have taken advantage of community-based projects for participation as the means rather than as the outcome of therapy. We will describe the characteristics of these approaches and focus on similarities and differences that support the key concepts of participatory processes: opportunities, strategies, experiences and outcomes that reflect new goals and directions.

THE LOCAL ENVIRONMENT MODEL: FROM NORWAY TO ANYWHERE?

Participation in physical activities for persons with disabilities in local communities is often a challenge. Both social and physical barriers may contribute to individuals with disabilities participating in less physical activity than the general population (Jirikowic and Kerfeld 2016).

The Local Environment Model involves: activity-based intensive participation, adapting environments and/or tasks, skilled professionals, group model, mutual engagement, and assessment and evaluation.

The local environment model (LEM) is a programme, designed and implemented at Beitostoelen Healthsports Centre (BHC) within the healthcare system in Norway. Norwegian disability policy stipulates inclusion in mainstream schools and kindergartens with free healthcare for all children, to facilitate physical activity participation for children with disabilities in their home, school and local community (Nyquist et al. 2016; Willis et al. 2018). The aim of this model is to enhance participation in community leisure activities for children and youth with disabilities by providing an intensive 3-week stay with individually adapted physical activities including assistive devices, and enough time and space to learn the preferred activities. The principles are generic and could be implemented in other environments or countries (Willis et al. 2018).

The LEM includes a preparation stage in the local community, intervention stage at BHC and follow-up stage back in the local community. Core components are derived from adapted physical activity (APA) theory (Sherrill and Hutzler 2008), situated learning theory (Standal and Jespersen 2008) and the International Classification of Functioning, Disability and Health (ICF) (WHO 2007). Core implementation drivers are enabled through careful staff selection and programme structure, didactics, facilitative administration and transformational leadership; thus, incorporating universal principles promoting community participation anywhere.

Who Can Participate?

All individuals with disabilities can apply to stay at BHC; 3 weeks in a group with eight other children and youth with disabilities and their caregivers, preferably from the same or neighbouring community. It starts with a wish by a young person with a disability to learn an activity to be performed among peers at home. However, to learn the activity, adaptations of the activity, the learning process or an assistive device may be required. For example, visual impairment may be a barrier to use a sit-ski independently, so a bi-ski might be the appropriate assistive device for this activity. During 3 weeks of intensive practicing both the children and their caregivers will have to learn how to manoeuvre the bi-ski.

Participation Experiences of the Local Environment Model

One month prior to their stay, children, youth and adults are asked about their activity preferences and a team from BHC visits their local communities to tell them about the centre and programme. At BHC, the participant and caregiver enter a liminal phase where there are different rules and responsibilities than at home. The preferred activity and the learning process are adapted, so that the participant can perform the activity in their own way with the assistance they need.

At the centre there is a new kind of freedom where children and youth, for once, experience not standing out, because everybody 'has something' and all others also struggle with similar challenges. Others may need more help than they do themselves, or, may be they need exactly what another individual happens to be good at. In this way participation in the group enhances participation by practicing participation in a safe and including environment. During the last week of the stay, the local service providers such as therapists, assistants and teachers, are invited to the centre for 2 to 3 days to learn how to facilitate implementation of the new activities in the community of the children and youth. Three months after the stay, the team from BHC again visit the local community of the individuals to evaluate what has happened at home. This support focuses on physical and social environmental factors that may be barriers or facilitators for participation in preferred activities among peers in the local community. Success factors are sought to learn from and bring to other groups at the centre. Many activities are continued in local communities 1 year after leaving BHC Baksjøberget et al. (2017).

COMMUNITY-BASED ACTIVITIES: AFTER-SCHOOL CLUBS AND SUMMER CAMPS

I can now kick and catch a ball, but they still won't let me join in

– John, aged 7, with Developmental Coordination Disorder (DCD);
Green and Martini (2017, p. 195)

The importance of developing interventions that are participatory in nature rather than assume that a participatory outcome will be achieved, is exemplified in John's lament. John set his goals for therapy to be able to kick a goal (football/soccer). When John attended for a therapy review, he described how, despite now having the ability to throw, kick and catch a ball, the other kids at his school did not let him join in their games. His, and other students', comments reflect the need for interventions that engage children and young people in opportunities within the contexts that are meaningful to them and in which they desire to take part, because having the component physical skill is not sufficient to enable participation.

Situating opportunities within the school environment or in after-school clubs is one method. Based on the opportunities these settings could offer, we set up after-school clubs for children with movement difficulties in local community centres. The first project placed these clubs in a local sports centre as a clinical service. The success of this was evidenced with most children transitioning from the 'sports club for children with movement difficulties' to regular sports activities such as gymnastics and swimming provided at the centre. Situating the clubs in a 'regular community setting' provided opportunities to meet with the various instructors to consider strategies to involve the child within regular sessions with peers.

Following on from these sports clubs, an after-school club for children with DCD was set up in community gyms. The Cognitive Orientation to daily Occupational Performance (CO-OP) approach was the basis for the therapeutic intervention, embedded within a 'Detective club' (Green and Martini 2017). Removing the therapeutic context by selecting venues that children typically attend for after-school activities was deemed essential to programme success. These venues had space for parents to join in club activities or go for coffee/tea and socialise. While we did measure and report on traditional therapeutic targets of goal attainments set by the children and their parents (Green and Martini 2017), the consequences of these clubs extended far beyond these aims. Session records show the following examples:

- Following a club using frisbees, children asked to take frisbees home and arranged to meet up on the weekend in the park.
- After one child had learnt to ride a bike in the club, he and his father were able to go for a bike ride – their first positive shared experience. Two weeks later, the whole family went for a ride.
- A group of 5 and 6-year-olds requested several play dates outside of the club, and one family coordinated a weekend sleepover for the children.

A similar model of situating therapy within non-therapy contexts is evident in the 'themed' day camps for children with hemiplegia or unilateral cerebral palsy: circus-themed in Australia and magic-themed camps in Israel and United Kingdom (Green and Ziviani 2017). The magic-themed programme has held the camps in regular community settings including theatres and community arts centres. In these camps, the process of participation was valued as important as the movement skills outcomes. This is reflected in the thank you letter written and signed by all the students in our first Israeli camp in 2010:

> We had 10 wonderful days. We also laughed as our teachers helped us learn new skills. We wanted to thank you for giving us this opportunity. Thank you for pushing us. Thank you for not giving up on us; and Thank you for not feeling sorry for us. Thank you from all of us.

The young people from this camp created their own Facebook page and organised magic shows in each other's schools. Following this camp, we recruited the older graduates as paid trainers in subsequent camps, providing an opportunity for them to share experiences, gain work experience, have some fun and a 'just right challenge'. As one teenager stated: 'Thank you for turning my disability into an ability.'

VIRTUAL COMMUNITIES

Exponential developments in computer technologies and applications have had a phenomenal impact across all aspects of 21st century lifestyles; in Western societies and in less well-developed economies. Use of the internet, computer gaming and social media are common activities for children and adolescents (Council on Communication and Media 2013). This has shifted the nature of play and leisure for many individuals and increased opportunities for accessing educational, work and social activities. Technology has also influenced rehabilitation tools and processes. Studies of virtual reality (VR) and virtual reality-related technologies (such as participation in active video gaming) for children with disabilities have considered outcomes related to motor performance or physical activity participation

(Hickman et al. 2017). In addition, social media provides opportunities for education and learning (Asuncion et al. 2012).

Virtual Reality

Emerging evidence shows potential for participation through and with technologies across multiple areas including virtual play for children with disabilities (Reid 2002); and as valued leisure activities for young adults often excluded from many 'mainstream physical presence' leisure activities (Weiss Bialik and Kizony 2003). These virtual environments provide opportunities for participation that have value in themselves.

Online gaming has increased as a popular activity for children and adolescents in the past decade. Recreational use of the internet including social media is now reported to be greater than the time spent in school or with friends (in the 'real world') with 8- to 10-year-old's spending up to 8 hours per day and adolescents up to 11 hours per day (Council on Communication and Media 2013). These changes in the dynamics of play, gaming and leisure, open up opportunities for young people with disabilities to access mainstream activities, but may also pose some hazards for young people at greater risk of addictive disorders (Paulus et al. 2018).

Virtual and online shopping is an area for participation that provides, on the one hand, opportunities to shop and purchase needed and desired goods. On the other hand, however, physical elements of shopping (in the real world) and accompanying social interactions may be lost.

Social Media

In Chapter 7, the importance of being connected to a social community was highlighted; having friends and being able to spend time together, sharing experiences and conversations, as well as providing and receiving emotional support, are critical to all people. Individuals with severe movement impairments and complex communication difficulties are at risk of social exclusion for many reasons. Social media provides access to social participation in many different ways and may have particular benefit for those in regions with less developed services for individuals with disabilities. Mobile technologies are increasingly available across the globe and virtual environments (Asuncion et al. 2012) offering enhanced access to information and an ability to engage with important topics. They also allow individuals to develop and maintain friendships and build social connectedness with a community; albeit one that without an immediate physical presence.

Access to physical social contexts and environments may be limited by environmental barriers as well as communication impairments (Chapter 7). Research exploring the impact on young people with communication disabilities, living in rural Australia, of learning to use social media, showed increased social connections, increased frequency and nature of communication and surprisingly, also improved speech intelligibility and literacy (Raghavendra et al. 2015). These findings were echoed in work by Hynan and colleagues (2014) in a qualitative study of young people using augmentative and alternative communication in metropolitan areas in the United Kingdom; highlighting capacity of social media to enable social connectedness and perceived opportunities for self-determination.

With opportunities, may also come hazards. Online (cyber) bullying is on the increase, and its impact on children without disabilities a concern (Best Manktelow and Taylor 2014). Children with special educational needs, particularly those who have fewer friends and who are alone at (real-world) playtime or who have intellectual and/or developmental disabilities, are vulnerable to being bullied

(Rowley et al. 2012) or to suffer cyberbullying (Didden et al. 2009). While it is not known whether young people with disabilities are more exposed to cyberbullying than their peers, they may lack the emotional resilience, communication and/or practical skills to manage these events. Raghavendra et al. (2015) and others emphasise the importance of providing parents and service provides with the knowledge and skills to facilitate access and use of social media. It is also likely they require tools to identify and manage cyberbullying.

SPECIALISED PROGRAMMES

Specialised Teaching with a Focus on Dance Classes for Children with Cerebral Palsy

A variety of adaptive and inclusive programmes for persons with cerebral palsy are increasingly available. Among those, dance classes are becoming more common in community, arts, education and health provider programming. The variety of dance forms and approaches to dance instruction may:

- include individuals with and without disability;
- be limited to participants with specific diagnoses, or a variety;
- require participation of family members, or assistants;
- involve a performative aspect;
- include trained physical and occupational therapists;
- be based on social dance experiences such as ballroom dancing; or
- focus on specific dance forms such as improvisational dance or Western classical ballet.

A common characteristic of dance programmes is enjoyable participation in a social group which is thought to enhance the quality of life of participants. One important aspect of dance programmes is that while the participant may be attending for the enjoyment of learning to dance in a supportive group environment, the instructor can design the class with a variety of objectives. While this might include learning movement for self-expression and socialisation, the specialised dance teacher or therapist may design and teach classes with specific rehabilitative and social interaction objectives. López-Ortiz et al. (2012) provides an example of this duality, where participants in a Western classical ballet-based dance class, designed to address movement impairment in cerebral palsy in a joyful participatory activity, was perceived by the participants as 'fun' and not therapy. The social participatory aspect of dance is a normalising experience for individuals with cerebral palsy.

The physically therapeutic aspect of dance classes for those with conditions like cerebral palsy is worth exploring since motivation for regular physical therapy decreases as children grow into adolescence and adulthood. Terada and colleagues (2017) have shown improvements in aerobic capacity for adults with cerebral palsy with severe movement limitations following participation in wheelchair dance. The non-competitive and creative nature of dance may provide a more rewarding experience for individuals for whom competitive sport and or 'routine' exercise are less appealing. Furthermore, the organisation of movement in classical ballet may help build an organised internal model of the body that is available for coordination of movement beyond the ballet class (López-Ortiz et al. 2012). Thus, therapeutic objectives are inherently integrated within the programme and leveraged, while the intrinsic expressive content in dance activities adds a psychosocial therapeutic dimension.

Harnessing the physicality of participation in a dance class requires knowledge of dance teaching methods and motor control deficits in cerebral palsy. This combined knowledge enables the teacher/therapist to target specific rehabilitation objectives within the framework of dance movements.

López-Ortiz et al. (2018) mapped categories of dance skills from the neurophysiological point of view into body structures and functions, activities and participation,which may guide the design of dance interventions targeting specific health outcomes. Using this framework, the trained ballet teacher or therapist may apply Western classical ballet teaching methods to address rehabilitation in a targeted manner.

Self-expression and socialisation are viewed as intrinsic by-products of participation in a dance class, occurring naturally as part of the process of dance.

Psychosocial dimensions in a dance class, however, can also be deliberately targeted as desired, in combination with the physical dimension. Since Western classical ballet is an expressive and creative performing art, the participants in the programme may be offered the opportunity to share and demonstrate their newly acquired skills to others by performing a class demonstration in the dance studio or in a theatre.

KEY ASPECTS OF SPECIALISED PROGRAMMES

Participatory interventions can provide new and valued opportunities and experiences, strategy generation and self-management and importantly, outcomes showing aspirations for new goals and directions. Opportunities to influence societal attitudes towards disability may also occur. Mapping the different examples provided against the concepts of participation and key ingredients of change processes, we see each offers essential opportunities for choice, social interaction and personal growth. The non-intrusive therapeutic aspects of these interventions, embedded within traditional skill-based acquisition programmes such as sport, dance, drama, 'specialist' clubs are appealing. These examples emphasise group dynamics in which learning of new and challenging skills is a shared experience, and personal achievement is valued, as well as respected, regardless of the initial starting point. Positive outcomes are evidenced in children as young as 4 years of age who report success through engagement and encouragement of their peers. Digital media also provides opportunities for participation across education, work, leisure and daily activities. The next section considers some of the key aspects of participatory interventions and opportunities illustrated through the examples provided.

Building Skills

Our examples illustrate situated learning among peers (Chapter 2). Time and space is available for massively repeated trials and practice, until the participants reach their goals and master individual objectives and preferred activities in real and virtual (e.g. social media) environments. Across the physical programmes, the principles of adapted physical activity pedagogics are evident, with adaptation of the activity as well as of the social and physical environment (Sherrill and Hutzler 2008). Group settings allow the child and family to see other children and families who experience the same daily challenges. These opportunities strengthen the courage or resolve to go beyond some of their own boundaries and thereby build activity competence required to be able to perform the preferred activity together with peers: in the words of one 11-year-old, to 'compete on a level playing field'.

Peer support and healthy competition in meaningful activities (e.g. importance of winter activities for Norwegian families) is evident across the programmes. Peer learning is probably the most important ingredient in the learning process. Nothing matches learning from others who are also learning the same skills (Standal and Jespersen 2008) and peer recognition of achievements is valued more highly than 'adult feedback' (Green and Martini 2017).

Involvement of caregivers may also be important, as in the bi-ski example in which caregivers not only feel the wind and speed, but what it is like to let go of control and trust the person steering the bi-ski. Caregivers must steer an empty bi-ski up and down the slope till they develop a feeling of mastery. Finally, the care givers steer the bi-ski with their own child or youth in it, a powerful emotional experience: breath-taking joy mixed with some fear. It is the combined skill development of youth and caregiver that makes for successful outcomes. Laughter and tears are always seen, especially among the caregivers but also among the staff. Goal attainment is always realised in moments of happiness (Willis et al. 2018) and the shared experience of over-coming challenges contributes to this stretching of achievement beyond expectation.

Social Learning

Bringing together people from the same community can facilitate social contact in the local environment after programmes end. Individuals participating in the BHC programmes in Norway, have continued to do physical activities together for 15 years, through to adulthood. Similarly, families participating in the Detective Club and Magic Camp programmes continue to be in contact 10 years later; organising varied shared activities.

For some young people, participation in these programmes will have been the first time they have met 'someone like me', and experienced being the assistant instead of always being the one who needs assistance. These learning situations in regular environments allow for special adaptations to be developed which are acceptable and in tune with the desires of the individuals involved. Being in a context where all the participants 'have something' provides the possibility to be one of many, and not standing out as the only one with a disability, for example, at the local school. The groups can enable feelings of belonging which may last far beyond the time at BHC, the clubs, camps and dance classes; contributing to self-acceptance and the development of an identity.

Empowerment

Mastering new activities or improving earlier learnt skills creates a feeling of empowerment. The story of the Vietnamese dance workshop highlights the value of enjoying for 'enjoyments' sake'. Participation practice in physically and socially safe environments may enhance feelings of mastery, perhaps sufficient to feel safe enough to go beyond former boundaries, and thus experience a new sense of self. Participation and involvement of family members who also experience empowerment and mastery, has shown to be of great benefit to being able to support children and transfer the performance of the preferred activities to the local environment at home (Willis et al. 2018). These community-based settings for participatory interventions contribute to empowering the whole family. Dance classes, magic shows and sports events in communities of diverse races, ethnicities and socio-economic backgrounds, along with per-formances to others within dance studios, public schools, on stage or in public events are good examples of where social empowerment has been realised. These also assist local service providers in promoting transfer of participation from therapy and rehabilitation centres to local school and community settings.

LINK TO VIGNETTE 18.1
'From Overcoming to Enjoying', p. 217.

Challenging Attitudes about Disability

Being the only one with a disability at the local school often gives the child and youth a certain role. They may be the one whom everybody pities, or the teacher may organise classmates to be with him or her during breaks. Or, the opposite might happen, namely teasing and exclusion. For example, speech difficulties may make people think that the person has an intellectual disability, leading caregivers and assistants to think that they know best what kind of assistance the child or youth with a disability needs.

Such attitudes are systematically challenged in community-based projects and activities which positively reframe capabilities by showcasing the skills, attributes and humanity of the individuals and groups. The transactional influences for learning and participation, among therapists and individuals with disabilities, shifts exponentially with shared enjoyment as illustrated in the vignette (18.1) providing a Vietnamese story.

Cultural Adaptation

Participatory interventions are also possible – if not even more feasible – in low resource settings. One example is a dance project developed to promote social interaction for children with intellectual disabilities in a Chilean orphanage (Green and Ziviani 2017). The children joined the dance project to support creative movement opportunities, choreographing scenarios to music of their choice, culminating in a performance of an 'army tank' to the Led Zeppelin band's Kashmir. On return to the United Kingdom, this experience was emulated in an after-school programme run in collaboration with a dance company for students from a local secondary (high) school and those in a special educational facility. This project and the research we undertook illustrated how positive shared experiences may also influence attitude change and open opportunities for children (Green and Ziviani 2017).

The principles from the LEM, developed in the Norwegian mountains, show capacity for adaptation to different healthcare systems and cultures to facilitate leisure participation. The intensive training could be organised as day camps with different frequencies, length of sessions, and times during the day (Sorsdahl et al. 2019). Willis et al. (2018) have described how the LEM may be transferred from Norwegian mountains to a summer-land on the other side of the globe.

PARTICIPATION AS PERFORMANCE

Participation in activities that have therapeutic benefits, for the sheer pleasure of participating as well as for any new skills achieved, do not need to be linked directly to rehabilitation services. The Amici Dance Theatre Company, instigated by Wolfgang Stange in 1980, is an integrated group of *able-bodied* and *disabled* artists and performers. With regular workshops and public performances in the United Kingdom and worldwide, the company have challenged concepts and attitudes of disability (https://www.turtlekeyarts. org.uk/amici-dance-theatre-company). Similarly, the Kaos Choir (https://www.thekaosorganisation.com/), an integrated group of hearing and hearing-impaired children aged 4–18 years, made headlines when they opened the 2012 Olympic games in the United Kingdom. Ability Unlimited is a New Delhi-based dance company exclusively for individuals with disabilities as both teachers and artists; aiming for active participation in Indian society (https://www.theguardian.com/world/2007/aug/01/india-disability).

Some children with motor impairments in the Chicago classical ballet programmes have participated in the annual performances of *The Nutcracker* by the Joffrey Ballet. Ballet classes have been implemented in Valencia, Spain with support of the Universidad Cardenal Herrera, the city ballet company, Ballet de la Generalitat, and a local community ballet school. Recently, the ballet programme was offered in a culturally sensitive manner at the main state rehabilitation centre of Mérida, Yucatán, México, CREE-Mérida, for a population of children with cerebral palsy of Mayan ethnicity.

CRITICAL ELEMENTS OF PARTICIPATORY INTERVENTIONS

The examples given in this chapter illustrate the key points of participatory processes: opportunities, strategies, experiences and outcomes that lead to the future with new goals and directions. Willis et al. (2018)

define 10 crucial elements contributing to meaningful participation experiences for children and youth with disabilities:

- personal preferences;
- enjoyment;
- experiencing mastery;
- experiencing freedom of choice;
- belonging in a group, and developing an identity;
- environment-focused elements;
- authentic friendships among equal peers;
- the opportunity to practice participation;
- role models with different functional levels, and family support; and
- the activity-related element of learning in a context with enough time and space for as many trials and repetitions as needed.

All these elements are evident in the examples provided; contributing to meaningful leisure in children and youth with disabilities. Participation as a lived experience incorporates subjective elements that may have meaning and value for individuals that are not seen by onlookers. Positive exposure and shared experiences are a driving force behind the United Kingdom's Disability Matters e-learning programme and the community projects referred to in this chapter.

In participatory interventions, it is the 'intervention' itself that engages the person in meaningful participatory experience.

These participatory interventions support learning and development within the social situations of relevance to individuals and communities, consistent with situated learning theory (Standal and Jespersen 2008). These opportunities for social engagement, as part of natural interactions rather than therapeutically designed interventions to support social skill acquisition, allow children and young people to reconstruct their identity; reframing being, being there and being involved within the social worlds of their peers and community.

Utilising socially-mediated environments of mixed ability for teaching and learning of new skills, provides a very different medium for enabling and encouraging young people. The sense of social belonging and meaningful social interactions are illustrated clearly in these examples. The importance, however, of participation in individual or solitary activities has often been overlooked in the literature; the positive values of solitude overlooked, or perhaps mistaken for loneliness. Little is known of the benefits of choice for 'blissful solitude' and/or participation in personal spaces. These opportunities for individual participation may (or may not) be enhanced through virtual and digital media when access to physical spaces for personal contemplation and enjoyment are limited in time as well as space. Furthermore, we have seen within these community-based projects, that these programmes have supported young children, youth and adults with a belief that encourages the creation of new goals.

CONCLUDING THOUGHTS

What we see encapsulated in participatory interventions is the empowerment of self, when learning is situated in relevant and meaningful contexts and environments. Ownership of 'I did this', or 'I learnt this' rather than 'My therapist helped me to do this' are essential differences in the language of these programmes. Mastery of a dance movement such as an 'elevé' presented by your dance teacher, is quite a different perspective of a skill from 'able to transfer weight from the heels to toes'.

Opportunities for choice in the focus of the activities (e.g. drama, sport, craft) and mode of delivery (e.g. clubs, camps, online) are more likely to be available in some cultures. However, virtual communities and social media open up access for meaningful participation across cultures and socio-economic groups as technology is increasingly accessible.

SUMMARY OF KEY IDEAS

- Participatory interventions offer opportunities for new experiences embedded within activities; valued as part of typical experiences within culturally relevant communities.
- Outcomes of participatory interventions are evident with the variety of new opportunities that emerge that were not anticipated at the outset.
- Participatory interventions should lead to empowerment, resilience and a sense of hope with enhanced expectations for the future.

REFERENCES

Asuncion JV, Budd J, Fichten CS, Nguyen MN, Barile M, Amsel R (2012) Social media use by students with disabilities. *Acad Exch Q* **16**: 30–35.

Baksjøberget PE, Nyquist A, Moser T, Jahnsen R (2017) Having fun and staying active! Children with disabilities and participation in physical activity: A one year follow-up study. *Physical & Occupational Therapy in Pediatrics* **37**: 347–358.

Best P, Manktelow R, Taylor B (2014) Online communication, social media and adolescent wellbeing: A systematic narrative review. *Child Youth Serv Rev* **41**: 27–36.

Council on Communications and Media (2013) Children, adolescents, and the media. *Pediatrics* **132**: 958–961.

Didden R, Scholte RH, Korzilius H et al. (2009) Cyberbullying among students with intellectual and developmental disability in special education settings. *Dev Neurorehabil* **12**: 146–151.

Green D, Martini R (2017) Group approaches in childhood. In: Dawson D, McEwen S, Polatajko H (Eds.) *Enabling Participation Across the Lifespan: Advancements, Adaptations and Extensions of the CO-OP Approach.* Washington: Amer OT Assoc Pubs.

Green D, Ziviani J (2017) The Arts and Children's Occupational Opportunities. In: *Occupation-Centred Practice with Children: A Practical Guide for Occupational Therapists*, 2nd edn. West Sussex: Wiley-Blackwell, pp. 311–328.

Hickman R, Popescu L, Manzanares R, Morris B, Lee SP, Dufek JS (2017) Use of active video gaming in children with neuromotor dysfunction: a systematic review. *Dev Med Child Neurol* **59**: 903–911.

Hynan A, Murray J, Goldbart J (2014) "Happy and excited": perceptions of using digital technology and social media by young people who use augmentative and alternative communication. *Child Lang Teach Ther* **30**: 175–186.

Jirikowic TL, Kerfeld CI (2016) Health-promoting physical activity of children who use assistive mobility devices: a scoping review. *Amer J Occupat Therap* **70**(5).

King G, Rigby P, Batorowicz B (2013) Conceptualizing participation in context for children and youth with disabilities: an activity setting perspective. *Disabil Rehabil* **35**: 1578–1585.

López-Ortiz C, Gladden K, Deon L, Schmidt J, Girolami G, Gaebler-Spira D (2012) Dance program for physical rehabilitation and participation in children with cerebral palsy. *Arts Health* **4**: 39–54.

López-Ortiz C, Gaebler-Spira DJ, McKeeman SN, McNish RN, Green D (2018) Dance and rehabilitation: a systematized review of the evidence for cerebral palsy. *Dev Med Child Neurol* **61**(4): 393–398.

Nyquist A, Moser T, Jahnsen R (2016) Fitness, fun and friends through participation in preferred physical activities: achievable for children with disabilities? *Int J Disab Dev Edu* **63**: 334–356.

Paulus FW, Ohmann S, von Gontard A, Popow C (2018) Internet gaming disorder in children and adolescents: a systematic review. *Dev Med Child Neurol* **60**: 645–659.

Raghavendra P, Newman L, Grace E, Wood D (2015) Enhancing social participation in young people with communication disabilities living in rural Australia: outcomes of a home-based intervention for using social media. *Disabil Rehabil* **37**: 1576–1590.

Reid DT (2002) Benefits of a virtual play rehabilitation environment for children with cerebral palsy on perceptions of self-efficacy: a pilot study. *Pediatr Rehabil* **5**: 141–148.

Rowley E, Chandler S, Baird G et al. (2012) The experience of friendship, victimization and bullying in children with an autism spectrum disorder: associations with child characteristics and school placement. *Res Autism Spectr Disord* **6**: 1126–1134.

Sherrill C, Hutzler Y (2008) Adapted physical activity science. In: Borms J (Ed) *Directory of Sport Science: A Journey Through Time: The Changing Face of ICSSPE*, 5th edn. Leeds: Human Kinetics, pp. 89–103.

Sorsdahl AB, Moe-Nilssen R, Larsen EM et al. (2019) Long-term change of gross motor function in children with cerebral palsy; an observational study of repeated periods of intensive physiotherapy in a group setting. *Euro J Physio* 1–7.

Standal ØF, Jespersen E (2008) Peers as resources for learning: a situated learning approach to adapted physical activity in rehabilitation. *Adapt Phys Activ Q* **25**: 208–227.

Terada K, Satonaka A, Terada Y, Suzuki N (2017) Training effects of wheelchair dance on aerobic fitness in bedridden individuals with severe athetospastic cerebral palsy rated to GMFCS level V. *Eur J Phys Rehabil Med* **53**: 744–750.

Weiss PL, Bialik P, Kizony R (2003) Virtual reality provides leisure time opportunities for young adults with physical and intellectual disabilities. *Cyberpsychol Behav* **6**: 335–342.

WHO (2007) *International Classification of Functioning, Disability and Health: Children and Youth Version: ICF-CY*. Geneva: World Health Organization.

Willis CE, Reid S, Elliott C et al. (2018) A realist evaluation of a physical activity participation intervention for children and youth with disabilities: what works, for whom, in what circumstances, and how? *BMC Pediatr* **18**: 113.

Our participatory experiences and contributions can be unique and powerful. In the following vignette an experience is described in which dance is the medium for learning and participatory joy. As you read, look for the transactional influences among the people in the story and consider who has learned what.

From Overcoming to Enjoying (Vietnam)

Yen-Thanh Mac

The moment I saw this picture (Fig. V18.1), I could not stop crying. Because of my false assumptions, I had almost taken away 'one of the most enjoyable moments' in the lives of these friends. I really care for them, I keep encouraging them to overcome obstacles, but I forgot about joy.

This is what happened:

Initially, I and a doctoral student planned to organise a dance performance involving friends living with cerebral palsy. We wanted to celebrate World Cerebral Palsy Day, 2017: this would be a public

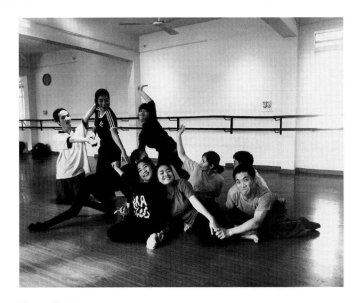

Figure V18.1

performance. I wanted to prove to many people that 'cerebral palsy' does not mean 'brain failure', as translated in Vietnamese. They have abilities, even dance, although many able-bodied people would never think this possible. I believe that dance is more a question of attitude than physical skill.

Ultimately, we could not create this public performance for World Cerebral Palsy Day, but we conducted a workshop which we hoped would help our friends to reduce spasticity and enhance their confidence. We invited several professional dancers to support us and we enjoyed a 5-day creative movement workshop having fun; giving back love for our bodies, through moving, playing and developing more possibilities to move.

After the workshop, a dancer suggested a performance of my friends in a contemporary dance show that included her students. Instead of being happy (because this was what I had planned originally), my mind and my heart were in conflict. I really care about my friends. I worried that people would look at what was missing, what did not work; that the performance would be seen as a 'fundraising event' and the viewers may look down on my friends.

However, when my friends asked me if the performance could happen, I fully respected their wishes. I decided to 'be an observer and supporter only' of the rehearsal and show. Surprisingly, I found my friends seemed happier than during the workshop. The dancer told me the secret statements she used to inspire my friends:

> Every physical movement is dance, which stimulates energy that generates all the activities on Earth …
> Please do not see you are 'people living with disability', [that] you are 'special' with limits you need to try to overcome. I just appreciated your unique movements as I appreciate 'able-bodied' people's unique movements.

The performance received much positive feedback. The audience could see that all of the dancers supported and listened to each other; respecting each other's limits and abilities.

Learning from my mistake, I have realised that dancing is not for proving that people living with limitations can do something like typical people do. Dancing is for enjoying. By focusing on differences and limitations more than on similarities and potential we build barriers and contribute to oppression, in dance and other areas of life.

PART V
Future Challenges

Childhood Disability and Participation in the 21st Century

Peter Rosenbaum

> Many years ago, I was reviewing the progress of an ex-preterm 4-year-old with significant visual impairment and cerebral palsy who would now be classified in level II on the Gross Motor Function Classification System (GMFCS). He was the youngest of a large sibship, with an experienced mother. The boy had just recently learned to pull to stand and cruise holding onto the furniture. When I asked how he was doing, his mother replied, 'He's getting into a lot of mischief. That's good, isn't it!'
>
> Thirty-five years later I still recall this mother's insightful observation as a thunderbolt: the idea – new to me at that time – that a child's self-directed activities (labelled with the adult notion 'mischief') were such an important step for the child. I recall being embarrassed at how much more attuned his mother was than I to this evidence of developmental progress. The word 'participation' had yet to be applied in our field, but she knew it, recognised it, and valued it!

As is evident throughout this book, the idea of 'participation' is now recognised as an essential goal for all of child and youth development. Embedded in the World Health Organization's (WHO) International Classification of Functioning Disability and Health (ICF; WHO 2001) framework, this concept is a cornerstone of modern thinking in the field of developmental disability. This begs the questions: Why are we just discovering this now? What came before this focus on participation?

The simple answer is that our 20th century biomedical thinking impelled us to apply the 'right' therapies, directed at addressing and hopefully correcting what we now refer to as 'impairments' in 'body structure and function'. The assumptions were that therapies would improve function; that functioning would move toward 'normal' performance; activity and therefore participation would follow, made possible by improvements in basic functioning of the 'impaired' body. At that time, we were not thinking about or assessing 'participation', and consequently we simply do not know whether our therapies did in fact promote children's participation. We did not think of it, so we did not look.

There remain strong differences of opinion between proponents of 'therapies' to achieve 'nice' (in their view hopefully 'normal') functioning, and people who encourage and empower kids and parents to 'do', without a primary focus on doing things 'right'. An interesting illustration of contrasting views involves the 1988 study by Palmer et al. In this early intervention randomised controlled trial (RCT), 48 infants (12–19 months of age) with 'mild' to 'severe' (sic) spastic diplegia were randomised to receive either 12 months of neurodevelopmental (NDT-based) physical therapy or 6 months of NDT therapy preceded by 6 months of an infant stimulation ('Learning Games') programme. The latter intervention included motor, sensory, language and cognitive activities of increasing complexity. After 6 months, the infants in the Learning Games arm of the trial had higher mean motor scores than those in the NDT group, and were more likely to be able to walk. These differences persisted after 12 months of therapy. Even more interesting was the observation that the infant stimulation group also had a higher mean cognitive quotient than the NDT-based group. The authors concluded that 'The routine use of physical therapy in infants with spastic diplegia offered no short-term advantage over infant stimulation. Because of the limited scope of the trial, our conclusions favouring infant stimulation are preliminary.' It should be noted both that these findings were unexpected, and that the study had not been designed to assess the infant stimulation intervention; rather the latter programme was meant to provide a 'comparison' – and presumably less effective – alternate treatment.

At the time this study appeared – in the context of our strong belief in the importance of 'therapies' – there was much consternation. Most of us saw a glass half empty – therapy didn't do what we expected, and this was a blow to our beliefs. In hindsight, we ought to have seen a glass half full: promoting early exploratory behaviour enhanced children's *development* in several spheres. Here was an as-yet unrecognised example of the value of early 'participation'.

In the mid-late 1980s, there was a general belief among service providers that young children with diplegia who were wanting to stand and walk – usually up on their toes, with a crouched gait, with internal femoral rotation – were demonstrating 'poor gait and posture', and that this should be prevented lest it create musculoskeletal problems. A similar concern has been expressed about 'allowing' children with diplegic cerebral palsy to W-sit, though to our knowledge there is no evidence that this adaptive sitting posture causes any problems to children who do it. Thus, parents were discouraged from allowing their children to develop their motor abilities in these ways, at least in the NDT-based interventions popular at that time (and even today). One can imagine that the toddlers in the infant stimulation arm of the Palmer et al. (1988) study, being 'allowed' to develop and practice their motor skills without this proscription, learned a great deal by using their spontaneous mobility and stability to explore and get into 'mischief'.

Our current interest in children's participation forces clinicians to confront the tensions between the goals of 'therapy' (addressing impairments at the level of body structure and function) and the promotion of child development, including participation. Palmer et al.'s (1988) study illustrates clearly how our beliefs at the time constrained us to see only one side of the story, and miss the significant messages revealed by the data. We have argued elsewhere (Rosenbaum 2009; Rosenbaum and Gorter 2012) that professionals concerned with variations in child development, manifested in the neurodisabilities, need to pay more attention to the 'developmental' aspects of children's predicaments and see our interventions as having the goal to promote and enhance children's 'being, belonging and becoming' (Brown et al. 1997; Raphael et al. 1999). We have also expressed great concern that the idea of valuing only 'normal' functioning, while limiting other ways of doing things, is far too restrictive.

> *We strongly believe that we need to value and respect variation (Rosenbaum 2006).*

If one accepts these premises – and there is an increasing embrace of these ideas in many places, but not all (Jindal et al. 2017) – there are important implications for our clinical, research and 'political' activities regarding how we think, counsel, intervene and advocate to promote the fullest development of young people whose lives are complicated by impairments and are therefore unfolding differently.

CLINICAL IMPLICATIONS

At the clinical level – prioritising child development over specific functional details of children's lives – it is now obvious that all our recommendations to families must identify 'participation' and 'engagement' as primary goals. For parents, this means encouraging, supporting and allowing their children with impairments as much latitude as possible to learn to do things for themselves. This is of course how typically developing children progress – by tireless repetition of things important to them (and typically developing children don't ask for permission – they just do things!). Think of how relentlessly young children practice activities like climbing, or drawing, or language skills. These activities, and a thousand others, are considered by adults to be 'play' – but they are in fact the 'work' of children learning mastery over the routines of their daily lives, be these activities of daily living or the skills of their favourite pastimes.

To have anywhere near the same opportunities for participation, children with impaired development may need to have their environments engineered for them and be empowered to try out and practice their emerging skills in their own way. This means that as professionals counselling families we need both to offer parents encouragement to allow their children to engage in activities in whatever way they can, and to provide examples of what we mean. Powerful illustrations may include describing to families the immense impact on children's development of the use of augmentative interventions such as powered mobility (Rosenbaum 2008). When young children with mobility restrictions are empowered – literally and figuratively – their world opens up to them in ways that are often very dramatic, as illustrated by Butler's groundbreaking studies (Butler 1986; Okamoto and Butler 1986).

> LINK TO VIGNETTE 19.1
> *'A Newcomer to Canada', p. 227.*

In the early 1980s I regularly followed Jessica, a bright, engaging 6-year-old with what we now would call GMFCS level IV cerebral palsy. Her parents were early adopters of powered mobility, which Jessica used at home, in her integrated classroom and in the community. One day in clinic her mother proudly reported the following story: A few days earlier Jessica's power chair would not start; her mother asked her if she had been riding her chair across the lawn and through the sprinkler; Jessica denied this; her mother took the cover off the motor and saw water pour out; and Jessica was grounded for one day for lying! Jessica's mother was very pleased at this evidence of her daughter's typical behaviour and at her own opportunity to provide developmentally appropriate sanctions for what she saw to be her daughter's age-appropriate 'mischief'. 'Participation and engagement'? This mother got it!

Consider the implications of giving children free rein in the way described in the reflection above. First, and most obviously, they learn a great deal about themselves: for example, what they can do, what gets them into trouble, and the social consequences of what adults call bad behaviour. The second implication is essentially the corollary of the first. When children are supported to be engaged and to participate in life in ways that are meaningful to them, their parents,

When children are given free rein, they learn a great deal about themselves.

families, teachers, health professionals and even ordinary members of the community can see capacity and capability in people too easily characterised (at least traditionally) by a catalogue of terms like 'impairments', 'disabilities', 'handicaps'. Often the way things are done by kids with impairments is different from the ordinary – but that only confirms the enormous variation in our human capacities. There is a strong likelihood that by expecting things to be done 'typically' we miss what young people, growing up with different experiences of life, might in fact achieve if we give them the opportunity to express their abilities in their own ways.

Do you remember to ask parents what they want to boast about their kids?

This leads to a third implication for all professionals – the importance of helping parents build on their children's strengths and interests. We need to ask parents what they want to boast about, and what their kids are interested in. Then it becomes our responsibility to support and advise and advocate for the children and families to have opportunities to accomplish those goals. After finding out what kids want to do but cannot, we need to understand why that is not happening and identify what adaptations will enable the child and family to experience those activities. Modelling this for parents sends a powerful message to them and their families – and the communities in which they live and play – that with a bit of imagination and advocacy, all of us can support children's development and their 'being, belonging and becoming'.

RESEARCH IMPLICATIONS

Let us consider again the Palmer et al. (1988) study in the light of current ICF-based ideas, and ask 'What if?' First, what might the design of that study look like today? What questions might be addressed? What outcomes would we want to explore? How differently might even the same study have been reported (perhaps celebrated) had children's development and 'participation' been the stated goals of the trial?

Leaving these rhetorical questions for readers to consider, the author and his colleagues are involved in a study designed to share the ideas presented in this chapter with parents new to the journey of childhood disability. The five-workshop intervention is being evaluated for how well we are able to influence parent self-reports of their wellbeing and mental health, their sense of competence and their perceptions of their parenting style and skills – at baseline, at the end of the workshops, and then 3, 6 and 12 months later. Once proof of concept has been established we will undertake an RCT of this ENVISAGE programme and assess both parent outcomes and measures of child development prospectively over at least 2 years.

A second consideration in modern research in the field of developmental disability is the imperative to assess children's participation as either a primary or a secondary outcome. There is a burgeoning literature (see Chapter 12) on concepts regarding what participation looks like and the many tools available to assess it. To these outcomes one would now want to add an understanding of parents' perceptions of their children's strengths, and to know the extent to which, as their children manifest their participatory interests and engagement, parents' views of their child's capabilities (and hopefully of their own) become more positive. The field of clinical child disability research is ripe for these kinds of enquiries.

IMPLICATIONS FOR KNOWLEDGE TRANSLATION, COMMUNITY EDUCATION AND POLICY-MAKING

Finally, as leaders in the field of childhood disability and advocates for participation of children and youth with impairments, we must seize every opportunity to be 'knowledge brokers' and to inform the community of these new ways of looking at child development. Unless, like the authors writing in this book, people are deeply immersed in the evolving field of childhood disability, they have no reason to be aware of the seismic shifts in our thinking in the past 20 years, and how the scope of our activities and counselling has expanded.

For example, we are increasingly aware of the limitations of the biomedical approaches to trying to 'fix' developmental impairments with therapy alone; we know and espouse the ICF language and concepts; we understand what participation means and how to promote it. It must, however, be stated unequivocally that community leaders who are not (yet) familiar with these new ideas may have difficulty supporting parent-and-family-led initiatives that advocate, for example, for fully accessible community-based integrated playgrounds to allow access to their kids to participate equally. This is simply not part of people's traditional thinking about interventions for children with 'disabilities'.

It is therefore exciting to appreciate that in Australia the National Disability Insurance Scheme (NDIS) is embracing these modern ideas:

> Why do we need the NDIS? People with disability have the same right as other Australians to determine their best interests and to have choice and control over their lives. The NDIS recognises that everyone's needs and goals are different. The NDIS provides people with individualised support and the flexibility to manage their supports to help them achieve their goals and enjoy an ordinary life.

> – Australian Government (undated)

CONCLUSION

We have come a very long way in the past 30 years in how we think and act in the field of 'childhood disability'. There are good reasons to believe that parents and families embrace this broader, strengths-based way of thinking about child development in the context of 'disability'. As this book shows clearly, the deeper dives into concepts like 'participation' are allowing us to expand – and to change – the discourse in ways we believe are transformative. A lot has been accomplished, but much remains to be done. All of us who advocate for children and families – whether as clinicians, teachers, parents, researchers, policy-makers or legislators – must keep sharing ideas about participation as an essential life goal for everyone, and then track the continuing excitement as the lives of children with impairments, and those of their families, are enriched.

SUMMARY OF KEY IDEAS

- There remain strong differences of opinion between proponents of 'therapies' to achieve 'nice' (hopefully 'normal') functioning, and people who encourage and empower kids and parents to 'do', without a primary focus on doing things 'right'.
- The 'developmental' aspects of children's predicaments remind us that our interventions need to promote and enhance children's 'being, belonging and becoming' (i.e. their overall development) – and to celebrate the immense developmental variability with which children accomplish their goals.
- As the anecdotes in this chapter illustrate, the 'unit of interest' in our interventions in childhood disability must be the family, whose embrace of these concepts will empower children to be as fully engaged in life as possible.
- We need parents' help (their boasting, at our invitation) to know what their children want to do and might even be good at! Children's engagement in life, in ways that are meaningful to them, allows them to develop confidence, competence and a sense of self; equally importantly, it allows others to see these qualities 'despite' the children's impairments.

REFERENCES

Australian Government (undated) *About the NDIS* [online video]. Canberra: National Disability Insurance Agency, https://www.ndis.gov.au/about-us [Accessed 17 September 2019].

Brown I, Raphael D, Renwick R (1997) *Quality of Life – Dream or Reality? Life for People with Developmental Disabilities in Ontario*. Toronto: University of Toronto, Centre for Health Promotion.

Butler C (1986) Effects of powered mobility on self-initiated behaviors of very young children with locomotor disability. *Dev Med Child Neurol* **28**(3): 325–332.

Jindal P, MacDermid JC, Rosenbaum P, DiRezze B, Narayan A (2017) Perspectives on rehabilitation of children with cerebral palsy: exploring a cross-cultural view of parents from India and Canada using the international classification of functioning, disability and health. *Disabil Rehabil* **40**(23): 2745–2755.

Okamoto GA, Butler C (1986) Physical medicine and rehabilitation: powered mobility for very young disabled children. *West J Med* **144**(6): 733.

Palmer FB, Shapiro BK, Wachtel RC et al. (1988) The effects of physical therapy on cerebral palsy. A controlled trial in infants with spastic diplegia. *N Engl J Med* **318**(13): 803–808.

Raphael D, Brown I, Renwick R (1999) Psychometric properties of the Full and Short Versions of the Quality of Life Instrument Package: results from the Ontario province-wide study. *Int J Disabil Dev Educ* **46**: 157–168.

Reddihough DS, Meehan E, Stott NS, Delacy MJ, Australian Cerebral Palsy Register Group (2016) The National Disability Insurance Scheme: a time for real change in Australia. *Dev Med Child Neurol* **58**(Suppl 2): 66–70.

Rosenbaum P (2006) Variation and "abnormality": recognizing the differences. *J Pediatr* **149**: 593–594.

Rosenbaum P (2008) Effects of powered mobility on self-initiated behaviours of very young children with locomotor disability. *Dev Med Child Neurol* **50**: 644.

Rosenbaum P (2009) Putting child development back into developmental disabilities. Editorial. *Dev Med Child Neurol* **51**(4): 251.

Rosenbaum PL, Gorter JW (2012) The "F-words" in childhood disability: I swear this is how we should think! *Child: Care, Health Dev* **38**(4): 457–63.

WHO (2001) *International Classification of Functioning, Disability and Health: Short Version*. Geneva: World Health Organization.

As you read Asma's story, consider the intergenerational cultural differences that are at play: Asma is both 'the next generation' and one living life in a 'new cultural context' to the previous generation. The dilemmas and conflicts that arise for her, her family and for service providers, are brought into focus. How can Asma embrace her participation endeavours – involvement in future study, work, leisure and independent living – while remaining engaged with her culture? How might we support her to negotiate accommodations that are acceptable to her and others in the various situations and that might result in changes to attitudes and actions in her contexts?

A Newcomer to Canada (Canada)

Dana Anaby

Asma, a 16-year-old adolescent with a physical disability, attends a mainstream local high school. Her family emigrated from Southeast Asia to Canada 8 years ago and live in an ethnically diverse low-income neighbourhood in Montreal, mostly consisting of South Asian newcomers from India, Bangladesh and Sri Lanka and others; for example, Haiti. Asma has younger twin brothers and very dedicated parents who value their culture, tradition and religion. They are interested in culturally oriented activities such as going to the mosque and playing cricket. Asma is currently in Grade 10 and has a part time educational aid (personal assistant). She uses a walker to move around at school and home but uses a powered wheelchair for longer distances, accessing it with her right hand via a regular joystick. Asma is a highly motivated young woman who strives for full participation in various activities and settings and hopes to lead an independent life. Her aspirations, however, are not always aligned with the cultural values and expectations of her family and her immediate community. Asma feels that this disconnect is limiting her personal and social development.

At school, Asma is interested in joining the student council and put her name forward for nomination; however has never been elected by her peers to be a member of any team. It seems that her peers do not know how to interact with her, despite her good communication skills. Asma often stays in class during recess and lunch time instead of gathering with peers. It also seems that teachers and educational aids do not always know how to assist her or address these issues. Moreover, Asma's parents are quite concerned about her taking leadership roles in the school; particularly those that do not necessarily align with their cultural viewpoints and gender-specific norms deemed acceptable. They often say: 'in our culture, this role is not appropriate for a girl'. For Asma, taking such a role is an opportunity to expand her social network and practice new advocacy skills.

Asma, who is nearing adulthood, is interested in taking more control over her medical appointments and wants to be able to communicate her needs and concerns with her paediatrician. She feels she can provide information (e.g. clinical reports) and answer questions about her health more accurately than her parents currently do, and believes this will prepare her for the transition to adult healthcare. Asma is not sure; however, how to go about this, nor what tools or programmes are available to guide her.

Asma likes art, in particular photography. After school, she spends most of her time in her room listening to music, looking at art books and downloading photos to her iPad (tablet), which she won in a debate competition at school. She has become knowledgeable about fine art and art history including Southeast Asian art. Asma wishes she could be more socially active in her community, but is not sure how. While community art programmes are available, instructors' knowledge about ways to adapt their programmes are limited. In addition, her parents do not believe that community involvement and socialisation will improve her functional skills and rehabilitation process. Asma is discouraged by this and is concerned this will make her even more isolated.

In the summer, Asma, who wears a hijab, is planning to find a part time job in order to save up enough money for a camera. She has no idea where or how to start and is concerned about reactions of her extended family, friends and neighbours, who at times assume responsibility for her care. Asma, on the other hand, seems to have high confidence in her abilities and values her independence. She is also aware that employers' perspectives towards her disability and their willingness to accommodate, could prevent her from finding a job at all. Her first attempt to apply for a volunteer position at a local contemporary art museum was discouraging; she felt she was denied the opportunity due in part for being as she describes: 'both a young South Asian woman and a person with a disability'. Asma hopes others will be more knowledgeable about her culture and skills and she strives to break any 'double stigma' affecting her participation in desired activities.

Evolution of Needs and Expectations: The Transformation of Disabled Individuals and Healthcare Providers

Bernard Dan, Karine Pelc and Michel Sylin

The way we look at disability, disabled children and young people, and their families has greatly changed in recent decades. This has led to a level of clinical complexity that was previously unknown or over-looked. Adapted service must take account of frailty and an updated perspective on autonomy. Dramatic technological advances for evaluation and management have reshaped practice. Concomitantly, and only partially because of this evolution, there have been major changes in cultural perception at multiple levels – the place of the child, representations of disability, professional-family relationships – and new responsibilities in a redrawn ethical framework. Changes in social dynamics and the recognition of multiple modalities of participation have created new expectations. More profound changes are expected towards valuing disabled individuals in society, and these can be anticipated to modify social structures.

In this chapter, we address what drives these changes in terms of technological and social progress and revisit the current models of disability from a systemic perspective centred on the dynamic interdependence of individual and society, with a special focus on participation.

PROGRESS: THE POWER OF DISSATISFIED HOPEFULNESS

Designing management for disabled children entails, for the greatest part, contemplating the future. Very often, this implies a perspective of gain of skills and function. 'Gain' is held to be related to appropriate guidance and intervention, but it is also in line with physiological development. The implicit assumption (regardless of disability) is that with the passing of time a child grows and gains in strength, proficiency and autonomy. The perspective of progress might even apply in degenerative conditions, be it for selected domains of functioning. For instance, it is often reasonable to set specific goals for functional improvement in children with Duchenne muscular dystrophy or leukodystrophy while otherwise facing increasing impairments (Synofzik and Ilg 2014; Suk et al. 2014).

This perspective replicates the general aspiration for progress that characterises most contemporary cultures (Nisbet 1994). Many of us see mankind as advancing, with accumulating knowledge replacing false beliefs, and new scientific findings translating into more effective interventions. This expectation is reinforced by many examples in the past. It is associated with a general fascination with technological change (Burbules 2016).

> *Progress implies a widespread attraction towards novelty.*

A focus on novelty may be associated with uncritical belief in the latest word and its corollary that 'what is not novel is insufficient', including previous practices, tools and versions of instruments or equipment used for diagnosis or management, and previous knowledge and expertise. The progress perspective in disabled children is associated with justified optimism; but also, with a pregnant perception of imperfection. The mixed feeling of permanent dissatisfaction while improvement is in sight reinforces the desire for new tools and practices, and contributes to questioning the limits of progress. What is currently being held as impossible (e.g. a cure for cerebral palsy), or a prognosis that appears defeatist (e.g. the child will not walk), is revised as reflecting ignorance, lack of imagination and of faith in progress. 'Reactionary attitudes' are seen as a risk, slowing progress.

Another consequence of the fascination with technology is that 'what can be done must be done' (Hofmann 2015). Dramatic technological advances have led to new societal expectations that do not necessarily contribute to the goals of management (Dan et al. 2017). The question 'whose needs are being served?' must guide clinical practice.

TECHNOLOGY FOR DIAGNOSIS AND TREATMENT

Increasingly accurate neuroimaging helps follow up experience-reliant neuroplasticity (Kolb et al. 2017). Advances in mathematical modelling are shifting the focus from localised brain functions to an understanding of distributed functions across widespread networks (Dan 2016). Technological developments and cost reduction afford genome sequencing (Tărlungeanu and Novarino 2018). Emerging gene therapies are becoming available to compensate for the failure that cause selected diseases (Gray 2013). Hopes for progress have thus very much brightened; yet, we must resist 'the tyranny of the idea of cure' when it is not possible and concentrate on alleviation and support (Mac Keith 1967), which is acquiring new meaning thanks to these developments.

Animal models (Harony-Nicolas and Buxbaum 2015) and stem cell modelling (Ardhanareeswaran et al. 2017) provide insights into potential compensatory mechanisms. The therapeutic potential of stem cells targeting the body structure and function level may eventually enhance person – environment fit and participation; to date, however, no valid therapeutic applications are available in developmental disorders, including cerebral palsy and autism.

Rapid progress in consumer electronics (e.g. smart phones) are benefiting many disabled persons. Devices are being used for supporting activities, and also assessment and therapy. Active video gaming allows the user to feel experiences similar to events and activities in real life (Bortone et al. 2018). Current simulation prioritises visual input over other afferent information that is relevant to both real life functioning and experiences, and issues of bidirectional transfer of skills or tasks between the virtual environment to the real world remain to be effectively addressed. Keen engagement into virtual reality must not overshadow the importance of (the need for) investing and designing natural as well as functional spaces (Green 2018). The facilities may also feature specific landmarks supporting wellbeing in general or sensory and cognitive processing, social interaction, or motor cognition through rehabilitative and therapeutic neuroarchitecture (Marcus and Sachs 2013).

A variety of brain stimulation modalities, whether invasive (e.g. deep-brain stimulation, vagal nerve stimulation), or noninvasive (e.g. transcranial magnetic stimulation or direct current stimulation) are being explored and refined. Our understanding of the precise neurophysiological effects remains incomplete, but the range of possible indications seems to expand in neurodevelopmental disabilities, perhaps combined with conventional rehabilitation approaches. Electrical stimulation can also be applied to muscles with impaired motor control in order to produce functional movements. This technique can increase strength and improve selective motor control and balance in children with cerebral palsy, though gains in activity and participation are yet to be clarified (Moll et al. 2017). Robotic exoskeletons are being developed to facilitate the production of movements in the hope that this translates into enhanced participation.

A common question to all these emerging management techniques concerns their place within support services. They may play a therapeutic role in repetition, consistent with a recent trend supporting training intensity (Tinderholt Myrhaug et al. 2014). In addition to therapeutic and educational purposes, some techniques offer, at least potentially, the option of objective assessment that would help evaluate the achievement of management goals. The assumption that the use of these techniques is motivating (e.g. engage in therapy, learning, participation) must be verified. Those that are usable outside the clinical facility greatly expand the space for management. Finally, issues of cost and obsolescence are anticipated to be limiting factors and make ethical issues even more complex.

ETHICAL ISSUES: A PRINCIPLED APPROACH

The ethical complexity of these issues can be addressed within the general analytical framework of bioethics, which includes the principles of autonomy, beneficence, nonmaleficence and justice (Beauchamp and Childress 2001). The principle of autonomy describes the person's right to make their own choices supported by informed consent and eventually surrogacy. Beneficence highlights the person's best interest and welfare. It also includes preventive healthcare. Nonmaleficence ('do no harm') also emphasises the person's interest, and particular quality of life, but applies when considering not to take action that would result in more harm than good. The fourth bioethical principle is justice, emphasising fairness and equity among individuals. It implies, for example, fair distribution of care by health professionals and by the health system. This principle raises difficult discussions, particularly when it involves scarce resource (Eyal 2014). Regarding new technologies, this principle requires developers and implementers to include cost-efficiency and local adaptation in their priorities, as exemplified by recent efforts in 3D printing of medical and orthopaedic equipment (Pavlosky et al. 2018).

Many clinicians consciously value these ethical principles, but most do not use them directly in clinical decision making (Page 2012). Hopefully, renewed interest for ethical thinking (Callahan 2005) will result in more ethical practice and better articulation between the 'personal' principles (autonomy, beneficence, nonmaleficence), and the 'societal' principle of justice.

PARTICIPATION: A PRINCIPLE OF SOCIETY

The difficulties of disabled individuals are measured against a set of norms. In Kens' story, expectations of behaviour form in a context where knowledge of the disability is hidden. These norms define the most prevalent ways of functioning in a society, and what the society expects from its members.

Many cultures have regarded disability as a property of the disabled individuals (Garland-Thomson 1997). In Kenya, Eddy's mother interprets his autism symptoms as possession by an evil spirit, despairing of his inclusion in society. A 'mythological' understanding regards disability as the manifestation of occult powers (punishment or ordeal). Alternatively, some cultures

LINK TO VIGNETTE 20.1
'Ken and the Natural Disaster', p. 236.

Disability is, to a large extent, defined by exclusion from societal norms.

LINK TO VIGNETTE 20.2
*'My Child is Possessed
by Evil Spirits', p. 238.*

attribute to disabled persons exceptional abilities to perceive inaccessible truths (Dan 2005). Such representations are not confined to remote times and space. When people question 'Why me? What have I done to deserve this?', they avow at least lip service to the assumption that there might be some metaphysical underpinning to their disability.

The much more prominent medical model considers disability as the consequence of health problems: experts identify a person's impairments and limitations and act to improve them. Both the mythological and medical models focus on the disabled person as the source of their problems.

In contrast, the social model considers that disability results from environmental conditions preventing disabled persons from participating fully in society, whether deliberately or inadvertently. The more comprehensive biopsychosocial model proposed in the International Classification of Functioning, Disability and Health (ICF) framework (WHO 2001) is championed in this book. It attempts to provide a holistic model of functioning and disability by integrating medical with social models (Solli and da Silva 2012). The ICF holds participation as a specific dimension in one's health condition.

The participation construct suggested in the ICF has had a profound influence on our understanding of both health and disability, with participation recognised as a paramount standard of the person's experience, values and even sense of meaning and purpose. Participation thus contributes to characterising the relevance of almost any therapeutic intervention, whichever other ICF dimension is primarily targeted. To give but a few examples, treatments to reduce spasticity or seizures, orthopaedic surgery (body function and structure), approaches that promote hand function or mobility (activity), classroom adaptation (environmental factors), or programmes enhancing fitness or facilitating lifestyle changes (personal factors), all get planned, performed and their effects monitored in view of ultimately enhancing a person's participation.

Participation was originally defined in the ICF as a person's involvement in life situations that are meaningful to them (WHO 2001). Each individual life is obviously replete with many different situations, and the individual also shows many possible types of involvement in them. The ICF provides a long list of life situations; for example, learning at home. In disability practice, however, the accent has been placed specifically on the individual's engagement in society, i.e. social participation. In this perspective, participation is a principle of society. The emphasis on social participation has proved useful in rehabilitation (Piškur et al. 2014). More generally, social participation has been shown to have a very strong relevance to subjective wellbeing. DDB Needham Life Style Surveys found that social engagement in meetings such as attendance to group activities or volunteering were associated with high levels of happiness, rated as equivalent to that associated with a doubling of income (Putnam 2000). It must also be noted, however, that high social engagement in groups with divergent activities, or excessive involvement; for example, having too many social roles, can generate stress due to conflicts between roles (Avison et al. 2007).

Participation can be understood in the light of the roles that individuals carry out in the society. Since the times of the ancient Greek philosophers at least, we have learned to recognise engagement in society as an essential human trait. Plato and Aristotle graphically called humans the 'city-state animal' (ζῷον πολιτικόν). Yet we are still puzzling about the fabric of society itself, about what it means in terms of social participation, and how this might clarify rehabilitation options for disabled individuals.

Surprisingly, it is difficult to suggest a simple definition of society. Society appears to be a complex dynamic system emerging from interactions between individuals (and groups) through reciprocal roles. These roles dedicate people to particular social structures, such as working in a factory, joining a fan club, chairing a parent support group, or attending clinic as a patient or a therapist. By playing social roles, individuals create, maintain and alter the social structures. Social roles are closely associated with cultural expectations. For example, we see in the person who acts as a physician the image we have of what a physician is, what we think she can do, and the context in which she does it. Within this system of interactions, individuals create their mental representations of each other's actions. In turn, these representations gradually come to dictate the reciprocal roles that members of the society play, resulting in social construction of reality (Berger and Luckmann 1966). For example, the 'patient' acts as a patient and entertains a particular, largely predefined, consensual repertoire of relationships with the person identified and acting as a therapist, and reciprocally. In other words, society pre-exists (as a system), and makes one exist. In turn, the reciprocally accepted social roles make society stable.

A person's social participation is a behavioural manifestation of their social role. Often, it reflects an actual behaviour; for example, when a patient expresses health-related discomfort, makes a medical appointment, waits for it, etc., all characteristic of a patient's role. In other instances, participation is a behaviour's outcome; for example, undergoing medical testing.

The concept of disability (one must not forget that it is not a real object) originates in the social role of the disabled. As a component of society, this social role is not easily prone to change. In mythological and the medical models of disability outlined above, the role of the disabled is assigned to the person through a curse/trial or a health problem, respectively. This cultural assignment is so robust that it often survives even where the social and ICF models have been influential (Falvo and Holland 2018).

Any individual can have a multitude of social roles in succession or concomitantly – choir boy, boy scout, son, brother, friend, student, football team supporter, patient, holiday maker, etc. Sometimes these roles interfere with each other, at other times they do not. There are also different modalities in manifestations of social roles, some focused on persons and some on the environment (Imms et al. 2017). One can participate in football with relevance to the game by building one's play or by watching. Characterising person-focused processes informs about the connection between personal factors and society through the person's interaction with and relation to other persons. Looking at environment-focused processes reveals how social roles are determined by external factors, which act as a transformative mover, generating participation as a product of the (ICF health condition) system.

One difficulty in (re)connecting the person with society through the ICF framework is that this model, while designed as holistic, tends to isolate the subject and compartmentalise the various components 'body functions and structures', 'activities' and 'participation' on the same level, separate from personal and environmental factors, which are regarded as contextual. It may be more useful to recognise that participation and environmental factors are inextricably linked as this is what society is all about. Personal factors are also closely linked to activities. They include the person's social assets (cognition, education, style of speech and dress, etc.) that promote social mobility, i.e. their cultural capital (Bourdieu 1979). When appraising a situation, choosing goals and planning management within the ICF framework, it may be helpful to recognise 'impairment' as the trigger component, 'participation' as the moving force in the system structured by 'environmental factors', and 'health' as one particular perspective rather than as the result of the system. In this view, the health condition (which occupies an overarching position in the ICF framework) appears as a subset in the general organisation of society, which is driven by participation.

Consequently, to value the individual in society, their participation should be valued for what it is – not despite impairment. This has major implications on society itself, as social participation thus becomes a means to change society and lift barriers (Piškur 2013). This empowerment must be afforded by society. As suggested by the World Health Organization, 'it is the collective responsibility of society at large to make the environmental modifications necessary for full participation of people with disabilities in all areas of social life' (WHO 2001, p. 28). In turn, societal developments will have an impact on social participation. These societal changes will influence how we educate, offer service and conduct research. A limitation of this system must be noted: the risk of reinforcing social categorisation and stereotypes, and thus further stigmatising

Participation should be valued for what it is, not despite impairment.

and alienating people with disabilities. In a society self-consciously characterised by neurodiversity (Baron-Cohen 2017), people with a disability have other social roles and must remain free not to be confined to the role of being disabled. This may call for an emancipating process.

AND NOW?

What is needed, as in many fields, is more research. This may sound like a pathetic truism, as it is the conclusion of so many research reports that must admit to difficulties in generalising findings (Mayston 2018). There appears to be unprecedented dedication of teams worldwide (with marked preponderance in Europe, North America and Australia) to study participation in children with neurodisability. Yet, the evidence base is often lacking, and many current attitudes are based on debated clinical opinion. It remains important to clearly identify challenges of overcoming beliefs, whether traditional in cultures as illustrated by the vignettes, or in the mainstream of societies in which those studies are set. There remains a tension between desire for immediate action and sound evidence, with immediacy taking the lead. Ongoing developments will hopefully enable researchers to provide answers to the open questions thanks to registers, single case designs, qualitative methods, and partnership with children and families when designing research agenda, carrying out studies and interpreting results.

REFERENCES

Ardhanareeswaran K, Mariani J, Coppola G, Abyzov A, Vaccarino FM (2017) Human induced pluripotent stem cells for modelling neurodevelopmental disorders. *Nat Rev Neurol* **13**: 265–278.
Avison WR, McLeod JD, Pescosolido BA (Eds) (2007) *Mental Health, Social Mirror*. New York: Springer, pp. 333.
Baron-Cohen S (2017) Editorial perspective: Neurodiversity – a revolutionary concept for autism and psychiatry. *J Child Psychol Psychiatry* **58**: 744–747.
Beauchamp TL, Childress JF (2001) *Principles of Biomedical Ethics*, 5th edn. Oxford: Oxford University Press.
Berger PL, Luckmann T (1966) *The Social Construction of Reality: A Treatise in the Sociology of Knowledge*. Garden City, NY: Anchor Books.
Bortone I, Leonardis D, Mastronicola N et al. (2018) Wearable haptics and immersive virtual reality rehabilitation training in children with neuromotor impairments. *IEEE Trans Neural Syst Rehabil Eng* **26**: 1469–1478.
Bourdieu P (1979) Les trois états du capital culturel. *Actes Rech Sci Soc* **30**: 3–6.
Burbules NC (2016) Technology, education, and the fetishization of the "new". In: Smeyers P, Depaepe M (Eds) *Educational: Discourses of Change and Changes of Discourse*. Springer International Publishing, pp. 9–16.
Callahan D (2005) Bioethics and the culture wars. *Camb Q Healthc Ethics* **14**: 424–431.
Dan B (2005) Titus's tinnitus. *J Hist Neurosci* **14**: 210–213.
Dan B (2016) Beyond localizing neurology and psychology. *Dev Med Child Neurol* **58**: 4.
Dan B, Rosenbaum PL, Ronen GM, Johannesen J, Racine E (2017) Ethics in paediatric neurology. *JICNA* **17**: 71–75.
Eyal N (2014) Pediatric heart surgery in Ghana: three ethical questions. *J Clin Ethics* **25**: 317–323.
Falvo D, Holland BE (2018) *Medical and Psychosocial Aspects of Chronic Illness and Disability*, 6th edn. Burlington, MA: Jones & Bartlett Learning.
Garland-Thomson R (1997) *Extraordinary Bodies: Figuring Physical Disability in American Culture and Literature*. New York: Columbia University Press.
Gray SJ (2013) Gene therapy and neurodevelopmental disorders. *Neuropharmacology* **68**: 136–142.
Green D (2018) Designing "free" spaces for children with disabilities. *Dev Med Child Neurol* **60**: 730.
Harony-Nicolas H, Buxbaum JD (2015) Animal models for neurodevelopmental disorders In: Mitchell KJ (Ed) *The Genetics of Neurodevelopmental Disorders*. Hoboken, NJ: Wiley, pp. 261–274.
Hofmann BM (2015) Too much technology. *BMJ* **350**: h705.

Horridge KA, Dew R, Chatelin A et al. (2019) Austerity and families with disabled children: a European survey. *Dev Med Child Neurol* **61**: 329–336.

Imms C, Granlund M, Wilson PH, Steenbergen B, Rosenbaum PL, Gordon AM (2017) Participation, both a means and an end: a conceptual analysis of processes andoutcomes in childhood disability. *Dev Med Child Neurol* **59**: 16–25.

Kolb B, Harker A, Gibb R (2017) Principles of plasticity in the developing brain. *Dev Med Child Neurol* **59**: 1218–1223.

MacKeith R (1967) The tyranny of the idea of cure. *Dev Med Child Neurol* **9**: 269–270.

Mantwill S, Monestel-Umaña S, Schulz PJ (2015) The relationship between health literacy and health disparities: a systematic review. *PLoS One* **10**: e0145455.

Marcus CC, Sachs NA (2013) *Therapeutic Landscapes: An Evidence-Based Approach to Designing Healing Gardens and Restorative Outdoor Spaces.* Hoboken, NJ: Wiley.

Mayston M (2018) More studies are needed in paediatric neurodisability. *Dev Med Child Neurol* **60**: 966.

Moll I, Vles JSH, Soudant DLHM et al. (2017) Functional electrical stimulation of the ankle dorsiflexors during walking in spastic cerebral palsy: a systematic review. *Dev Med Child Neurol* **59**: 1230–1236.

Nisbet R (1994) *History of the Idea of Progress*, 2nd edn. New York: Routledge.

Page K (2012) The four principles: can they be measured and do they predict ethical decision making? *BMC Med Ethics* **13**: 10.

Pavlosky A, Glauche J, Chambers S, Al-Alawi M, Yanev K, Loubani T (2018) Validation of an effective, low cost, Free/open access 3D-printed stethoscope. *PLoS One* **13**: e0193087.

Piškur B (2013) Social participation: redesign of education, research, and practice in occupational therapy. *Scand J Occup Ther* **20**: 2–8.

Piškur B, Daniëls R, Jongmans MJ et al. (2014) Participation and social participation: are they distinct concepts? *Clin Rehabil* **28**: 211–220.

Putnam RD (2000) *Bowling Alone: The Collapse and Revival of American Community*. New York: Simon & Schuster; Chapter 20.

Servais L, Gidaro T (2019) Nusinersen treatment of spinal muscular atrophy: what do we know and what do we still have to learn? *Dev Med Child Neurol* **61**: 19–24.

Solli HM, da Silva AB (2012) The holistic claims of the biopsychosocial conception of WHO's International Classification of Functioning, Disability, and Health (ICF): a conceptual analysis on the basis of a pluralistic-holistic ontology and multidimensional view of the human being. *J Med Philos* **37**: 277–294.

Suk KS, Lee BH, Lee HM et al. (2014) Functional outcomes in Duchenne muscular dystrophy scoliosis: comparison of the differences between surgical and nonsurgical treatment. *J Bone Joint Surg Am* **96**: 409–415.

Synofzik M, Ilg W (2014) Motor training in degenerative spinocerebellar disease: ataxia-specific improvements by intensive physiotherapy and exergames. *BioMed Res Int* **2014**: 583507.

Tărlungeanu DC, Novarino G (2018) Genomics in neurodevelopmental disorders: an avenue to personalized medicine. *Exp Mol Med* **50**: 100.

Tinderholt Myrhaug H, Østensjø S, Larun L, Odgaard-Jensen J, Jahnsen R (2014) Intensive training of motor function and functional skills among young children with cerebral palsy: a systematic review and meta-analysis. *BMC Pediatr* **14**: 292.

WHO (2001) *International Classification of Functioning, Disability and Health (ICF)*. Geneva: World Health Organization.

In Ken's story we see how critically disruptive environmental events impact all people, but particularly those with neurodisability. One dilemma in Ken's story is the tension between a cultural preference for diagnostic privacy and the need to share to gain understanding; in this setting participation is doing as socially expected. The experience of exclusion from an evacuation centre becomes a turning point for Ken's mother.

Ken and the Natural Disaster (Japan)

Naru Fukuchi and Motohide Miyahara

Ken, aged 8 years old, was diagnosed with autistic spectrum disorder (ASD) without learning disability when he was 6 years old: he is obsessive about using only his possessions; he throws heavy tantrums; he has acoustic hyperesthesia; and only eats bland-tasting food. He goes to regular school and studies in a regular class because his intelligence quotient (IQ) is not low enough to qualify for a special class. Although he has some troubles in his school life, he could manage his feelings with support of the school nurse and by becoming absorbed in video games at home.

To see a child psychiatry specialist, Ken's parents drove him 130 km inland from their home on the Pacific coast in north eastern Japan. After seeing Dr Fukuchi and receiving the diagnosis of ASD, Ken was treated at a local psychiatric clinic with medication to control his tantrums and hyperactivity. Ken and his family had developed a range of strategies and were coping with daily challenges until the tsunami.

A massive earthquake and tsunami hit Japan in 2011. With other residents in the affected area, Ken and his family escaped the tsunami and evacuated to a shelter in a school gym, that was full of evacuees. Most evacuees suffered from agitation and hyperarousal, so they couldn't care for each other.

There were no partitions between families in the shelter, so they could easily hear what other people said. Ken couldn't avoid the noise, and because he had severe acoustic hyperesthesia, this environment was taxing for him. Initially, Ken remained silent and still, overwhelmed by the unexpected disaster and the sudden dramatic changes in life. Ken wrapped his head in a blanket, shut out all information and didn't respond to anything for a few days.

The shortage of food meant that Ken had to eat whatever the other evacuees were eating. Although his mother tried to feed him, he didn't respond and completely refused any food. When supporters kindly brought food for Ken to share, he suddenly threw it down and screamed loudly. From this incident, other evacuees started to look at Ken's family members with annoyance and began to avoid them.

Someone gifted a video game with the relief goods for evacuees and it was set up in a break room in the shelter. Ken started playing it all day and didn't want to yield to others. Some days later, a leader of the shelter scolded Ken severely because he didn't allow others to use video games. Ken threw a strong tantrum; he shouted, hit others and banged his head on the ground. Finally, he broke the video game, so other children couldn't play it anymore. After that, people in the shelter spread rumours about Ken, and other children teased and bullied him, provoking him to tantrums.

Since medical supplies were completely stopped by the disaster, Ken couldn't take his medications to control his tantrums and hyperactivity. Ken's parents could talk to a local paediatrician in the shelter, but he couldn't provide appropriate treatment: there are few child specialists, child psychiatrists and paediatricians who understand developmental disorders in rural areas in Japan.

Ken's family members didn't want to tell the people around them that Ken had ASD, because they were ashamed of his symptoms. They thought others would not understand, but would see his symptoms as 'selfish behaviours'. Ken's behaviour in the shelter must have been related to his ASD and lack of medication, but other evacuees couldn't understand it and they couldn't overlook his behaviour. After the incident with the video game, it was so difficult for Ken's family to stay in the shelter that they decided to live in their car. Following the Great East Japan Earthquake and Tsunami, a lot of families with disabled members stayed in their cars for similar reasons.

Because of the lessons learned from these experiences of the disaster, people in the area have been promoting public education on developmental disabilities. Ken's mother told Dr Fukuchi that she wanted the local paediatricians to learn more about ASD, and contributed to the development of an ASD support book. Dr Fukuchi has been contributing to public education and assists in the disaster zones in northeastern Japan. He seeks out opportunities to share his knowledge, skills and experiences with people all over the world.

The following vignette illustrates how the way in which we interpret and explain what we see drives our choices and perceptions of opportunity. In Eddy's mother's story, the explanations she has of his behaviour as, rude and then as possession, lead to a search for a particular cure. Without that cure she describes a sense of despair about his ongoing isolation.

My Child is Possessed by Evil Spirits (Kenya)

Joseph K Gona and Charles R Newton

Eddy is a 7-year-old boy from urban Mombasa County in Kenya. He is a boy with typical autism. Eddy screams a lot and is very aggressive. Eddy has lost his speech and seems to have lost sense of reality. He keeps to himself.

> I gave birth to Eddy as a healthy bouncing boy. But when he got to the age of around 3 years I started noticing funny behaviours. He could not respond when I called him by name. I thought he was rude, so I used to punish him. At school, teachers started complaining that Eddy's behaviour has changed. He had become very aggressive, was not joining others in play. I took my child to hospital, but the situation became worse. The hospital people did not give me answers to the problem of my child.

The mother of Eddy became so frustrated and the journey to look for a cure started.

> I was so desperate to see that my child got healed. I suspected my child had been possessed by evil spirits. You know here in Mombasa, there are many cases of evil spirits being directed to children by evil people. I have gone to all places, to 'wagangas' (witch doctors), herbalists, sheikhs and imams to pray for my child. No hope of cure and my child will ever be isolated.

Cultural and Contextual Challenges in Resource-Poor Countries: The Case of Sub-Saharan Africa

Joseph K Gona, Karen Bunning and Charles R Newton

This chapter explores participation for children with neurodisability in sub-Saharan Africa. It focuses on disability as a socio-cultural construct, with the interplay between the person and their environment. Factors associated with traditional beliefs, poverty and scarce resources compound the challenges of participation; for not only the child, but also the caregiver. Finally, there is a review of some approaches designed to promote community participation.

INTRODUCTION

The greatest number of children with disabilities live in low- and middle-income countries, with sub-Saharan Africa contributing about 45% (Bitta et al. 2017). Culture influences the place that children with disabilities and their families occupy in society. It affects how the individual with a disability is perceived and responded to by other people. It determines the formation of attitudes and the behaviours that externalise those inner feelings and judgements. Ultimately, culture impacts on the range and types of opportunities that develop social relationships, receive an education, acquire employment and a sustainable livelihood. Made up of the values, beliefs, attitudes and behaviours shared by a group of people, culture is not static, it is dynamic, continuously changing. The same is true of living with a disability as disability is a socio-cultural construct. Bidirectional influences are present between the developing child and the changing environment, which may affect the extent to which participation is achieved.

CHALLENGES

Cultural Beliefs

In many sub-Saharan Africa countries, where there is limited understanding of childhood-onset neurodisability and inadequate coverage of health, educational and social services (Bunning et al. 2014). Traditional beliefs and actions have persisted (Bunning et al. 2017). Representations of disability have tended to be negative and typically associated with an undesirable condition (Gona et al. 2011), although variations have been reported. For example, people with physical disabilities are seen as pacifiers of evil spirits (Gona et al. 2011), while autistic spectrum disorders (ASDs) are attributed to evil spirits, witchcraft and curses (Gona et al. 2015). Some of the distaste associated with disability in sub-Saharan Africa may lie in the cultural explanations that imply breach of social conventions, such as in Botswana (Shumba and Abosi 2011), Ghana (Anthony 2011) and Kenya (Bunning et al. 2017); and external, preternatural forces, for example, in Kenya (Gona et al. 2015), Malawi (McKenzie et al. 2013) and Namibia (Souza Tedrus et al. 2013). Another explanation concerns the will of God (Stone-MacDonald and Butera 2012). These explanations may imply that disability is a punishment from a celestial being, or indeed linked to fate, which may be associated with some form of acceptance.

LINK TO VIGNETTE 20.2
'My Child is Possessed by
Evil Spirits', p. 238.

Fearful images and dehumanising language associated with disability, may not only hinder acceptance of the child who has a disability, but undermine possibilities and opportunities for that child. Vignette 21.1, 'When Ben Smiled', illustrates the challenges associated with explaining and understanding disability and the influence on expectations for outcomes. Research in Kenya revealed that children with disabilities are viewed as both a burden to the community and sub-human beings, as exemplified by the lifeless ki-vi class of nouns in Swahili language used to refer to them (Gona et al. 2018).

LINK TO VIGNETTE 21.1
'When Ben Smiled', p. 245.

Poverty

Culture, however, is not a single determining factor in the lives and participation of children with neurodevelopmental disabilities. Poverty is an ever-present challenge. In sub-Saharan Africa, the majority of citizens experience a reduced standard of living compared to people in high-income countries (Ingstad and Whyte 2007). Thus, the challenges encountered by children with disabilities and their families are shared by all (Mitra et al. 2011). This includes poor access to health provision (Peters et al. 2008), low school attendance (Kuper et al. 2014), limited employment rates and low wages (Muzunoya and Mitra 2012). Persons with disabilities in resource-poor countries encounter lower educational and labour market outcomes and are more likely to be poor than those without disabilities (Trani 2010). In Africa alone, less than 10% of children with disability were reported as attending school (UNESCO 2015). It is often the case that families of children with disabilities spend relatively more on healthcare than those without disabled members (Mitra et al. 2011). In Sierra Leone, families with a child with severe disabilities spend an average of 1.3 times more on healthcare than families without a person with a disability (Trani 2010). Disability and poverty are integrally connected (Department for International Development 2004) and families face many daily struggles.

Disability and poverty are integrally connected.

Stigma and Discrimination

In a context of poverty and limited resources, fuelled by traditional beliefs about disability causation, social relations, community attitudes and actions may be affected (Eide and Ingstad 2013). Stigma describes the negative attitudes evinced towards a particular group of people who are viewed as displaying certain characteristics that both discredit and discount the person (Goffman 1963). Stereotypes of what a member of the group is like are generated. This leads to prejudicial treatment by others whenever a person is associated with that stereotype (Werner et al. 2012), as illustrated by Mama Shuku's experience in Vignette 4.1, 'I Will Not Kill My Child'. The disabled child's perceived lack of fit within the local community, and the 'affiliate' stigma experienced by those closest to the child, are major factors in their participation. In the face of aversive responses from others, caregivers and families may adopt a protective stance towards the child (Gona et al. 2018). However, the urge to keep the child safe may come at the cost of inclusion.

LINK TO VIGNETTE 4.1
'I Will Not Kill My Child',
p. 46.

The child's social participation frequently depends on the support of the primary caregiver, typically the mother. The time and energies associated with care and support in everyday living activities affects the extent to which participation opportunities may be taken up (Bunning et al. 2017). In particular, the physical burden of supporting a child with disability has repercussions for movement within and beyond the community. With inadequate transport systems in sub-Saharan Africa, unmade roads with rough or unstable surfaces, and a lack of physical aids and adaptations (e.g. wheelchairs), mobility becomes a problem, particularly for those children with multiple disabilities. The sheer difficulty of movement becomes a barrier to not only the child's social participation, but also that of the caregiver.

PARTICIPATION

There is limited information on the meaning of participation to children and their caregivers in sub-Saharan Africa. Nelson et al. (2017), examining the views of children, caregivers and community members in Malawi, identified seven main spheres of participation. These included household work that contributed to family life; social interaction and being with other people (e.g. chatting with neighbours, sharing family stories); social activities, such as unstructured play (e.g. ball games, skipping); organised activities with a definite purpose (e.g. church service, football match); activities of daily living (e.g. bathing, eating meals with the family); education and schooling (travel to school, reading, writing); and entertainment (e.g. watching television, listening to the radio). It appears that with regard to participation, both children with and without disabilities want similar opportunities to take part across varied life situations (Nelson et al. 2017). However, children growing up with disabilities tend to experience a narrower existence with fewer prospects for social participation and engagement in daily activities; for example, household, educational and recreational activities (Bedell et al. 2013; Hansen et al. 2014). Investigating Canadian children with physical disabilities, Law et al. (2006) attributed improved patterns of participation to underlying values and cohesion in the family unit, as well as supportive and 'resource-ready' environments that were considered accessible, non-discriminatory and socially responsive (Law et al. 2006). This is echoed by Bedell et al. (2013) who highlighted the importance of community action to support participation (Bedell et al. 2013).

In sub-Saharan Africa the challenges of participation for children with developmental neurodisability are compounded by limited home resources, inadequate transport (Hansen et al. 2014) and cultural stigma associated with disability (Bunning et al. 2017); inadequate information and poor availability of support (Bunning et al. 2014). The mothers interviewed in Hansen et al.'s study (2014) in Zambia, identified other family members and members of the local community as alternately facilitating, and impeding, their child's social participation (Hansen et al. 2014). Invited and supported participation appeared to be associated with general acceptance of the child's condition. Respondents identified their local church particularly as a place of inclusion, where children could take part in services. However, where the family becomes fragmented, adversely affected by the stresses of caring for a child with disabilities in a context of limited resources and community stigma, participation may be affected. As a result, many children and their caregivers experience social deprivation and isolation (Bunning et al. 2017; Gona et al. 2014).

Participation challenges are amplified by limited resources, cultural stigma and inadequate supports.

> *Involving caregivers in home-based interventions is linked to positive participation outcomes for children.*

Focused and improved attention to the child at home was viewed as providing a model of positive practice to others and therefore linked to improved participation for the child (Nelson et al. 2017). In particular, the chance to improve the child's mobility through therapy exercises as part of community-based rehabilitation was identified as positive help (Hansen et al. 2014). Furthermore, the active involvement of caregivers in home-based interventions appears to be important, not only to the child's development, but to the caregiver's perception of the child and uptake of participation opportunities (Bunning et al. 2014; Gona et al. 2014).

Beyond the homestead, intervention targeted at the community may support improved acceptance and participation. A key feature of the 'resource-ready' environment (Law et al. 2006) and critical to acceptance, participation and inclusion, is the understanding and support of neighbours, friends and members of the community (Hansen et al. 2014). Disability awareness initiatives, as included in community-based rehabilitation and inclusive development guidelines, support the notion of 'empowerment' (WHO 2011). Through activities that encourage people to question their views of disability, while also increasing their contact with people with disabilities, previous beliefs and stereotypes may be challenged (Moore and Nettelbeck 2013). Gona et al. (2018) reported how adults with disabilities, as experts-by-experience, shared their personal narratives with community groups in a rural part of Kenya, which triggered a reassessment of how disability was understood. Learning from people with disabilities underpins Allport's (1954) early 'contact hypothesis' whereby increased interactions between the devalued group and others promotes more positive attitudes and decreases prejudice (Armstrong et al. 2017). In this way, the environment is rendered 'resource ready' (Law et al. 2006).

Of course, achieving participation for children growing up with disabilities is not simply a matter of engineering more positive attitudes and responses in the community; actions are needed to alleviate the stresses within the family; for example, financial, psychosocial and physical (Hansen et al. 2014). Self-help groups are used as a vehicle to promote the wellbeing and livelihoods of a range of users and involve a variety of activities. Self-help groups bring together people with something in common, providing opportunities for sharing experiences and insights, exchanging information and developing self-esteem. Project SEEK is concerned with the development and maintenance of self-help groups for caregivers of children with developmental disabilities (https://www.uea.ac.uk/health-sciences/research/projects/seek). Through empowering activities focused on income generation, mutual psychosocial support, and access to education and health services, the membership moves collectively to improve their home situation and to promote the presence of their child in the community. The activation of caregivers and families as agents for change offers a route to improving the participation of children with neurodisability.

> *Activating caregivers and families as agents for change is powerful.*

CONCLUSIONS

Participation of children with neurodisability is challenged by poverty, scarcity of information giving rise to ignorance about the causes, inadequate coverage of services, and the stigma associated with such conditions. Certain traditional explanations of disability associate it with negative images or undesirable events. The stigmatising of individuals who share specific characteristics and who are perceived as different, can lead others to discriminate against them. In short, they become a discounted group. Some caregivers may assume a protective stance towards the child to minimise the risk to the child and family, or alternatively conceal the child because of shame. Both courses of action may result in separation from the surrounding community and low uptake of participation opportunities. Initiatives exist that are designed to help circumnavigate the negative and frequently isolating consequences of childhood-onset neurodisability, for the child, caregiver and family. However, real and lasting change requires a deliberate, comprehensive and enduring approach that tackles the constructs associated with traditional beliefs and empowers caregivers, and the children themselves in finding a place in their own communities.

SUMMARY OF KEY IDEAS

- Caring for a child with neurodisability in income/resource-poor regions brings many challenges.
- The role of the local community is crucial to participation.
- Experts-by-experience can help the shaping of attitudes.
- Change is most effectively achieved through community-based solutions.

REFERENCES

Allport G (1954) *The Nature of Prejudice*. Oxford: Addison-Wesley Publishing.

Anthony J (2011) Conceptualising disability in Ghana: implications for EFA and inclusive education. *Int J Incl Educ* **15**: 1073–1086.

Armstrong M, Morris C, Abraham C, Tarrant M (2017) Interventions utilising contact with people with disabilities to improve children's attitudes towards disability: A systematic review and meta-analysis. *Disabil Health J* **10**: 11–22.

Bedell G, Coster W, Law M et al. (2013) Community participation, supports, and barriers of school-age children with and without disabilities. *Arch Phys Med Rehabil* **94**: 315–323.

Bitta M, Kariuki SM, Abubakar A, Newton CRJC (2017) Burden of neurodevelopmental disorders in low and middle-income countries: A systematic review and meta-analysis. *Wellcome Open Res* **2**: 121.

Bunning K, Gona J, Newton C, Hartley S (2014) Caregiver perceptions of children who have complex communication needs following a home-based intervention using augmentative and alternative communication in rural Kenya: An intervention note. *Augment Altern Commun* **30**: 344–356.

Bunning K, Gona J, Newton C, Hartley S (2017) The perception of disability by community groups: Stories of local understanding, beliefs and challenges in a rural part of Kenya. *PLoS One* **12**: e0182214.

Department for International Development (2004) *The Effects of Poverty in Poor Countries*. London: Department for International Development.

Eide AH, Ingstad B (2013) Disability and poverty – Reflections on research experiences in Africa and beyond. *Afr J Disabil* **2**: 31.

Goffman E (1963) *Stigma: Notes on the Management of the Spoiled Identity*. Harmonsworth: Penguin Publishers.

Gona JK, Mung'ala-Odera V, Newton CR, Hartley S (2011) Caring for children with disabilities in Kilifi, Kenya: what is the carer's experience? *Child Care Health Dev* **37**: 175–183.

Gona JK, Newton CR, Hartley S, Bunning K (2018) Persons with disabilities as experts-by experience: using personal narratives to affect community attitudes in Kilifi, Kenya. *BMC Int Health Hum Rights* **18**: 18.

Gona JK, Newton CR, Rimba K et al. (2015) Parents' and professionals' perceptions on causes and treatment options for Autism Spectrum Disorders (ASD) in a multicultural context on the Kenyan Coast. *PLoS One* **10**: e0132729.

Gona JK, Newton CR, Hartley S, Bunning K (2014) A home-based intervention using augmentative and alternative communication (AAC) techniques in rural Kenya: what are the caregivers' experiences? *Child Care Health Dev* **40**: 29–41.

Hansen AMW, Siame M, van der Veen J (2014) A qualitative study: barriers and support for participation for children with disabilities. *Afr J Disabil* **3**: 112.

Ingstad B, Whyte S (2007) Disability connections. In: Ingstad B, Whyte SR (Eds) *Disability in Local and Global World*. Berkeley: University of California Press, pp. 1–29.

Kuper H, Monteath-van Dok A, Wing K et al. (2014) The impact of disability on the lives of children; cross-sectional data including 8,900 children with disabilities and 898,834 children without disabilities across 30 countries. *PLoS One* **9**: e107300.

Law M, King G, King S, Kertoy M, Hurley P, Rosenbaum P (2006) Patterns and predictors of recreational and leisure participation of children with physical disabilities. *Dev Med Child Neurol* **48**: 337–342.

Mark W, Cheung R (2008) Affiliate stigma among caregivers of people with intellectual disability or mental illness. *J Appl Res Intellect Disabil* **21**: 532–545.

McKenzie JA, McConkey R, Adnams C (2013) Intellectual disability in Africa: implications for research and service development. *Disabil Rehabil* **35**: 1750–1755.

Mitra S, Posarac A, Vick B (2011) *Disability and Poverty in Developing Countries: A Snapshot from the World Health Survey*. Washington: Human Development Network, Social Protection. http://documents.worldbank.org/curated/en/501871468326189306/Disability-and-poverty-in-developing-countries-a-snapshot-from-the-world-health-survey [Accessed 26 September 2019].

Moore D, Nettelbeck T (2013) Effects of short-term disability awareness training on attitudes of adolescent schoolboys toward persons with a disability. *J Intellect Dev Disabil* **38**: 223–231.

Muzunoya S, Mitra S (2012) Is there a disability gap in employment rates in developing countries? May 2012. Available at SSRN: https://ssrn.com/abstract=2127568.

Nelson F, Masulani-Mwale C, Richards E, Theobald S, Gladstone M (2017) The meaning of participation for children in Malawi: insights from children and caregivers. *Child Care Health Dev* **43**: 133–143.

Peters DH, Garg A, Bloom G, Walker DG, Brieger WR, Rahman MH (2008) Poverty and access to health care in developing countries. *Ann N Y Acad Sci* **1136**: 161–171.

Shumba A, Abosi O (2011) The nature, extent and causes of abuse of children with disabilities in schools in Botswana. *Int J Disabil Dev Educ* **58**: 373–388.

Tedrus GM, Fonseca LC, De Pietro Magri F, Mendes PH (2013) Spiritual/religious coping in patients with epilepsy: relationship with sociodemographic and clinical aspects and quality of life. *Epilepsy Behav* **28**: 386–390.

Stone-MacDonald A, Butera G (2012) Cultural beliefs and attitudes about disability in sub-Saharan Africa. *Rev Disabil Stud* **8**: 62–77.

Trani J (2010) *Disability In and Around Urban Areas in Sierra Leone*. London: Leonard Cheshire International.

UNESCO (2015) *Education For All, 2000–2015: Achievements And Challenges*. Paris: United Nations Educational, Scientific and Cultural Organization.

Werner S, Corrigan P, Ditchman N, Sokol K (2012) Stigma and intellectual disability: a review of related measures and future directions. *Res Dev Disabil* **33**: 748–765

WHO (2010)*Community-Based Rehabilitation Guidelines*. Geneva: World Health Organization.

In the following vignette, we see a clash of cultures influencing understanding of the cause and nature of Ben's difficulties and shaping expectations for Ben. Ms Mutolo's experience provides insight into the experience of disability and exclusion – exclusion to protect (from bullying) and exclusion because of a restricted context. As you read this story, consider the nature of the opportunity to be involved that Ben finds, and how we might build on that.

When Ben Smiled (South Africa)

Juan Bornman

Ms Mutolo attended the local primary health clinic for her regular antenatal check-up, upon which the nurse told her to go to the hospital with the ambulance that was waiting to also take a critically ill patient. She was reluctant, as her due date was still far off and she was not in labour. After a 2-hour ambulance ride, she was monitored at the hospital. A young doctor told Ms Mutolo, through a nurse translator, that the traditional remedy which she was taking, was slowly killing the baby and that she would not be able to give birth naturally. Ms Mutolo strongly denied taking traditional medicine, and said that she wanted to go home as she was concerned about her other five children at home who did not know where she was. She was forced by the nurse to sign a consent form and taken to theatre under threat.

Ben Mutolo[1] was born by caesarean section on 3 June 2011. His mother noticed that he was not crying and doctors took him from the room to resuscitate him. When she saw her baby the next day for the first time, the doctor told her her baby had needed blood which he collected from the blood bank with his own car due to the critical condition of her baby. The doctor also told her the baby had sustained a brain injury and as a result would not develop normally and would be dependent on her for his whole life. Ben was discharged after 1 month in hospital. Ms Mutolo remained only 3 days.

I met Ben and his mother when he was 6 years old. His father had left the family, who were now living in a two-roomed house, without electricity. They rent out one of the rooms for an income. Ms Mutolo does not work and stays at home to care for Ben. She is unable to obtain a child support grant for any of her six children (aged between 6 and 15 years), because she is a Mozambican citizen living in South Africa and her children do not have birth certificates.

Upon asking Ms Mutolo to explain Ben's strengths she said 'No strengths. What good will come from this child the way he is?' When asked about any family history of disability, Ms Mutolo said 'It cannot be called a disability because it was caused by somebody's negligence'.

Ms Mutolo said that Ben is currently healthy, after having been very sickly during the first 3 years of his life and often requiring medical attention. On probing she indicated that he frequently has seizures: 'His whole body shakes. Almost every day, and at night too. Sometimes even three times per day.' On asking her what she does when this happens, she explained that she picks him up, she sits down and then holds him tightly to her own body in an upright position to calm him down, until he eventually stops shaking. The traditional healer explained to her that the seizures happen because her husband put a spell on Ben as he brought bad luck to the family and therefore the treatment must be more spiritual, and cannot be delivered in a hospital.

Ben does not have opportunities to interact with other children, apart from his siblings. His mother says that she tries to keep other children away from him, as they make fun of him. She has noticed some children acting out a seizure and then laughing loudly. She would like him to interact with other children, but thinks that, for his own good, it is better to not be with other children. Although she would have liked him to go to school, there is no school for children with disability in their village, and the principal at the mainstream school explained that Ben would have to first be toilet-trained before they could accept him. Ms Mutolo is not sure if this will ever happen, because he is fully dependent on her for all of his activities of daily living: eating, dressing and toileting. She also doesn't know how she will transport him when he grows bigger – at the moment she carries him on her back. The hospital have said that she could have a wheelchair for Ben, but the chair does not fit into their already over-crowded house.

She has noticed that he sometimes watches the neighbourhood children play from where he sits propped up in a wheelbarrow with pillows under the shade of the tree. And then he smiles…

Looking to the Future

Dido Green and Christine Imms

In *Participation: Optimising Outcomes in Childhood-Onset Neurodisability* we aimed to garner knowledge and experiences from around the world, to consider the central constructs of participation and how these may be realised across varying cultures and contexts.

In this brief final chapter, we consider the future for children and their families as their outlook continues to expand and brighten. This book proposes many avenues for practice and research, and here we focus on the five core topics of the book to highlight a few directions.

1 THE CONCEPT OF PARTICIPATION

Participation involves both attending and being involved in your own life as well as the lives of those around you. While health, education and community services are aimed at enabling those with childhood-onset disability to live good lives, we need to agree upon what 'participation' is to target resources and interventions and to systematically investigate how to influence it positively. This book aims to clarify the participation construct by carefully defining the two essential elements – attendance and involvement – and equally carefully, distinguishing these from related, yet distinct concepts.

A good life is participatory.

Through the book, we stress two key points. Firstly, being able to perform tasks as expected (or in the same way as others, or independently) is not the same as participation. Secondly, participation does not only apply to specific life situations. You can participate – that is, attend and be involved – in any life situation. In some situations, attendance is not in question; for example, if you need to get dressed then you must be present in the physical sense. However, involvement while dressing may vary, and can be supported, for example, by exercising choice regarding what to wear; this is distinct from having the skills and abilities to dress.

The 'attendance' construct of participation is relatively straightforward; however, understanding of 'involvement' is more complex. We have defined involvement as the experience of participation while attending. Further research about how best to understand, measure and influence this multi-dimensional involvement construct is needed now.

2 CONTEXTS OF PARTICIPATION

Participation can be understood as the intersection where the person meets the context – that is, participation occurs as a transactional exchange among objects, activities, places and individual/s over time. Participation is optimal when there is a good fit between the person and the context. While this might seem obvious, the challenge is to support individuals with impairments to have as broad a range of contexts as possible in which they can thrive. If there are too few contexts providing a 'good fit', individuals and the significant people around them, may experience isolation potentially leading to loneliness and ill health.

Thus, a question for the future is how do we study the experience of participation in context over extended periods of time? Taking a developmental perspective, we know that the contexts of infancy differ to those of childhood, adolescence and adulthood. What pattern of attendance and involvement is optimal over time? If sub-optimal participation occurs in some contexts, or for some periods of time, what is needed to ensure durable wellbeing?

3 MEASUREMENT OF PARTICIPATION AND RELATED CONSTRUCTS

The field requires tools for measuring participation attendance, involvement and the core related constructs. These measures must meet the needs of individuals across the varied life situations that they, and those around them, experience during their life spans. We need good quality measures so that we can plan how to distribute our resources for the best effect, and to evaluate if we have been effective. A high-quality measure is one that meets core psychometric requirements – that is, it measures the construct of interest, has ecological validity and is reliable – and is acceptable to those using the measure. Acceptability is crucial as measurement brings judgement, and how we implement measures can have a detrimental as well as a positive effect on the recipient.

We particularly lack measures of the involvement construct – the subjective component of participation. To develop these measures, we need to know if it is possible to measure involvement at multiple ecological levels – within the individual, the individual-in-context and between systems. Involvement is an abstract or latent construct, and measurement of latent constructs often involves the use of indicator variables. One challenge is to ensure the items that are intended to indicate involvement do not instead describe one of the related constructs such as self-determination. Another challenge is to consider what level of understanding is needed to self-report the idea of involvement. Because the experience of involvement might involve multiple elements (e.g. how you feel, what you are thinking and/or what you are doing), an interview rather than survey approach, may be more effective with children. When we conduct semi-structured interviews with children about their experience of involvement, we see that they usually enjoy telling their story and being supported to elicit a 'score' to rate their involvement.

4 PARTICIPATION FOCUSED INTERVENTIONS

The principal challenge here is for professionals and service users to shift their thinking and focus so that they start with the end in mind. That is, participation is considered first and foremost in goal setting, in intervention planning and in outcome measurement. We have growing evidence about how to influence participation outcomes through carefully tailored multi-strategy approaches. We also have emergent knowledge about how to implement participation as an intervention that aims to change outcomes in related constructs along with future participation. This work is complex and requires sophisticated research frameworks and analytical methods. However, for today's practitioners, the clear message is that supporting participation in context by situating therapy in the naturally occurring settings of the child and family is a powerful method for supporting a positive sense-of-self, skill building, improved body functions and preferences for future participation.

Situating therapy in naturally occurring settings can be a powerful method for supporting participation.

If participation occurs in all life situations, then therapy and education can be no exceptions. Participation in the therapy context will involve transactional exchanges among the activities, objects, place and people – including therapists – over time. While we have always known that the therapeutic relationship is a crucial element of successful encounters, working to improve engagement with and engagement in therapy may act to speed up goal achievement and/ or result in greater achievement of outcomes – or indeed better experiences of the therapy situations. Examining and improving engagement in intervention requires healthcare and education professionals to consider both what they do and how they are involved in the exchange.

In school settings, the focus has been on improving the inclusion of children with disability. Although the definition of inclusion is closely related to participation, it is often manifested for children with disability as their ability to spend time within mainstream school settings. This can equate to attendance, and may, or may not, address the issue of involvement in learning. Bringing together separate discourses in research and practice for building and evaluating interdisciplinary practices is essential.

5 SPECIAL CHALLENGES

In today's world we can easily connect our ideas and actions across diverse countries and cultures through travel and/or through information exchange across the web. Yet, simultaneously, we appear to be worlds apart when we consider the lived experience of those in resource poor settings in comparison to those in high resource settings within our own, or other countries. This presents a challenge and an urgent question: When working together, how do we rapidly change the experiences of participation restriction so often reported from low-resource settings?

An additional challenge for the field, relates to the participatory experiences of groups, within and between communities and cultures. Patterns of migration, acculturalisation and cultural displacement influence societal attitudes to 'difference' including expectations and opportunities provided for individuals with disabilities.

FINAL THOUGHTS

This book provides a reference for all those interested in enhancing opportunities and outcomes for children, young people and families where there is an individual with a childhood-onset neurodisability. By focusing on participation – what it is, where it occurs, how to measure it and how to influence it – we aim to support professionals in utilising the most recent developments in the field.

Looking to the future, Part V of the book set several challenges – challenges not merely due to restrictions of physical or socio-cultural environments – but also challenges to take the opportunities that new perspectives as well as technologies and advancements afford, to maximise participation of individuals with disabilities and their families across multiple contexts.

Index

Other titles from Mac Keith Press www.mackeith.co.uk

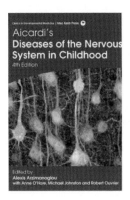

Aicardi's Diseases of the Nervous System in Childhood, 4th Edition
Alexis Arzimanoglou, Anne O'Hare, Michael V Johnston and Robert Ouvrier (Editors)

Clinics in Developmental Medicine
2018 ▪ 1524pp ▪ hardback ▪ 978-1-909962-80-4

This fourth edition retains the patient-focussed, clinical approach of its predecessors. The international team of editors and contributors has honoured the request of the late Jean Aicardi, that his book remain 'resolutely clinical', which distinguishes *Diseases of the Nervous System in Childhood* from other texts in the field. New edition completely updated and revised and now in full colour.

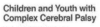
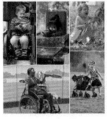

Children and Youth with Complex Cerebral Palsy: Care and Management
Laurie J. Glader and Richard D. Stevenson (Editors)

A Practical Guide from Mac Keith Press
2019 ▪ 404pp ▪ softback ▪ 978-1-909962-98-9

This is the first practical guide to explore management of the many medical comorbidities that children with complex CP face, including orthopaedics, mobility needs, cognition and sensory impairment, difficult behaviours, respiratory complications and nutrition, amongst others. Uniquely, contributors include children and parents, providing applied wisdom for family-centred care. Clinical Care Tools are provided to help guide clinicians and include a Medical Review Supplement, Equipment and Services Checklist and an ICF-Based Care: Goals and Management Form.

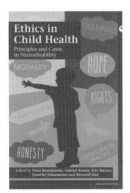

Ethics in Child Health: Principles and Cases in Neurodisability
Peter L. Rosenbaum, Gabriel M. Ronen, Eric Racine, Jennifer Johannesen and Bernard Dan (Editors)

A Practical Guide from Mac Keith Press
2016 ▪ 396pp ▪ softback ▪ 978-1-909962-63-7

This book explores the ethical dimensions of issues that have either been ignored or not recognised. Each chapter is built around an illustrative scenario and discusses how ethical principles can be utilised to inform decision-making. 'Themes for Discussion' at the end of each chapter will help professionals and policy makers put practical ethical thinking at the heart of care.

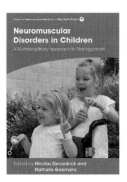

Neuromuscular Disorders in Children: A Multidisciplinary Approach to Management Nicolas Deconinck and Nathalie Goemans (Editors)

Clinics in Developmental Medicine
2019 ▪ 468pp ▪ hardback ▪ 978-1-911612-08-7
£85.00 / €96.05 / $115.00

This book critically reviews current evidence of management approaches in the field of neuromuscular disorders (NMDs) in children. Uniquely, the book focusses on assessment as the cornerstone of management and highlights the importance of a multidisciplinary approach. The large number of healthcare professionals involved in managing children with NMDs will find this a useful one-stop reference resource

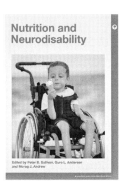

Nutrition and Neurodisability
Peter B. Sullivan, Guro L. Andersen and Morag J. Andrew (Editors)

A Practical Guide from Mac Keith Press
2020 ▪ 208pp ▪ softback ▪ 978-1-911612-25-4
£55.00 / €64.97 / $75.00

Feeding difficulties are common in children with neurodisability and disorders of the central nervous system can affect the movements required for safe and efficient eating and drinking. This practical guide provides strategies for managing the range of nutritional problems faced by children with neurodevelopmental disability. The easily accessible information on aetiology, assessment and management is informed by a succinct review of current evidence and guidelines to inform best practice.

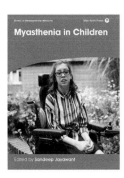

Myasthenia in Children
Sandeep Jayawant (Editor)

Clinics in Developmental Medicine
2019 ▪ 144pp ▪ hardback ▪ 978-1-911612-29-2
£65.00 / €73.50 / $80.00

Myasthenia is a rare, but underdiagnosed and sometimes life-threatening disorder in children. There are no guidelines for diagnosing and managing these children, especially those with congenital myasthenia, a more recently recognised genetic condition, but there have been significant developments in identification and treatment of myasthenia in recent years. This book will help clinicians and families of children with this rare condition direct management effectively.

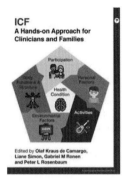

ICF: A Hands-on Approach for Clinicians and Families
Olaf Kraus de Camargo, Liane Simon, Gabriel M. Ronen and Peter L. Rosenbaum (Editors)

A Practical Guide from Mac Keith Press
2019 ▪ 192pp ▪ softback ▪ 978-1-911612-04-9

This accessible handbook introduces the World Health Organisation's International Classification of Functioning, Disability and Health (ICF) to professionals working with children with disabilities and their families. It contains an overview of the elements of the ICF but focusses on practical applications, including how the ICF framework can be used with children, families and carers to formulate health and management goals.

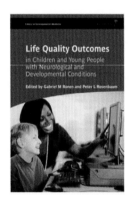

Life Quality Outcomes in Children and Young People with Neurological and Developmental Conditions
Gabriel M. Ronen and Peter L. Rosenbaum (Editors)

Clinics in Developmental Medicine
2013 ▪ 394pp ▪ hardback ▪ 978-1-908316-58-5

Healthcare professionals need to understand their patients' views of their condition and its effects on their health and well-being. This book builds on the World Health Organization's concepts of 'health', 'functioning' and 'quality of life' for young people with neurodisabilities: it emphasises the importance of engaging with patients in the identification of both treatment goals and their evaluation. Uniquely, it enables healthcare professionals to find critically reviewed outcomes-related information.

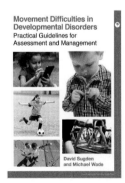

Movement Difficulties in Developmental Disorders: Practical Guidelines for Assessment and Management
David Sugden and Michael Wade

A Practical Guide from Mac Keith Press
2019 ▪ 240pp ▪ softback ▪ 978-1-909962-94-1

This book presents the latest evidence-based approaches to assessing and managing movement disorders in children. Uniquely, children with developmental coordination disorder (DCD) and children with movement difficulties as a co-occurring secondary characteristic of another development disorder, including ADHD, ASD, and Dyslexia, are discussed. It will prove a valuable guide for anybody working with children with movement difficulties, including clinicians, teachers and parents.

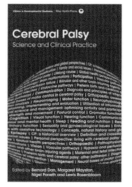

Cerebral Palsy: Science and Clinical Practice
Bernard Dan, Margaret Mayston, Nigel Paneth and Lewis Rosenbloom (Editors)

Clinics in Developmental Medicine
2015 ▪ 648pp ▪ hardback ▪ 978-1-909962-38-5

This landmark title considers all aspects of cerebral palsy from the causes to clinical problems and their implications for individuals. An international team of experts present a wide range of person-centred assessment approaches, including clinical evaluation, measurement scales, neuroimaging and gait analysis. The perspective of the book spans the lifelong course of cerebral palsy, taking into account worldwide differences in socio-economic and cultural factors. Full integrated colour, with extensive cross-referencing make this a highly attractive and useful reference.

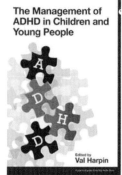

The Management of ADHD in Children and Young People
Val Harpin (Editor)

A Practical Guide from Mac Keith Press
2017 ▪ 292pp ▪ softback ▪ 978-1-909962-72-9

This book is an accessible and practical guide on all aspects of assessment of children and young people with Attention Deficit Hyperactivity Disorder (ADHD) and how they can be managed successfully. The multi-professional team of authors discusses referral, assessment and diagnosis, psychological management, pharmacological management, and co-existing conditions, as well as ADHD in the school setting. New research on girls with ADHD is also featured. Case scenarios are included that bring these topics to life.

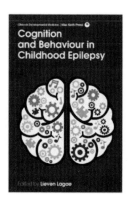

Cognition and Behaviour in Childhood Epilepsy
Lieven Lagae (Editor)

Clinics in Developmental Medicine
2017 ▪ 186pp ▪ hardback ▪ 978-1-909962-87-3

For many parents, cognitive and behavioral comorbidities, such as ADHD, autism and intellectual disability, are the real burden of childhood epilepsy. This title offers concrete guidance and treatment strategies for childhood epilepsy in general, and for the comorbidities associated with each epilepsy syndrome and their pathophysiology. The book is written by experts in the field with an important clinical experience, while chapters by clinical neuropsychologists provide a strong theoretical background.